INDIAN DIPLOMACY AND COVID RESPONSE

INDIAN DIPLOMACY AND COVID RESPONSE

INDIAN COUNCIL OF WORLD AFFAIRS

KNOWLEDGE WORLD

KW Publishers Pvt Ltd
New Delhi

Indian Council of World Affairs
New Delhi

ISBN 978-93-91490-87-4 Hardback
ISBN 978-93-91490-95-9 e-Book

Published in India by Kalpana Shukla

KW Publishers Pvt Ltd
4676/21, First Floor, Ansari Road
Daryaganj, New Delhi 110 002
Phone: +91 11 43528107
Marketing: kw@kwpub.in
Editorial: production@kwpub.in
Website: www.kwpub.in

Printed and bound in India

CONTENTS

LIST OF ANNEXURES

LIST OF CONTRIBUTORS

Harsh Vardhan Shringla

Dammu Ravi

Vinay Kumar

Vikram Doraiswami

Naveen Srivastava

Nagesh Singh

Arindam Bagchi

Anurag Bhushan

Jayant Khobragade

G Balasubramaniam

Devyani Khobragade

Dr S Janakiraman

Editorial / Research Team

Anupam Ray

Sumit Seth

Rajesh Uike

Kiran Khatri

Jyotsna Mehra

Dyutimoy Seal

Tarang Jain

Shreya Bose

Gaurav Dutta

Vivek Mishra

Ankita Dutta

INTRODUCTION

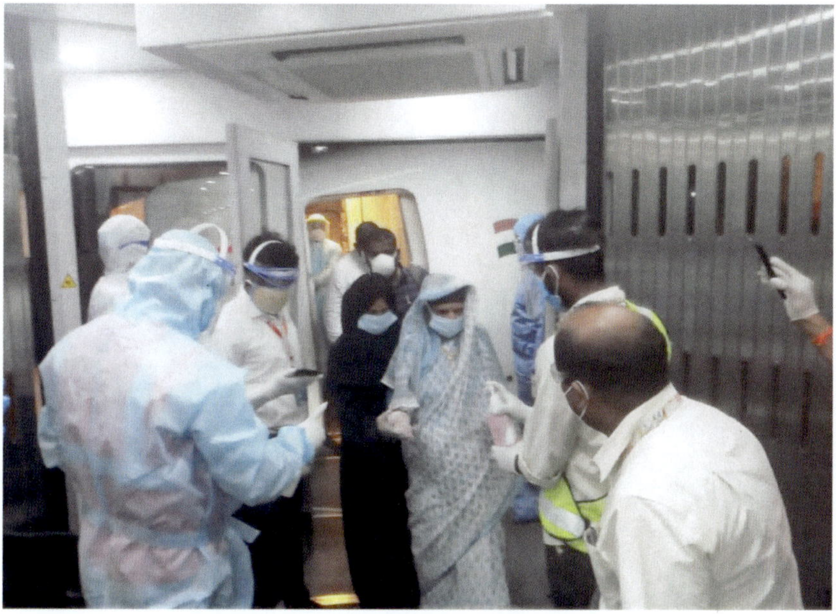

First two flights under Vande Bharat Mission bringing home
Indian citizens from UAE

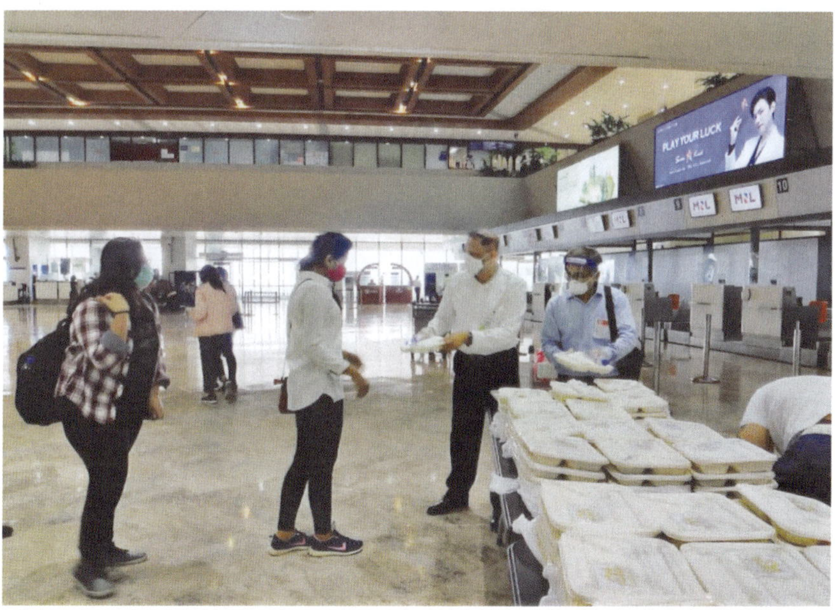

Vande Bharat Mission

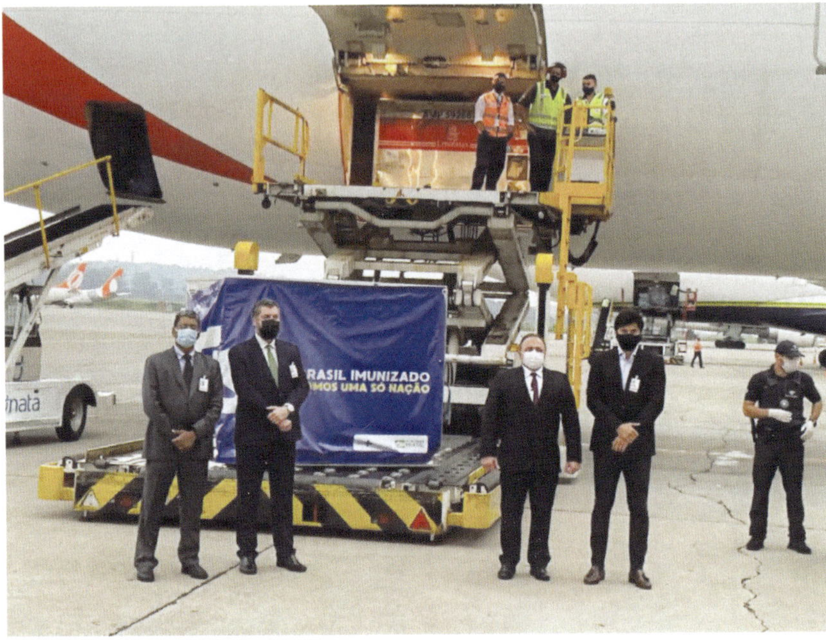

India delivers 2 million doses of Astra Zeneca vaccines to Brazil

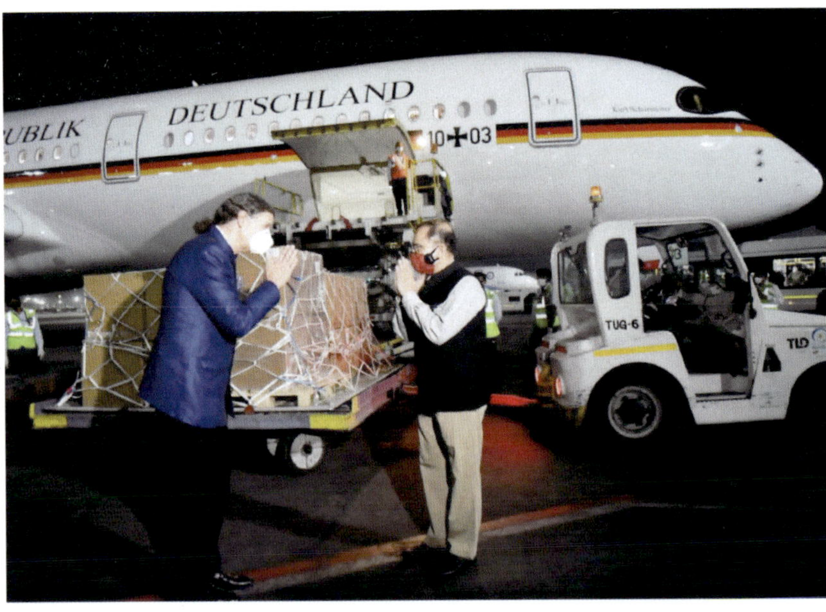

Procurement of 120 ventilators from Germany

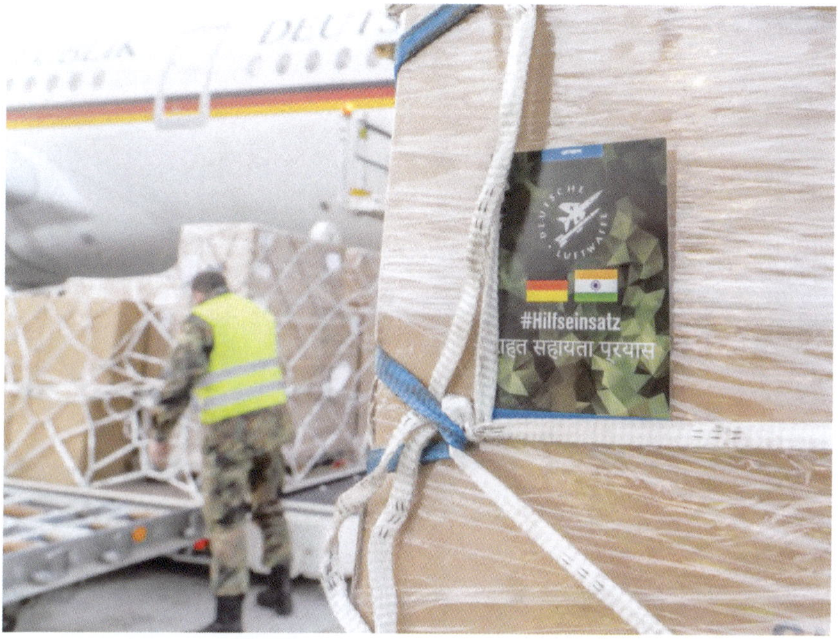

Procurement of medical and oxygen supplies from our partners abroad

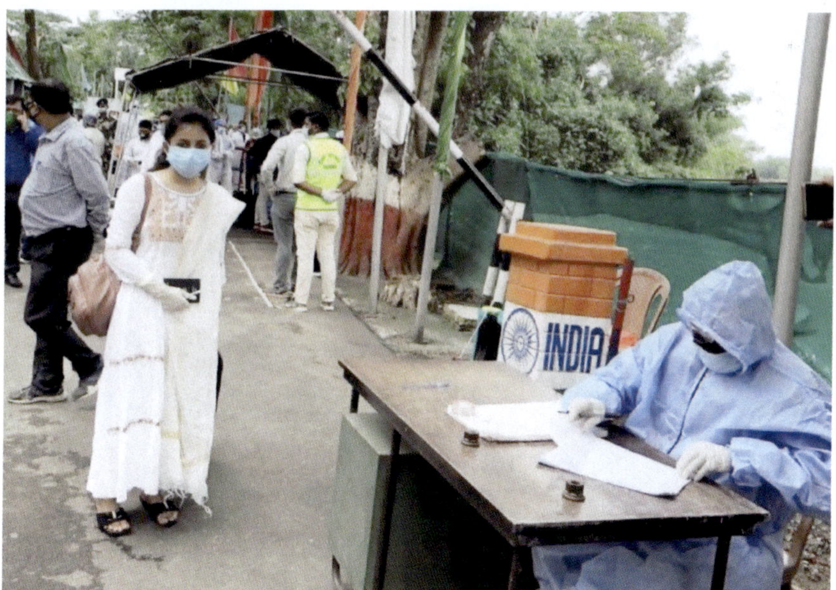

Indian citizens crossing over land border posts Dawki-Tamabil, Agartala-Akhaura, and Sutarkandi-Sheola

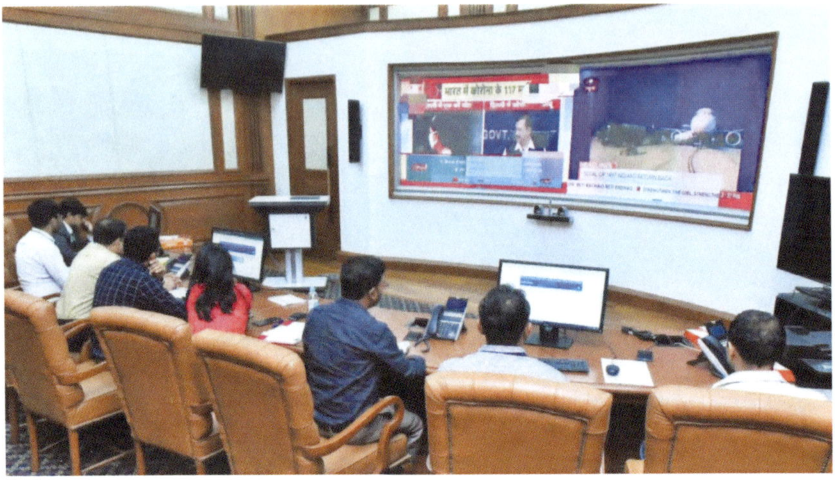

Ministry's COVID-19 Control Centre

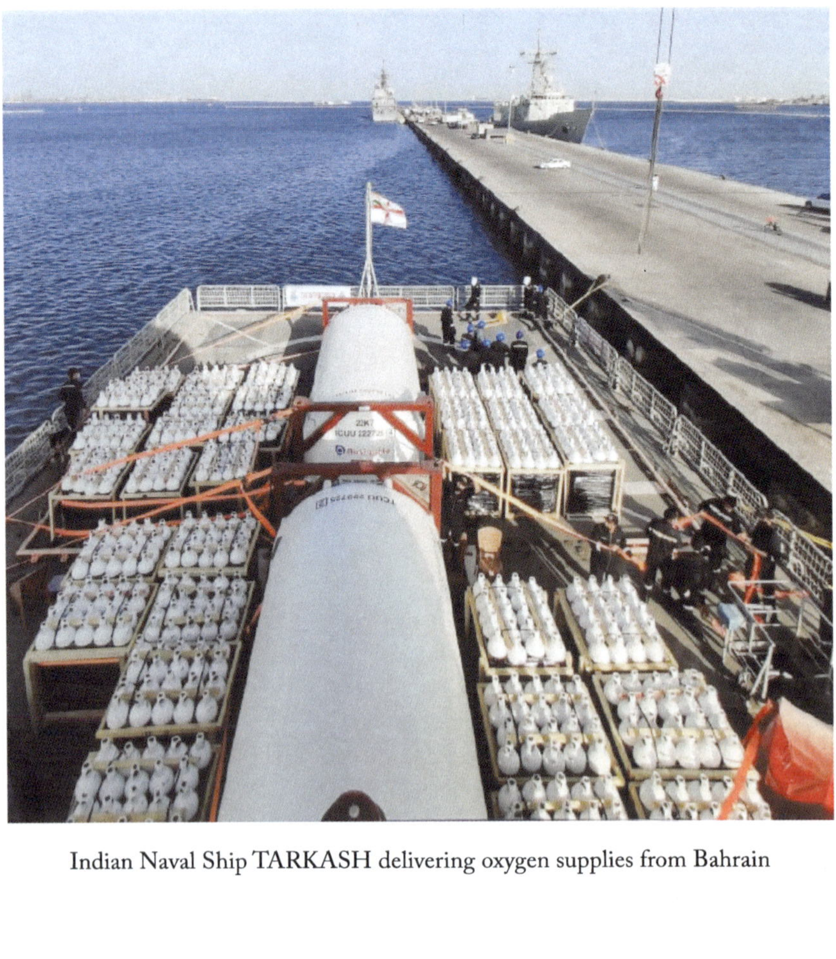

Indian Naval Ship TARKASH delivering oxygen supplies from Bahrain

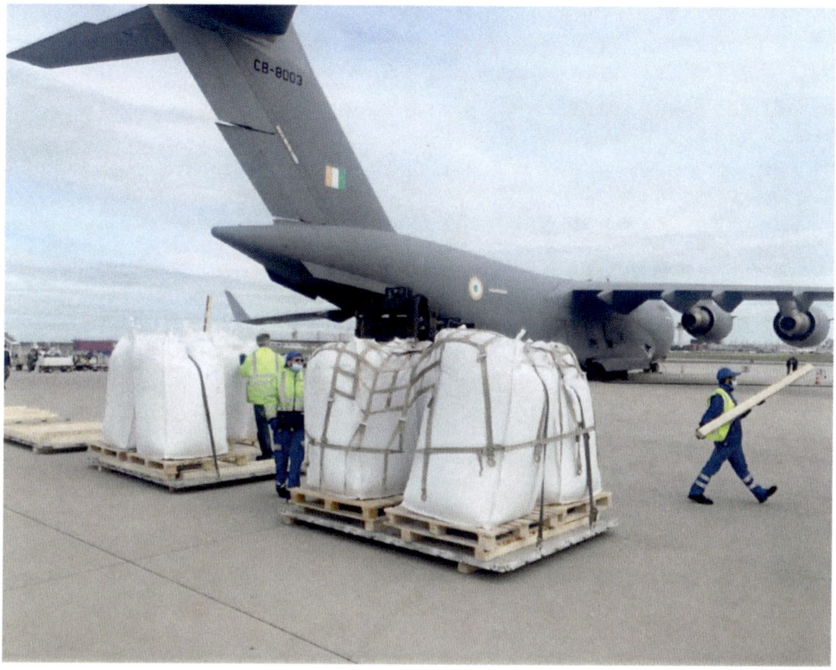

Indian Air Force deployed to airlift oxygen and medical supplies from partner countries

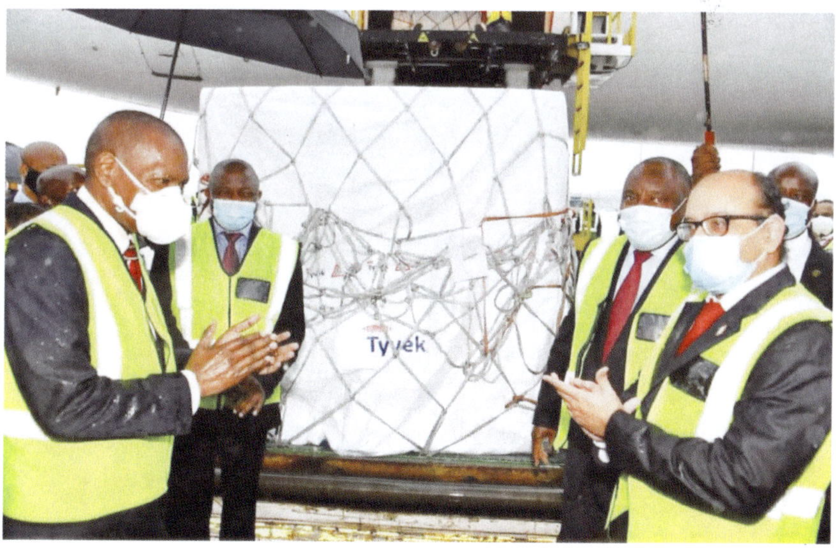

BRICS Cooperation: India delivered its first batch of vaccines to South Africa

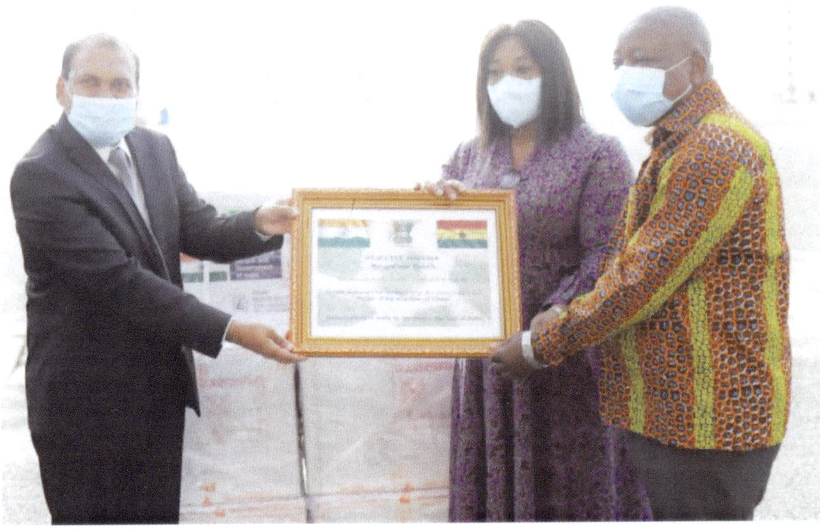

India delivered 50,000 doses of COVID vaccines to Ghana under Vaccine Maitri

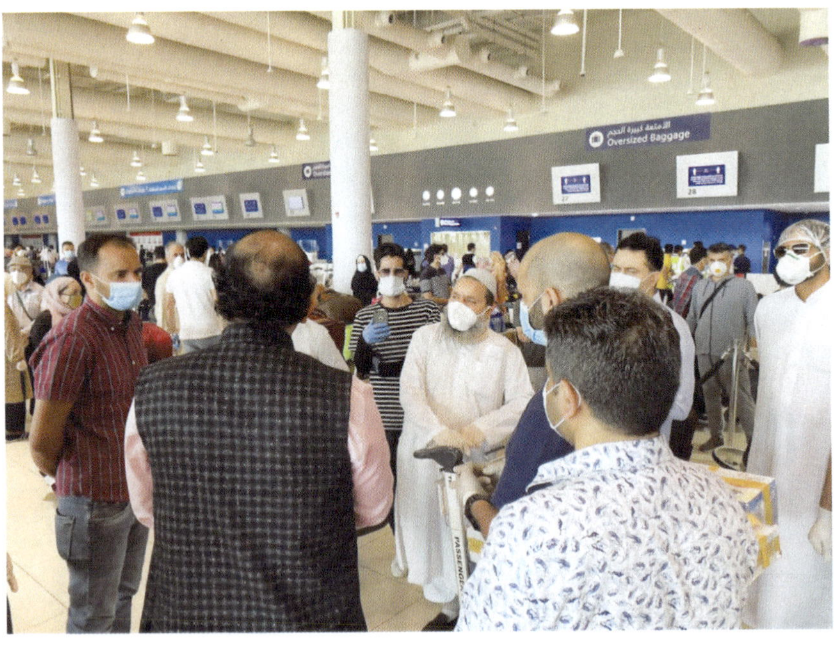

Mission Vande Bharat: First ever flight from Dubai to Srinagar bringing stranded Indians home

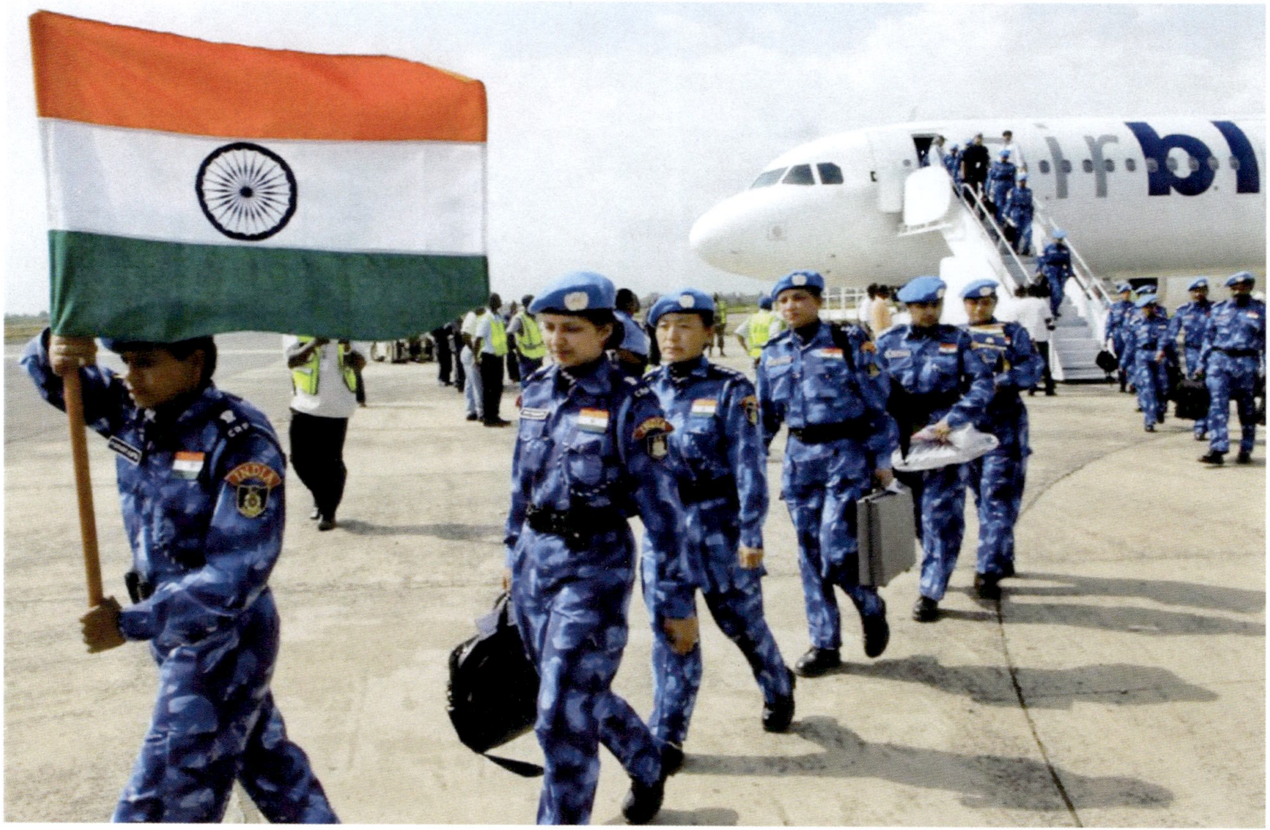

India donated COVID vaccines to United Nations Peacekeeping personnel

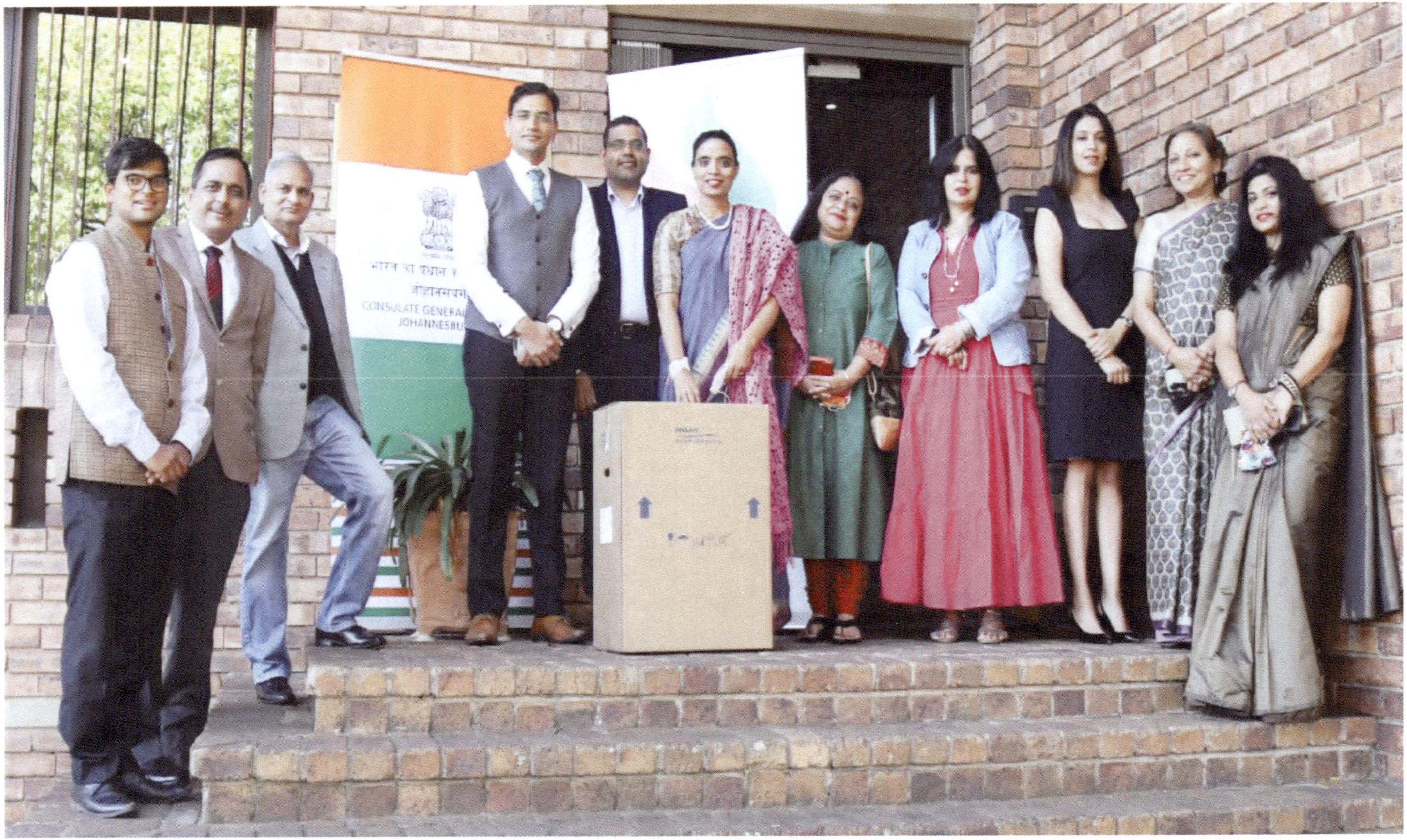

A consignment of oxygen supplies from the Indian community in South Africa delivered to India in its fight against the second wave of COVID-19

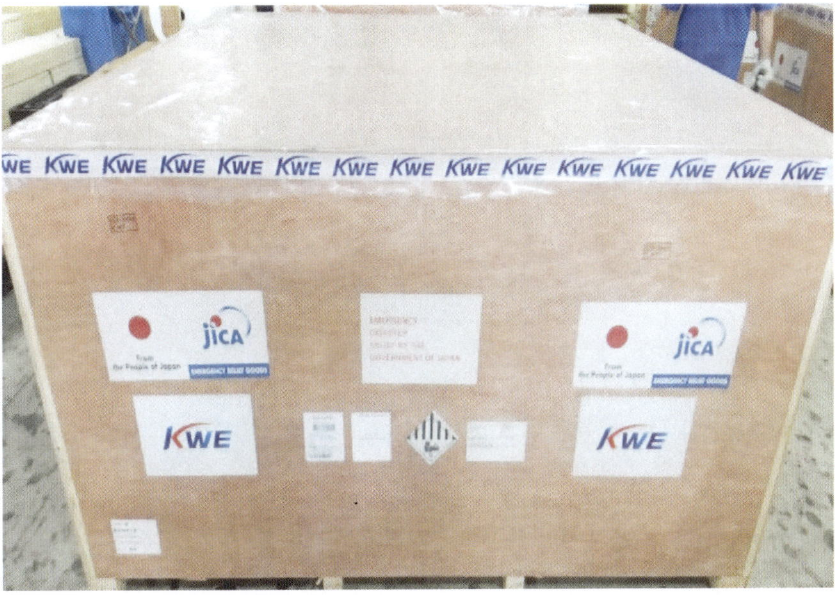

Japan's emergency assistance to India during the second wave of COVID-19

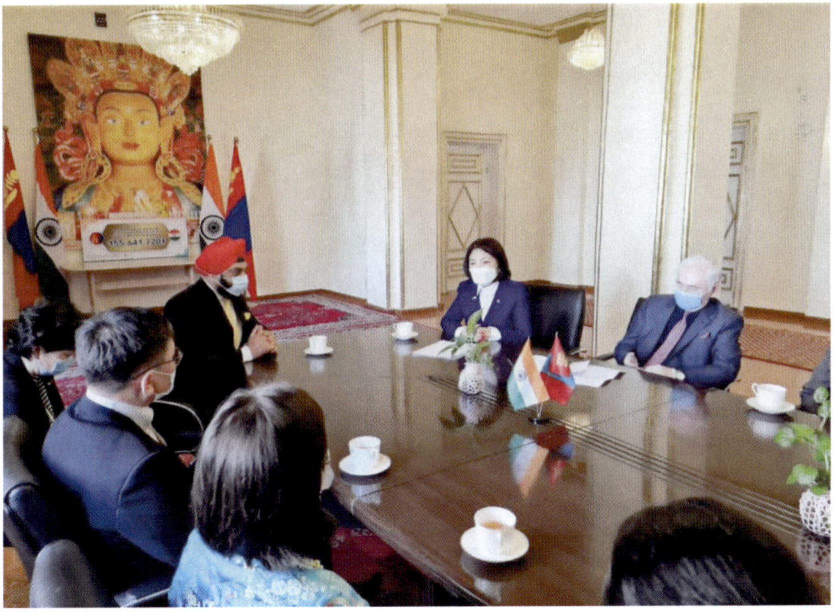

Head of India-Mongolia Parliamentary Group, Head of Mongolia India Business Council and Head of Centre for Indian Studies met to express solidarity with India & confirmed contribution of MNT 155 million to PM Cares Fund

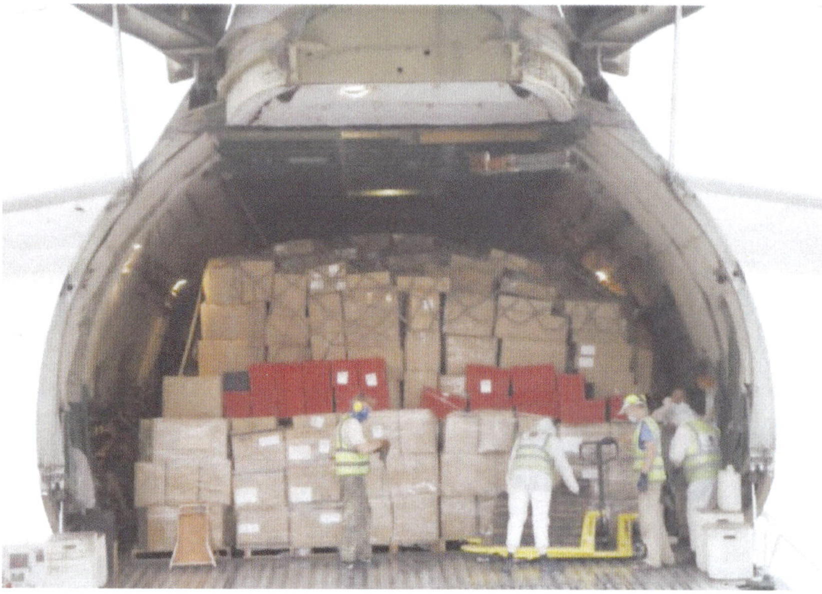

The Government of UAE's gift of ventilators and other medical supplies to India

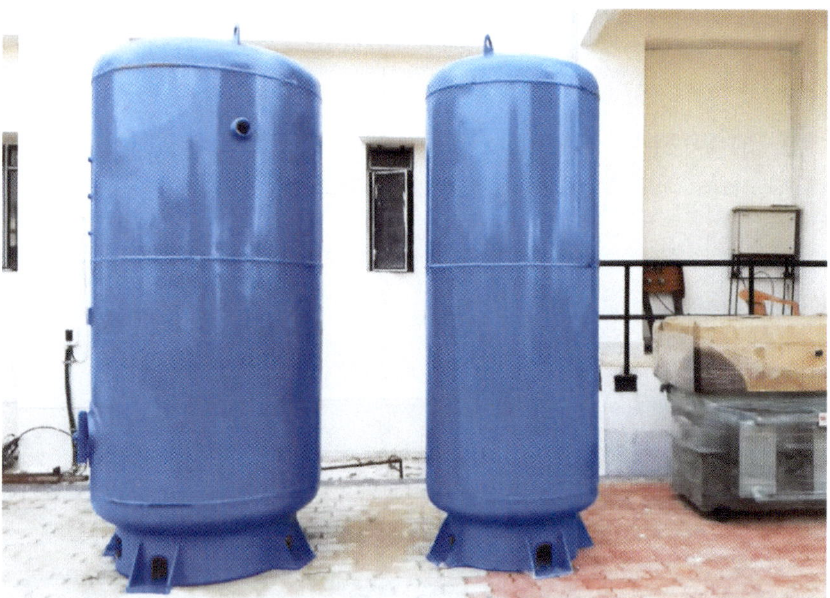

Government of Japan and UNDP partnered to ensure uninterrupted oxygen supply at hospitals in India's North Eastern Region

1

INTRODUCTION

The COVID pandemic has been the greatest shock to the international system since World War II. It was a health catastrophe that delivered an enormous economic shock.

The Ministry of External Affairs, like the rest of government and society, was faced with an unprecedented situation. India is a country with a global presence and global interests. It is a country with a major diaspora, with a globalised economy that is linked with global capital, technology, and trade flows. The disruptions caused by the pandemic therefore have had a significant and continuing effect

The purpose of this monograph is to detail and record the administrative and diplomatic response of the Ministry of External Affairs to this extraordinarily difficult challenge. The initial response, as it must be to all Black Swan events such as this, was necessarily ad hoc. However, as the pandemic persisted, the Ministry responded with a sui generis administrative model. This monograph attempts to identify the broad lines of that response. It does so with the intention of drawing lessons and identifying scalable and replicable components.

The following broad features of the response are to be noted:

1. The Ministry managed within existing resources. It is universally acknowledged that this Ministry has a lean staffing structure. The unprecedented pressures of the situation were met by the available leadership, manpower and resources.

This was achieved partly by delegation and outsourcing. The Ministry's leadership, at the level of EAM and Foreign Secretary, focused on identifying broad challenges, delegating authority, and creating empowered structures that could generate adequate solutions. This freed them to take strategic calls and devote attention to problems that were escalated to that level.

Authority was delegated in an unusual manner. Instead of trying to "fit" the challenge within an organisation that—like the rest of government—

is organised along jurisdictions and hierarchies, the Ministry adopted a matrix-structure like that of start-ups and big-tech companies. Existing chains of command were re-engineered and assigned specific pandemic related roles over and above their normal responsibilities. "Task forces", dealing with specific issues without being named as such, emerged. This created a surge capacity within the Ministry that allowed it to scale up literally overnight to meet completely unexpected challenges. As challenges waxed and waned, the Ministry was able to deploy and redeploy assets to deal with stresses.

2. Organisations that have matrix structures solve problems in a cooperative manner by bringing stakeholders together. The Ministry was able to quickly create networks that could link stakeholders to find solutions. Existing coordination mechanisms that integrated and mobilised the Ministry's global network of Missions and Posts were repurposed and plugged into national networks dealing with domestic problems. The evacuation, procurement and vaccine operations that linked central and state authorities with domestic and foreign players, state and non-state through embassies is a good example.

This facilitated a non-siloed approach when mounting "joint operations". The Ministry and Embassies were able to work harmoniously, efficiently, and effectively with armed forces, for instance, under severe constraints of time and operating freedom due to the restrictions and lockdowns.

The standalone COVID Cell that was created and headed by a senior officer acted as an in-house coordination center and clearing house.

The networks were simultaneously centralised and decentralised. They centralised information but decentralised action. It facilitated quick decision-making and rapid execution on a global scale.

This was achieved in part by using technology. The Ministry's e-Governance and IT Division created customised portals that allowed the networks to work in real time.

3. Policy was created "on the go." The matrix structure soon organised itself into a number of verticals. These are reflected in the chapterisation of the monograph. The verticals were able to identify and focus on problems and generate, in a cooperative manner, a number of procedures and policies that standardised responses and operating procedures on a

system wide basis. Uniformity in responses on a global scale therefore arose relatively swiftly.

4. The Ministry adapted rapidly to digital and virtual diplomacy in its outward facing operations. Virtual multilateral and plurilateral meetings commenced within a week of the lockdowns and were kicked off with G20 and South Asian leaders' meetings. At the operational level, the Ministry was involved in a Quad senior officials' coordination mechanism. This soon settled into a system of regular virtual and digital meetings to take forward the business of diplomacy.

5. The business of outreach and public diplomacy had to adapt to the disruptions and the uncertainty created by the pandemic. Countering misinformation on a global scale and its "weaponisation" required a 24/7 system to rapidly disseminate correct information and analyses.

6. A broad timeline of the response has been created. It attempts to list the administrative landmarks around which the Ministry organised its response. These began with the reports of the initial outbreak in China which reported the first COVID death in December 2019. The Government of India issued the first travel advisory on 17 January 2020, advising travellers to China to follow public health measures at all times. As the situation evolved the government issued another advisory on 25 January 2020, advising avoidance of all non-essential travel to China. As the COVID virus spread rapidly to other countries, visa restrictions were placed for nationals coming from Italy, Iran, South Korea, Japan and China. But due to spurt in cases, drastic measures were taken to curtail the spread of infections: From 13 March 2020, all existing visas (except diplomatic, official, UN/International Organisation, employment and project visa) were suspended, and visa free travel granted to OCI cardholders was kept in abeyance.

7. By then (12 March 2020) a COVID Cell headed by an Additional Secretary was created in the Ministry. On 24 March 2020, a nationwide complete lockdown was imposed with the hope that a strict lockdown would prevent the spread of the virus. The lockdown was initially meant to be imposed for 3 weeks but remained in force with extensions till end May. The COVID Cell became the central agency for responding to the exigencies created by the lockdown and the consequent disruptions. The Ministry's COVID Control Room had already started 24/7 operations

on 16 March 2020 and was scaled up rapidly to deal with requests from stranded Indians in various parts of the world, and in managing the evacuation of stranded foreign nationals in India.

8. Empowered Groups were created at the Government of India level to deal with the management of the pandemic. Additional Secretary (EA) represented the Ministry in this structure as it focused on procurement of PPEs, testing kits and other essential medical supplies. Additional Secretary (IO) was assigned the responsibility of liaising with other agencies on matters relating to vaccines.

9. In the next phase of operations, COVID Cell became the focal point for Vande Bharat Missions. Joint Secretary (AD) was assigned the task of liaising with Air India. JS eG&IT was enlisted as the point person for digital and information technology. Officers at the level of Additional Secretary/Joint Secretary were also assigned to deal with State Governments on Vande Bharat Mission related issues.

10. XP and PP Divisions were brought in to deal with outreach. Outgoing HADR was coordinated through DPA IV and the consented territorial divisions.

11. Subsequently, Vaccine Maitri was coordinated by AS (IO). JS (AD) dealt with the logistics along with concerned territorial Joint Secretaries.

12. The second wave of the mission saw the COVID Cell being scaled up to deal with incoming supplies. AS (EA) by then was embedded with the Empowered Group structure and worked with COVID Cell to coordinate incoming essential and lifesaving supplies. AS (IO) had also moved by then to a subsequent stage of vaccine diplomacy, including outreach to vaccine producers and facilitation of induction of vaccines.

13. The chapterisation reflects the broad verticals along which the Ministry's response was organised. These include Vande Bharat, Outbound evacuation, Procurement during the first and second waves, Outbound HADR and relief operations, Vaccines, Diplomatic Initiatives and Outreach. A separate chapter on how the Ministry's internal Administration division supported the response is included. Chapters were also added on the Role of Missions and working with the Armed Forces. A case study on working with an outsourcing partner, HLL Ltd, has also been included.

Digital diplomacy and outreach have been mentioned. The pandemic has serious geopolitical and geo-economics consequences. Geopolitical events such as the serious escalation of tensions on the border with China happened in the midst of lockdowns and disruptions. The Ministry and Missions continued with their core political and economic reporting and analysis functions. A comprehensive "fused" picture of the new realities was prepared based on inputs received from around the world.

14. The monograph was produced by a cooperative effort. Individual verticals contributed the sections that have been included. Editorial intervention has been restricted to a minimum.

Harsh Vardhan Shringla
Foreign Secretary

VANDE BHARAT MISSION

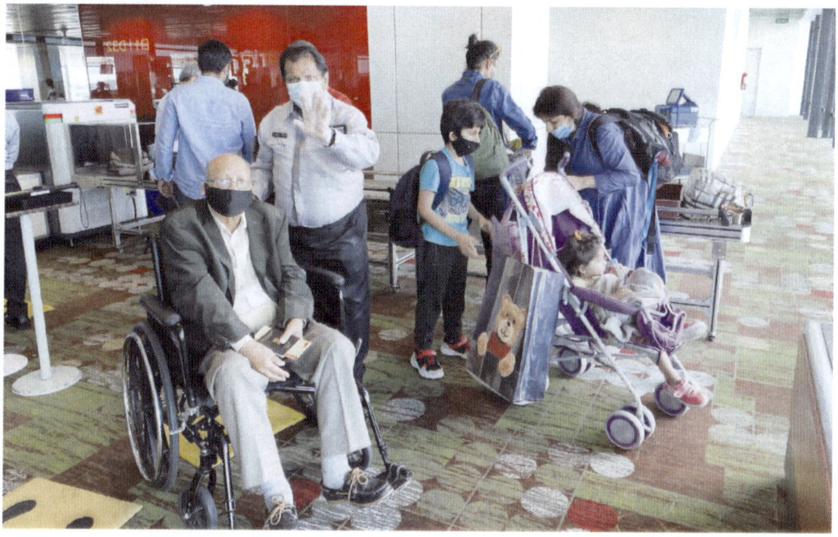

VBM Flight from Singapore to Mumbai with 243 passengers

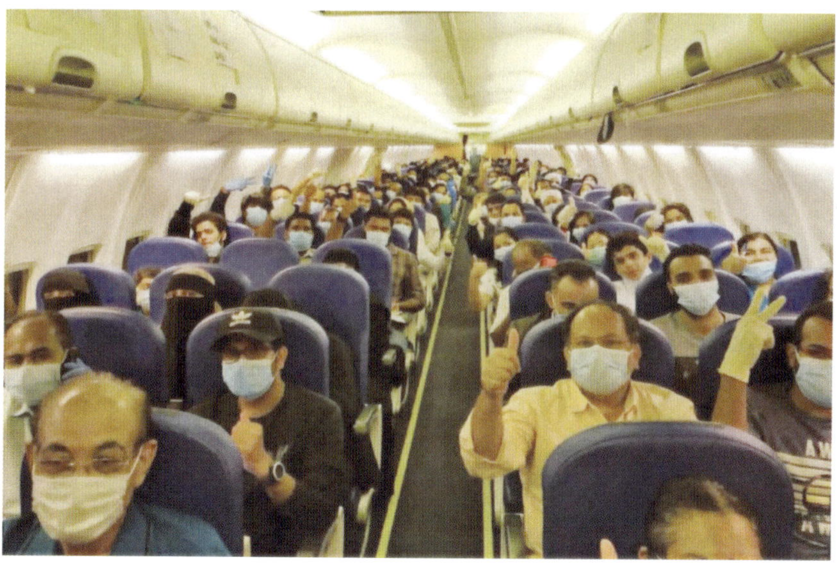

Second flight from Malaysia in Phase I of VBM—from Kuala Lampur to Kochi

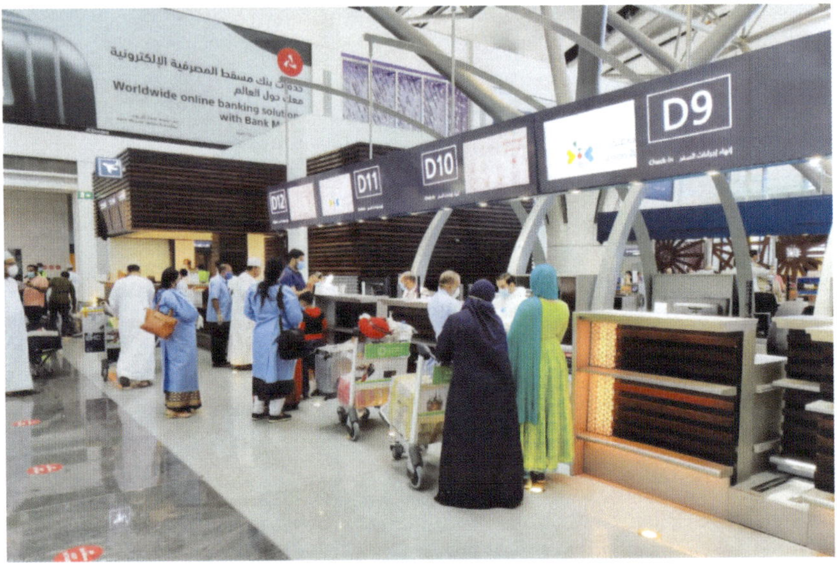

First special VBM flight from Oman with passengers including those with urgent medical needs, workers, stranded visitors, and people having family emergencies

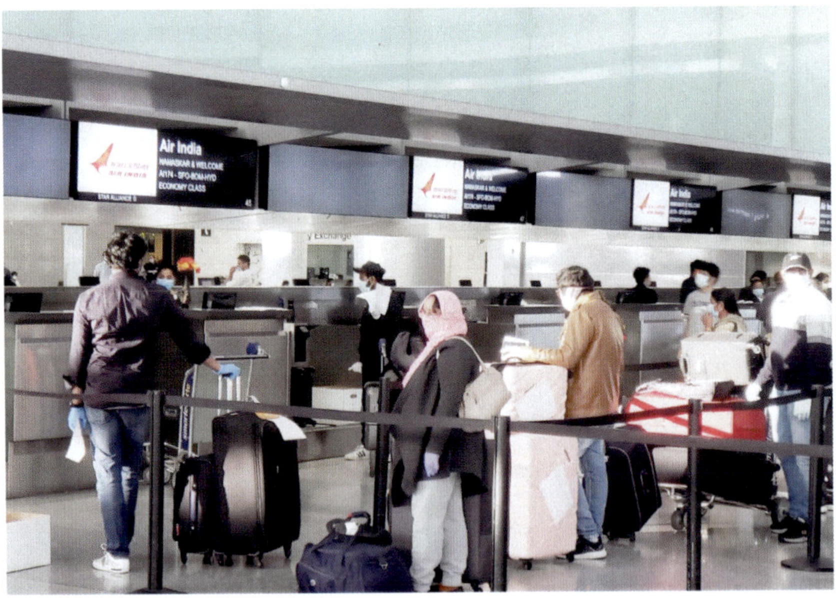

The US leg of VBM starts from San Francisco to Mumbai and Hyderabad

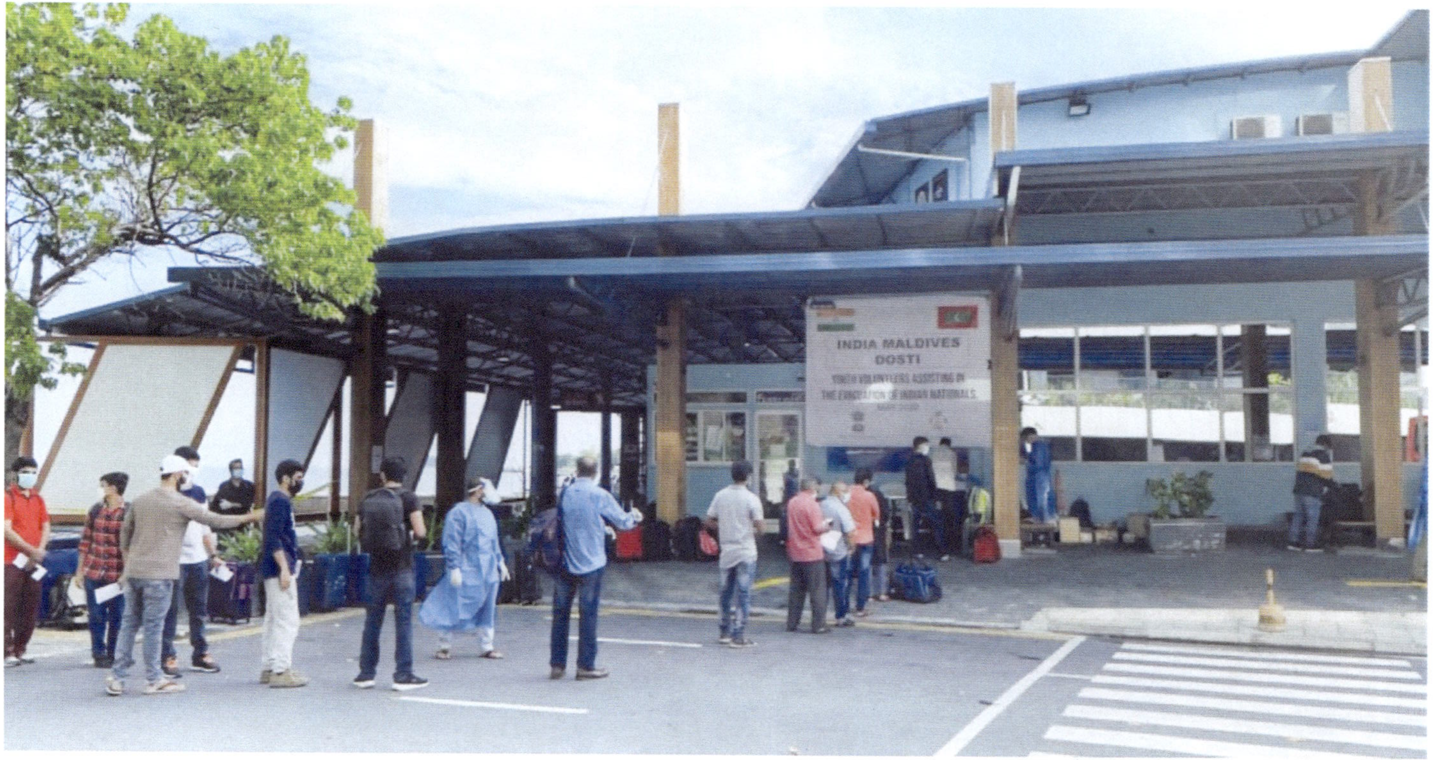
INDIA MALDIVES
DOSTI
YOUTH VOLUNTEERS ASSISTING IN
THE EVACUATION OF INDIAN NATIONALS

Indian nationals arriving at the Ferry Terminal in Malé to go through necessary checks and procedures as they prepare for evacuation by INS Jalashwa under Operation Samudra Setu as part of VBM

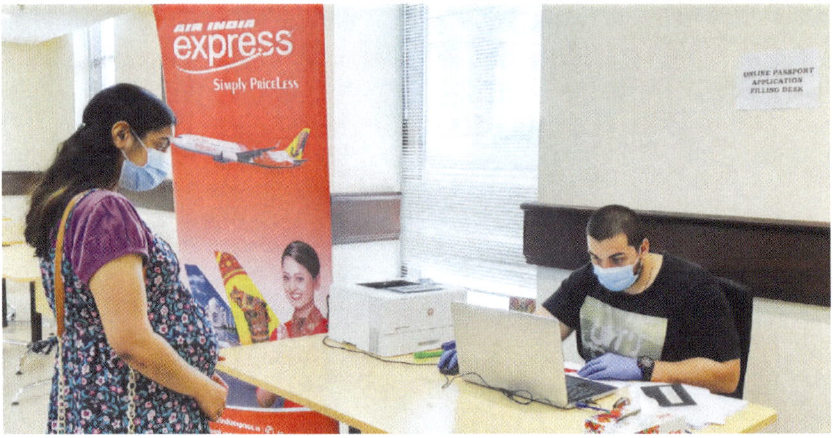

Preparations underway for first VBM Air India flight from Bahrain to Kochi to repatriate stranded Indians

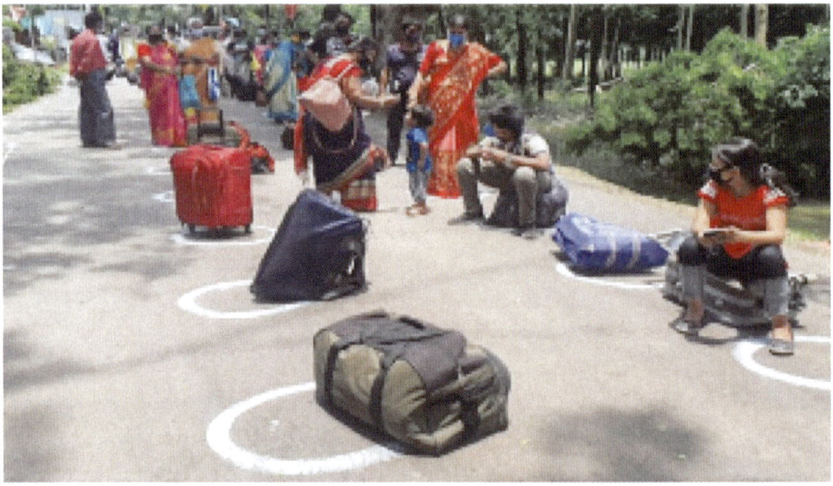

Around 200 Indian citizens largely from North East India crossed over through 3 land bounder posts (Dawlia-Tamabil, Agartala-Akhaura, Sutarkandi-Sheola) in late May 2020

2

VANDE BHARAT MISSION

GLOBAL LOCKDOWNS AND DISRUPTIONS

The pandemic triggered lockdowns and bans on movements across the world. At any given time, hundreds of thousands of Indians are travelling abroad. India also has one of the largest diasporas. Millions of Indians and Indian origin persons reside outside India. These include, amongst others, students, professionals, workers, and businessmen staying for varying lengths of time abroad.

The rapid spread of the virus in the first months of 2020 across the world created enormous anxieties and pressures. Country after country across the world imposed bans on travel and enforced lockdowns. This had the effect of stranding hundreds of thousands of Indians across the world. Internal travel bans in several countries created further complications.

Indian Heads of Mission (HoM) and Posts across the world were in close touch with stranded Indians and it became obvious that there was an urgent need to mount a rescue/evacuation operation to repatriate stranded Indians, and to enable movement of Indians and Indian origin persons across borders, to attend to emergencies and on account of other requirements.

During the initial days of the COVID pandemic, stranded Indians abroad became restive due to the rapid spread of virus in their countries of residence. Foreign governments imposed internal lockdowns, resulting in the shutdown of internal travel and international air travel. In some countries, medicines and hospitals were restricted for use by locals only, while expats were left to fend for themselves. Our HoMs echoed a sense of urgency to mount rescue/evacuation flights from India.

This necessarily had to be an interagency process involving multiple operational, agencies and stakeholders in India and abroad. It also had to take into account misgivings about allowing free movement across borders because of apprehensions that this would cause an exponential spread of the virus. The Ministry had a pivotal role in this interagency process because it was the first and principal point of contact with the hundreds of thousands of Indians stranded abroad.

"MAPPING" STRANDED INDIANS

In the first week of April 2020, EAM directed COVID Cell to formulate a plan of action to bring back Indians stranded on foreign soil. Foreign Secretary and COVID Cell thereupon embarked on an exercise to "map" Indians who wished to return. As per the inputs provided by our Missions, the tentative number of stranded Indians who desired to return to India was assessed to be more than 5 lakh. Forty per cent of this number, or about 2 lakh were from the Gulf countries alone.

DETERMINING TRAVEL PRIORITY

The process of ascertaining numbers was a first step. Given the large numbers and limitations in terms of mode and frequency of travel, a system of priorities that allowed the most 'compelling cases' to travel first had to be created. Foreign Secretary asked Heads of Mission and Posts to assess the levels of distress and desperation. COVID Cell sought further information from Missions and Posts, developed and circulated criteria for prioritising passengers. The criteria that were developed to prioritise order of travel can be seen at Annexure 1a.

24×7 COMMUNICATION CENTRE

The Ministry established a 24×7 communication centre to act as a single point of communication and a call centre for COVID related queries from around the globe. The communication centre utilised telephone, email, social media to answer queries, resolve problems, disseminate information and act as clearing house and coordination centre. Internal chains of command and jurisdiction were reoriented to increase bandwidth. Capacities were scaled up when required by "plugging-in" officers, including those with specific geographical responsibilities or expertise, when required.

APPROVALS

Based on inputs received from the ground, through the network of Missions and Posts abroad, a strategy was worked out and presented to EAM. This was presented on 13 April 2020 to the Inter-Ministerial Group in which the National Security Advisor and the Chief of Defence Staff participated. This Group agreed to proceed with the plan of action. Additional operational and policy inputs and details were added to the plan by the Committee of Secretaries and Group of Ministers (GoM).

This plan was presented by Foreign Secretary to the Prime Minister on 21 April 2020, in the presence of GoM (see Annexure 1i). Prime Minister directed that the plan be put into action in order to bring back stranded Indians in a phased manner—starting with the Gulf region—where a larger number of Indian workers had lost their jobs due to the lockdown, and therefore had no means to sustain their livelihood.

INTERAGENCY PROCESS

SOPs for handling passengers returning from abroad, including protocols for quarantine, etc. were drawn up in consultation with the Ministries of Health and Family Welfare, Civil Aviation and Home Affairs. State Governments, who were responsible for quarantine, were involved in the decision making through multiple video conferences.

The Ministry of External Affairs was given the direct responsibility of managing the process of implementing SOPs applicable to the return of citizens from abroad. Ministry of Civil Aviation handled the operational aspects of arranging flights in coordination with the Ministry. Security agencies, airport management systems, health authorities, multiple state level and municipal authorities and hotels were all involved in the coordination process.

The Ministry assigned a senior officer at the rank of Additional Secretary and Joint Secretary to each State. They became the single point of contact for the State authorities, which brought in settlement of the multitude of the issues. (See Annexure 1g)

COORDINATION WITH STATE GOVERNMENTS

Coordination with State governments was critical in ensuring that Indians returned to their domiciles in the most economic and quick manner. The Ministry accordingly had to devise a mechanism to coordinate with all State Governments. On 5 May 2020, Foreign Secretary briefed State Chief Secretaries about the VBM operations. Foreign Secretary therefore designated senior officers of the Ministry, at the level of Additional Secretaries (AS)/Joint Secretaries (JS), as nodal officers for coordination with specific States. These nodal officers acted as clearing houses and points of contact between state governments, the Ministry and Missions abroad. A WhatsApp group was set up bringing the State Coordinators from the Ministry, the Security Agencies, the Air India personnel and our Missions, which were literally operating as the ground handling and ticketing agents for the VBM flights.

The States were preoccupied with inter-State movement of migrant workers and were faced with the dilemma of allowing stranded Indians returning home, while migrant workers at home were still held back and facing hardships. States feared a political backlash for restraining movement of internal migrant workers while allowing VBM returnees.

VANDE BHARAT BEGINS

VBM flights commenced operations on 7 May 2020. State governments, Missions and all relevant Ministries/Departments adapted swiftly, just as the pandemic situation demanded.

The Ministry's Administration Division headed by Joint Secretary (Administration), coordinated the scheduling of flights, their frequencies and the destinations based on a continuous assessment of the demand for repatriation from different countries.

Missions collated and updated their databases about returning Indians on an hourly basis. Based on this projected demand, a consolidated list of flights required for each Phase, usually a period of one month, was prepared. Approval of the Foreign Secretary and EAM was obtained before conveying the requirements to Air India.

The Ministry worked with Air India in identifying the date and size of the aircraft. Missions and Posts also worked with local governments to obtain the necessary clearances and ground handling for the flights during lockdown conditions. During the actual repatriation, Missions physically deployed personnel to man the desks at airports, ensured access, during lockdowns and disruptions, for passengers trying to reach airports. The Missions also prioritised the returnees based on their immediate need and helped the airline even in selling the tickets to the needy.

Initially, most international arrivals were at Delhi and Mumbai airports with only a few international flights reaching other destinations within India. At the time, domestic air travel was also not available. As a result, there was strain on quarantine facilities in these two cities. To ease these pressures, select domestic airports across the country were made operational to cater specifically to VBM flights. This involved coordination with Ministry of Civil Aviation, Ministry of Home Affairs, Bureau of Immigration and State Governments. Thereafter, to assess demand, at the time of registration with Missions/Posts, passengers were asked to indicate their final destination within India. Based on this, State-wise demand was projected for repatriation requests from each country. At the time of scheduling in coordination with Air India, this data was used to press 'feeder' flights into service from Delhi and Mumbai to destinations in other States. Where necessary, feeder flights were organised within a State too, using smaller aircrafts. VBM flights reached a total of 32 airports across 19 States. Feeder flights also helped in ensuring minimal exposure of the passengers, thus ensuring strict compliance with extant health regulations.

Initially, Vande Bharat flights were operated by Air India flights only. Private sector Indian carriers—IndiGo, SpiceJet, GoAir and Vistara—soon joined Vande Bharat in order to meet the growing demand. They played a very useful role in linking high-demand locations such as West Asia and South East Asia, where these airlines had operated before the pandemic. These four Indian private carriers operated 545 international flights from 7 different countries during June-December 2020, repatriating around 80,000 stranded persons.

Foreign Secretary directed that COVID Cell develop an online portal that could act as a management information system for planning flights and also to record data of returning Indians. The portal would be a single information source accessible to the relevant agencies involved in the repatriation process. These included the relevant Ministries/ Departments, State Governments and Missions which were involved in the welfare of the returning persons. With the help of an experienced team of consultants, EG & IT Division designed, in-house, the Ministry's 'REPAT Portal'.

The Portal was designed to capture relevant data about returning Indians and categorise them according to domicile. Missions asked local stranded Indians through emails to provide data about themselves in pre-formatted Excel sheets that were linked to REPAT Portal.

A real-time picture thus developed that allowed COVID Cell, at the click of a mouse, to allocate aviation resources to routes that linked concentration of Indians abroad directly to specific destinations in different Indian states.

States were able to see data in real time and were able to plan for the arrivals of flights. The portal and the real-time data it provided was useful for state governments, immigration, and health officials to plan logistics such as screening, testing, quarantine and transportation for arriving passengers.

Passengers were required to give an undertaking to ensure that only those with compelling reasons boarded flights on a priority basis (Annexure 1b).

It was decided to name repatriation operations as 'Vande Bharat Mission' (VBM)—the biggest operation ever in the history of independent India. Air India had worked out 64 flights for Phase-I of the VBM and Missions worked out passenger manifests in advance.

Eventually, the repatriation flights were termed as international flights under bilateral 'Air Bubble' arrangements with 26 countries. By end-June 2020, as restrictions were gradually lifted, including on OCIs and foreign nationals, the registrations on the Ministry's Repat Portal went up significantly and exceeded 5 lakh. The number of flights was accordingly expanded.

During the 14 phases of VBM, as on 14 October 2021, a total of 56,03,992 passengers were repatriated back to India via air routes, 3987 via sea routes, and 5,02,151 via land routes – totaling 61,10,130.

A snapshot of flights and arrivals are at Annexure 1f.

Repatriation Summary Sheet	
Carrier	**Passengers**
Air India And Air India Exp	1884466
Deportee	2591
Amnesty	7344
Chartered	3705584
Other Foreign Carriers	4007
Naval Ships	3987
Land Border Crossings	502151
Total	6110130

CHARTER FLIGHTS

The growing demand for flights from Indians stranded abroad far outstripped Air India's capacity. It was therefore decided to allow charter flight operations from 26 May 2020 from various parts of the world. These were especially meant to bring back project related workers from the Gulf region, merchant shipping crews and cruise personnel, etc. who remained stranded at various ports, facing restrictions on their internal movement.

Ministry of External Affairs, in consultation with Ministry of Home Affairs and Ministry of Civil Aviation, proposed an SoP for charter flights, according to which, requests for charter flights were to be sent first to our Missions abroad, on whose recommendations the Ministry would then seek clearance from DGCA and States. The SoPs for operating charter flights can be found in Annexure 1e.

On the Ministry's recommendations, the SoP was further streamlined to facilitate chartered flights to operate from most regions except from remote areas of Latin American and Caribbean countries, and parts of Africa.

Chartered flights could thereafter directly coordinate with State governments and DGCA for obtaining clearances without the involvement of Missions and the Ministry. This simplified procedure helped to expedite the clearance processes, and several Indian associations/groups were able to hire the services of chartered flights smoothly, and brought back a large number of stranded Indians. Chartered flights organised directly by community associations were allowed, provided they adhered to specific and broadly defined rules set out in an SoP prepared by Ministry of Civil Aviation and processes implemented by the Ministry. By end-October 2020, the number of Indians repatriated through chartered flights reached 1.2 million, overtaking the number of passengers brought in by the VBM flights at that time.

Privately run Indian carriers and other foreign carriers also contributed capacities to increase the pace and the range of destinations being served.

As lockdown restrictions were eased in a calibrated manner, bilateral Air Transport Bubble arrangements were established with a few countries to allow limited commercial passenger services on reciprocal basis. Ministry of Civil Aviation established such air bubble arrangements with 26 countries—Afghanistan, Bahrain, Bangladesh, Bhutan, Canada, Ethiopia, France, Germany, Iraq, Japan, Kenya, Kuwait, Maldives, Nepal, Netherlands, Nigeria, Oman, Qatar, Russia, Rwanda, Seychelles, Sri Lanka, Tanzania, Ukraine, United Arab Emirates, United Kingdom, United States of America and Uzbekistan.

Ministry of Home Affairs issued SOP for travel on VBM and Air Transport Bubble flights on 22 August 2020.

OTHER FLIGHTS

Obtaining permissions for Air Ambulances involved delicate logistics and multiple approvals from Ministry of Health, Ministry of Home Affairs and the DGCA for cases of medical emergencies of Indian nationals located abroad for treatment. It also entailed document verification by Missions, and certification of receiving hospitals in India. Adhering to timelines was of great significance in such matters. Overall, about 100 patients were brought into the country by Air Ambulances for medical treatment.

Although VBM flights were gradually extended to cover other countries, remote areas of Latin American and Caribbean countries, West Africa and CIS countries could not be covered because of geographical distances and logistical hurdles. VBM operations to specific locations in those regions were not found to be economically viable. Gathering stranded Indians to a particular hub was explored but found not feasible. Plans to bring them to the US and placing them on VBM flights did not materialise for the same reasons as well as due to visa issues. However, KLM flights with extensive operations to the Latin American region (with Amsterdam as its hub) offered an opportunity for stranded Indians, as did Ethiopian Airlines with an extensive network in the African region.

Since return of Indians by foreign carriers required DGCA approval, the COVID Cell had to take it up for approvals on a case-by-case basis, notwithstanding DGCA's reluctance to encourage these options. In all, about 3000 stranded Indians were evacuated from Peru, Columbia, Bolivia, Panama, Chile, Venezuela, Mexico, Guatemala, Nicaragua, Honduras, Belize, etc. and from the Caribbean region—Antigua, Barbados, Guyana, Suriname, Trinidad and Tobago, Jamaica, St. Lucia, etc.

A number of Indians returned by amnesty flights from Kuwait and deportation flights from UAE, Saudi Arabia, Bahrain, Kuwait, Malaysia and the US. In these cases, the Ministry expedited necessary approvals and processes including fee waiver for emergency certificates.

IX 1344 Crash on 7 August 2020

Three months after the launch of Vande Bharat, on 7 August, a VBM flight, Air India Express IX 1344 operating on the Dubai-Kozhikode sector crashed. It overshot the runway in Kozhikode due to poor weather conditions. Of the 190 persons on board, all Indians, 21 were killed including 19 passengers and both the pilots. 169 persons survived of which 167 were injured.

Immediately after the accident, the Ministry set up a 24×7 control room with dedicated helpline numbers to provide information and assistance to the affected. The control room was manned by the Ministry's personnel and operated until 10 August 2020. It established real-time coordination among Kozhikode Airport, district administrations of Kozhikode and Malappuram districts, Ministry of Civil Aviation, DGCA, Embassy of India, Abu Dhabi, Consulate General of India, Dubai, and Air India control rooms established in Abu Dhabi, Dubai and Sharjah.

The Ministry focused on providing updated information to the families—both in Kerala and in UAE—of the passengers and crew. This involved coordinating with agencies on the ground to ascertain the status of each passenger and crew member based on the flight manifest and updating details of the hospitals where the deceased and the injured had been taken. Simultaneously, the VBM coordination team in the Ministry worked with DGCA, Embassy of India, Abu Dhabi, and Consulate General of India, Dubai to reschedule other VBM flights to ensure minimum disruption to the repatriation efforts. Kozhikode Airport was operational the next day, on 8 August 2020, and flights approved earlier were cleared to operate.

REPATRIATION BY LAND

In addition, the opening up of land border check-posts with Nepal, Bhutan and Bangladesh triggered a surge in the number of returnees by land routes, which by end-June 2020 reached over 1 lakh, taking the total returnees to 3.80 lakh.

MHA Standard Operating Procedure (SoPs) are available in Annexure 1c.

REPATRIATION BY SEA/SAMUDRA SETU

The Chief of Naval Staff called on EAM in April 2020 to discuss deployment of naval ships to support repatriation efforts. Subsequently, Foreign Secretary met with the Chief of Defence Staff, and Addl. Secy. (COVID) met the Deputy CIDS (Operations). The Department of Military Affairs provided the necessary support.

Several options and factions were considered including risks of exposing passengers to the virus during long journeys over several days in a closed environment and the narrow price differential between travel by ships and air travel from relevant destinations.

Eight naval ships subsequently, in an operation entitled 'Samudra Setu'—four ships for Male; two ships for Bandar Abbas in Iran; two ships for Sri Lanka—sailed out to bring stranded Indians home. Over 4,000 Indians—including fishermen and workers who could not afford to return by air—were repatriated by the sea route.

ROLE OF INDIAN MISSIONS ABROAD

Indian Missions abroad extended all possible assistance to the stranded Indians after COVID related restrictions were imposed. The assistance varied based on the needs of the people. Missions set-up 24×7 COVID emergency helplines for all kinds of assistance to Indian nationals in need. In some countries, Indian nationals were provided with masks and sanitizers, food kits, preliminary medical consultation, along with aid, boarding & lodging, and even tickets in the most deserving cases.

These initiatives were conducted by the Missions through the Indian Community Welfare Fund (ICWF) resources as well as through close cooperation with the local Indian community and their local associations.

An Indian Community Welfare Fund exists in all the Indian Missions and Posts abroad to assist Indians in distress. ICWF funds can be disbursed to distressed Indian nationals overseas on a means-tested basis for boarding/lodging, air passages to India, legal assistance, payment for small fines and penalties, transportation of mortal remains and emergency medical care. Cumulative ICWF disbursals during the pandemic amounted to INR 42 crore (until August 2021). More than 1.6 million individuals were assisted.

Some Missions sought the help of local places of worship such as Gurudwaras, as well as community centres for providing lodging and boarding, or created innovative makeshift arrangements for the same. In consultation with host governments, Missions also helped in timely dissemination of local government guidelines on health, preventive measures, and provided medical facilities, facilitated travel logistics. Missions also assisted in testing for symptoms and other facilitation at the airports at the time of an individual's departure to India. As an example, details of assistance provided by some of the Missions can be found in Annexure 1d.

Missions played an important role in arranging chartered flights in cooperation with local Indian communities and companies to repatriate their workers.

Even though the critical phase of repatriation of stranded Indians was mostly over by December 2020, Missions continued to oversee the smooth functioning and forwarding of the manifests of chartered flights, air bubble flights and other flights under VBM, as per the extant guidelines of the Government of India.

SKILLED WORKERS ARRIVAL DATABASE FOR EMPLOYMENT SUPPORT OR SWADES

The Government of India has a robust institutional framework for the welfare, safety and protection of Indian migrants working abroad. The e-Migrate system, Pre-Departure Orientation Programme, MADAD portal, Indian Community Welfare Fund, Pravasi Bharatiya Sahayata Kendras, helplines at Indian Missions and Posts, shelter homes, etc. are some mechanisms that assist Indian workers abroad. The experience of operating these systems and the data they provided proved useful during the pandemic.

The government launched the SWADES initiative for Indian nationals returning under VBM on 30 May 2020. SWADES is a joint initiative of the Ministry of Skill Development and Entrepreneurship, Ministry of Civil Aviation, and the Ministry of External Affairs. It created a database of returning Indian nationals based on their skill sets and experience. An online SWADES Skills card containing details of each returnee's work sector, job title, employment and years of experience was uploaded onto the database. The information collected via the skills card was used to facilitate placement opportunities by integrating this database with Skill India's ASEEM (Aatmanirbhar Skilled Employee Employer Mapping) portal. As of June 2021, more than 30,900 persons had registered their SWADES Skill cards. Job connects were established between 6,704 candidates and employers registered on ASEEM.

WUHAN EVACUATIONS

China was the first country to witness the outbreak of the pandemic starting December 2019. The Government of India closely followed pandemic related developments in China, and by the latter part of January 2020, it was evident that the situation was rapidly deteriorating. The principal focus of the outbreak was Hubei province and its capital city of Wuhan. A particular source of concern for the Government of India was the large number of Indian students in Hubei. Their families in India were, naturally, extremely concerned about their health and well-being.

Three special flights were organised—on 31 January 2020, 1 February 2020 and 26 February 2020—to evacuate Indians as well as nationals of our neighbouring and some other countries from Hubei province. The first two back-to-back rounds of evacuation were carried on board Air India flights, while the third round of evacuation was done on board an Indian Air Force C-17 Globemaster plane. All three rounds of airlifts took place from Wuhan.

These three flights together evacuated a total of 766 persons from Hubei, which included 718 Indians and 43 foreign nationals belonging to 7 different countries, as well as 5 officials from the Embassy of India in Beijing, who had traveled to Wuhan to manage the evacuation process on the ground (they traveled on-board the second and the third flights). The foreign nationals included 23 from Bangladesh, 9 from Maldives, 2 from Myanmar, 1 from South Africa, 1 from Madagascar and 1 from the United States of America. In addition, 6 Chinese citizens who were spouses and/or children of Indian nationals were also evacuated.

The first two flights evacuated a total of 647 Indians (324 on the first and 323 on the second, including 2 Embassy officials) and 7 Maldivian nationals (on the second flight). The third Indian Air Force flight airlifted 76 Indians (including 3 Embassy officials) and 36 foreign nationals. Among the foreign nationals evacuated on board this flight, there were citizens of the following countries: China (6), Bangladesh (23), Maldives (2), Myanmar (2), South Africa (1), Madagascar (1) and the United States (1).

India had committed to assisting China in tackling the challenges posed by the pandemic. Responding to a request from the Chinese side, the third evacuation flight operated by the Indian Air Force also delivered over 15 tonnes of medical assistance comprising masks, gloves and other emergency medical equipment for Chinese health-care professionals. These were handed over to the Hubei Charity Federation.

All the evacuees and the Embassy officials on their arrival in India were kept in government quarantine facilities near Delhi (Indian Army camp at Manesar and ITBP camp in Chhawla) for two weeks and tested for COVID twice. All of them tested negative and were thereafter sent to their respective places of stay in India for self-isolation for another two weeks.

These evacuations were a multi-agency effort led by the Embassy of India in Beijing and the East Asia Division of the Ministry of External Affairs in Delhi, supported by the Ministry of Civil Aviation, Air India, the Indian Air Force, Ministry of Health and Family Welfare and other government agencies.

The Embassy of India in Beijing continued to remain in touch with those Indian nationals who had decided to stay back in Hubei province through 24×7 hotline numbers, dedicated email and other social media channels. The Embassy, along with its Consulates, also continued to provide assistance to Indian nationals in other parts of China to help them cope with the pandemic.

STRUCTURAL RESPONSE

Senior Ministry officials at the level of Additional Secretary and Joint Secretary coordinated different elements of Vande Bharat.

Initially work was coordinated by COVID Cell. As the scope of the operation expanded and become more complex to include separate issues such as Charter flights, Deportee flights, Amnesty flights and Naval ships, capacities were scaled up by additional deployments at multiple levels and by activating a flat "matrix" within the Ministry that allowed mobilisation of resources residing in differing hierarchies and jurisdictions (Annexure 1h).

EVACUATION-OUTGOING

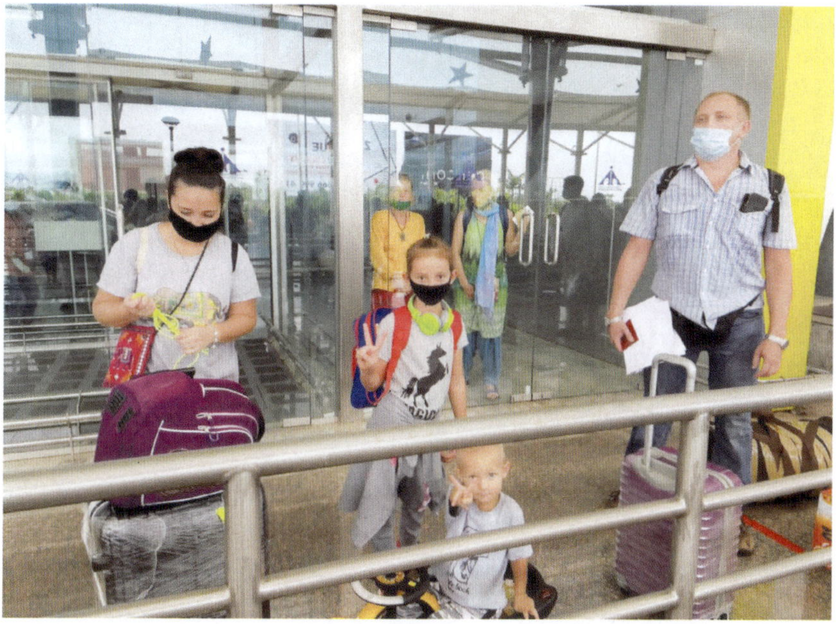

42nd relief flight from Goa on 13 June 2020 carrying 439 adults and 8 infants in Rossiya airlines to Russia

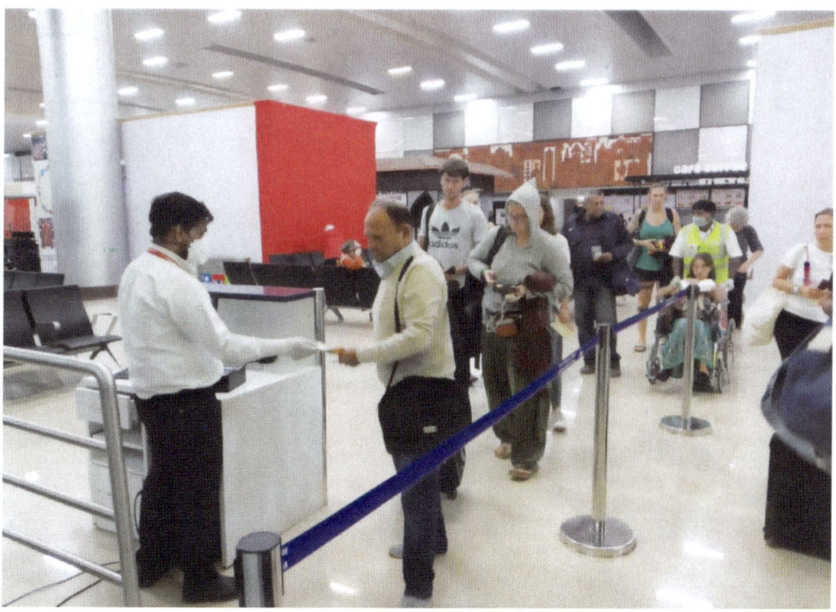

317 German and EU passengers departed from Goa International Airport to Frankfurt on 31 March 2020

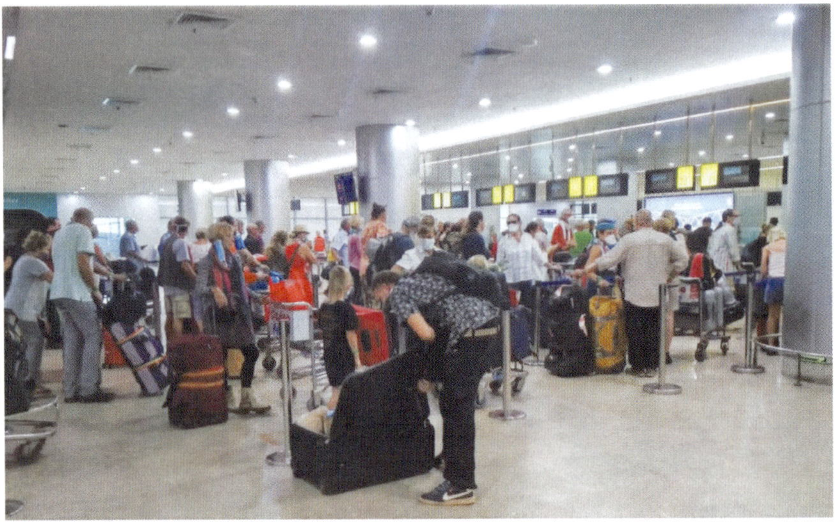

Goa Customs officers played a key role in evacuating 897 foreign tourists of different nationalities stranded in Goa amidst lockdown by attending to flights arriving and departing from/to Helsinki, Frankfurt and Doha in April 2020

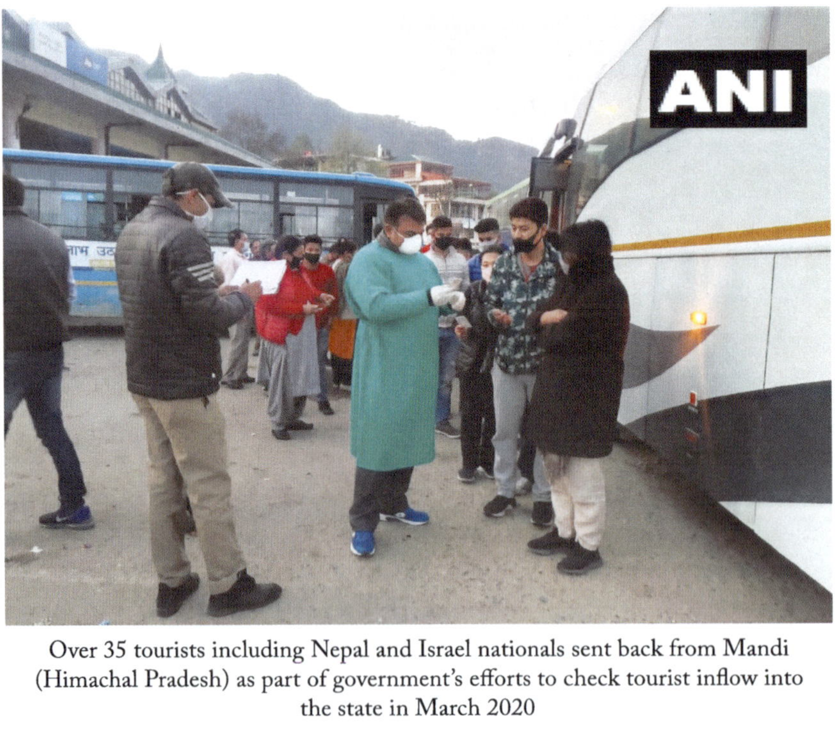

Over 35 tourists including Nepal and Israel nationals sent back from Mandi (Himachal Pradesh) as part of government's efforts to check tourist inflow into the state in March 2020

3

EVACUATION-OUTGOING

The international disruptions and the national lockdown also had the effect of stranding a large number of foreign nationals in India. These foreign nationals were in India for various purposes such as tourism, work, family visits, etc. Like Indians stranded abroad, the foreign nationals in India desired to travel back to their homes.

As in the case of inbound Vande Bharat movements, the outbound movement of the stranded foreign nationals posed an enormous logistical challenge. India is a large country and domestic travel, particularly to remote areas, can be a complicated matter. The lockdown, domestic (with effect from 25 March 2020) and international, amplified many of these complications and generated completely new sets of difficulties.

The task of coordinating the domestic and outbound movement of these foreign nationals was assigned to Chief of Protocol and COVID Cell.

The problem they were confronted with had many dimensions. It was difficult to obtain an accurate estimate of the number of foreign nationals stranded. Initial estimates, based on visa and entry data, placed it in six figures. They were in multiple locations in a continental sized country. They were from different nations (from at least 50—and almost certainly more) and therefore were headed to a large number of countries and locations within countries.

Most of them wanted to return home at the first possible chance.

Locating and "mapping" them was an initial challenge. Arranging their transport to locations in India from which they could be transported out was another challenge. Navigating the lockdown and the travel requirements in lockdown conditions created another set of difficulties. Finally, they had to link up with aircraft that would then take them home.

A large number of players, national and international, were involved in this massive evacuation exercise. State and district level authorities, union government agencies, service providers in the hospitality, travel and health sectors were some of those involved. Delhi has 154 Embassies and many of these Embassies, and other international governmental and non-governmental agencies, were, naturally, involved in the process.

Each Embassy and nationality was essentially a separate case. Each diplomatic Mission had its own unique challenges. A number of smaller foreign Missions and Consulates, with lesser capacity, required more handholding and assistance than others.

The outbound population had to be "mapped" in cooperation with diplomatic Missions in New Delhi. Anecdotally speaking, it involved locating and contacting "Russians in Goa, Israelis in Himachal Pradesh, Americans in many parts, Germans doing yoga in Rishikesh, Swedish nationals on Bengal-Jharkhand border", etc. Many of them were travelling individually. Others were in groups of varying sizes. Several did not have mobile phones or were otherwise difficult to locate.

Chief of Protocol, and Protocol Division, with assistance from COVID Cell, was the nodal point where the many chains of command, lines of effort and logistical chains involved in this evacuation intersected. A multidirectional coordination effort was required to deal with the demands of this exercise. In one direction, Chief of Protocol and COVID Cell liaised and worked with the local diplomatic corps. They were also the point of interaction with the other agencies in the Government of India that required to be involved such as the Ministry of Home Affairs, Ministry of Health and Family Welfare, and the Ministry of Civil Aviation. They also had to establish contact and work with several state governments and with district administrations across the country. Coordination was required in managing logistics, in navigating the regulatory and policy frameworks, in developing solutions to unique problems, and in "last-mile delivery." All of this was accomplished in a very short time-frame with no precedents to fall back upon.

Once their whereabouts were ascertained they had to be staged in collection points and then transported to airports from which they could be flown out. This was an extremely complicated exercise as Ministry had to work with each nationality and Embassy to develop a unique solution. The initial arrangements were necessarily ad hoc in nature. There was no set pattern to the movements and arrangements. Some groups were able to arrange transportation on their own. Others used buses and vehicles that reached them - for instance from Delhi. In many instances, Ministry had to assist in locating transportation resources.

State government and local authorities were requested for help across the country in mobilising logistical and other resources that were required to move these groups.

An accompanying set of problems related to movement authorisations and passes in lockdown conditions. Curfew passes were required not just in Delhi but in several locations in India. Curfew relaxations also had to be obtained to allow movement within and across state boundaries. This posed yet another set of difficulties. The basic unit of administration in India outside urban areas and municipal bodies is the district. Until procedures and SoPs emerged, district administrations were the key enablers in the movement of the foreign nationals. For instance, a group traveling from Himachal Pradesh to Delhi would have to drive across Punjab and Haryana to reach Delhi. They would have to traverse several districts in each state. In the rapidly evolving situation at that time, travelers had to navigate multiple checkpoints under separate chains of command as they crossed distinct boundaries. Similar movements happened simultaneously. As an illustration, other groups were moving from Goa, across various districts of Maharashtra, to Mumbai while the Himachal-Delhi movement was happening.

Chief of Protocol and COVID Cell rapidly evolved a system to deal with these issues. Close cooperation was required with the Home Ministry and State, district and police authorities. Senior officials including Foreign Secretary intervened where required. This coordination effort was literally conducted around the clock as large numbers of movements were taking place in a large number of states at any given time. Bottlenecks and obstacles appeared and had to be dealt with. Reports and feedback flooded in and interventions were made on a nationwide scale to keep the transportation of these outbound foreign nationals on track. SoPs, developed jointly with other agencies, quickly emerged to deal with a variety of situations. For example, COVID Cell started a system of issuing letters that were accepted by local authorities.

Another set of SoPs had to be developed rapidly to deal with the exit formalities of these nationals. The Ministry worked with Foreigners

Division of the Ministry of Home Affairs and Immigration authorities to develop the flexibility that were required to manage the orderly departure of foreign nationals from airports.

No outbound evacuation on this scale had ever been organised. Hundreds of incoming and outgoing flights to evacuate these passengers, whether commercial, charter or other, had to be facilitated. Plans had to be worked out with civil aviation authorities, the embassies and the transportation service providers. Last mile problems were common and required troubleshooting and interventions, often at very high levels. Last minute requirements of overflight and flight clearances was another common problem. Applicability of quarantine requirements for aircrews had to be worked out. As in other cases of interagency cooperation, channels of communication swiftly emerged to deal with these problems.

Movements of large numbers of people can be expected to—and did—create other problems. For instance, short-term accommodation at points of departure was sometimes an issue. Restrictions on movement of people meant that many services that travellers require were disrupted. Humanitarian and medical situations arose. In all of these and more, Ministry assisted foreign Missions and others to find solutions.

After the surge in outbound evacuations was managed, a slower stream of outbound movements continued. Foreign nationals often utilised outward Vande Bharat Flights from India to travel out.

SoPs had to be developed to deal with issues such forced overstay on account of the lockdowns.

By October 2020, about 110,000 foreign nationals belonging to 120 countries were safely evacuated out of India.

HUMANITARIAN ASSISTANCE AND DISASTER RELIEF

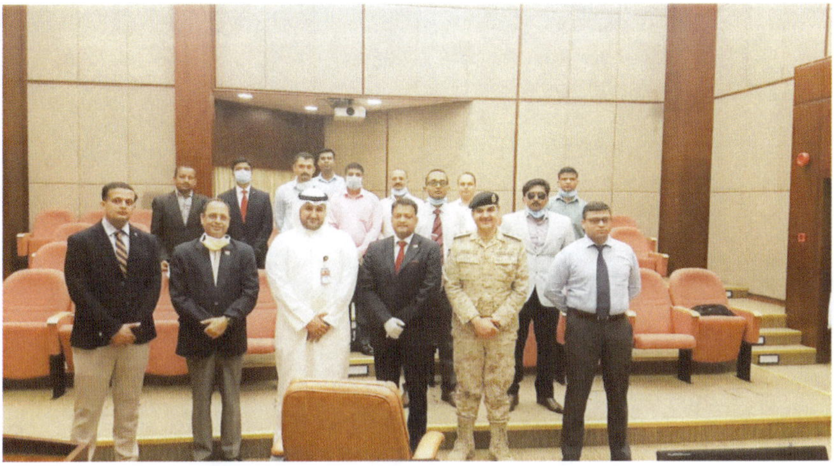

Indian Rapid Response Team in Kuwait
at Jabel Al Ahmed Hospital for capacity building and interaction

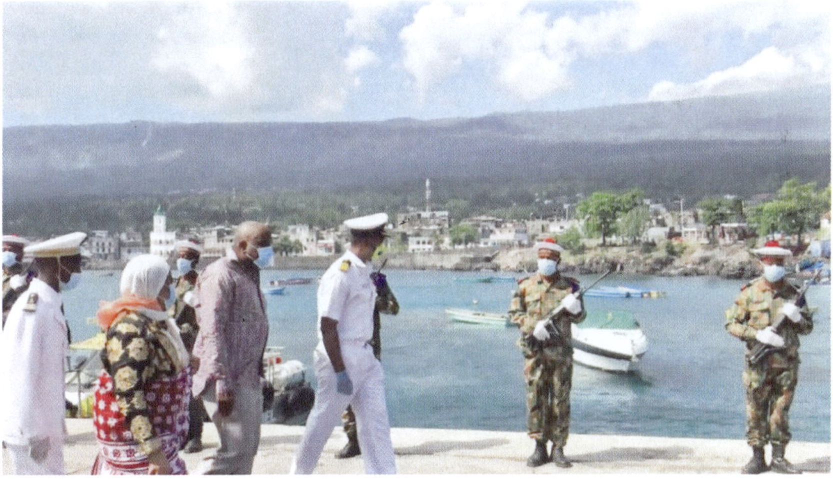

INS Kesari with a consignment of COVID related essential medicines for the people of Comoros, in addition to doctors and paramedics, entered Port of Moroni in Comoros on 31 May 2020 as part of Mission Sagar

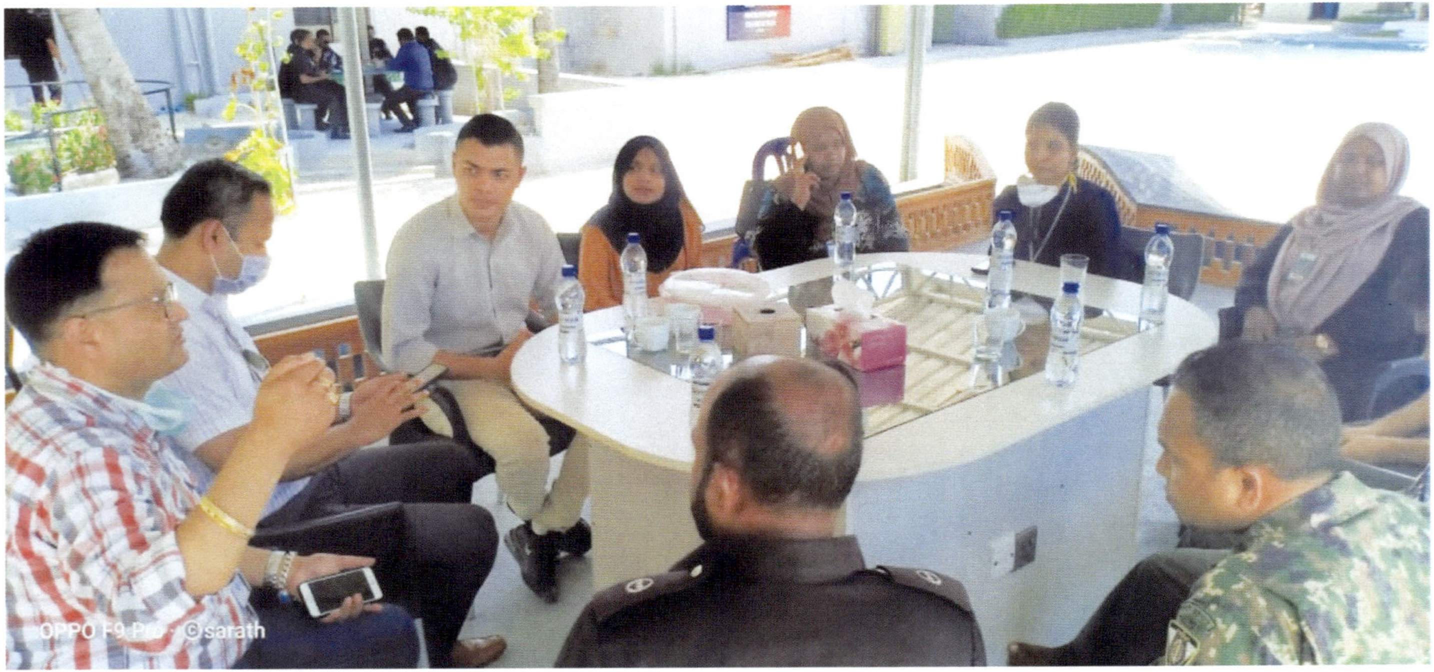

The composite COVID medical relief team from India exchanged best practices and protocols with the Medical team in Maafushi prison in Maldives

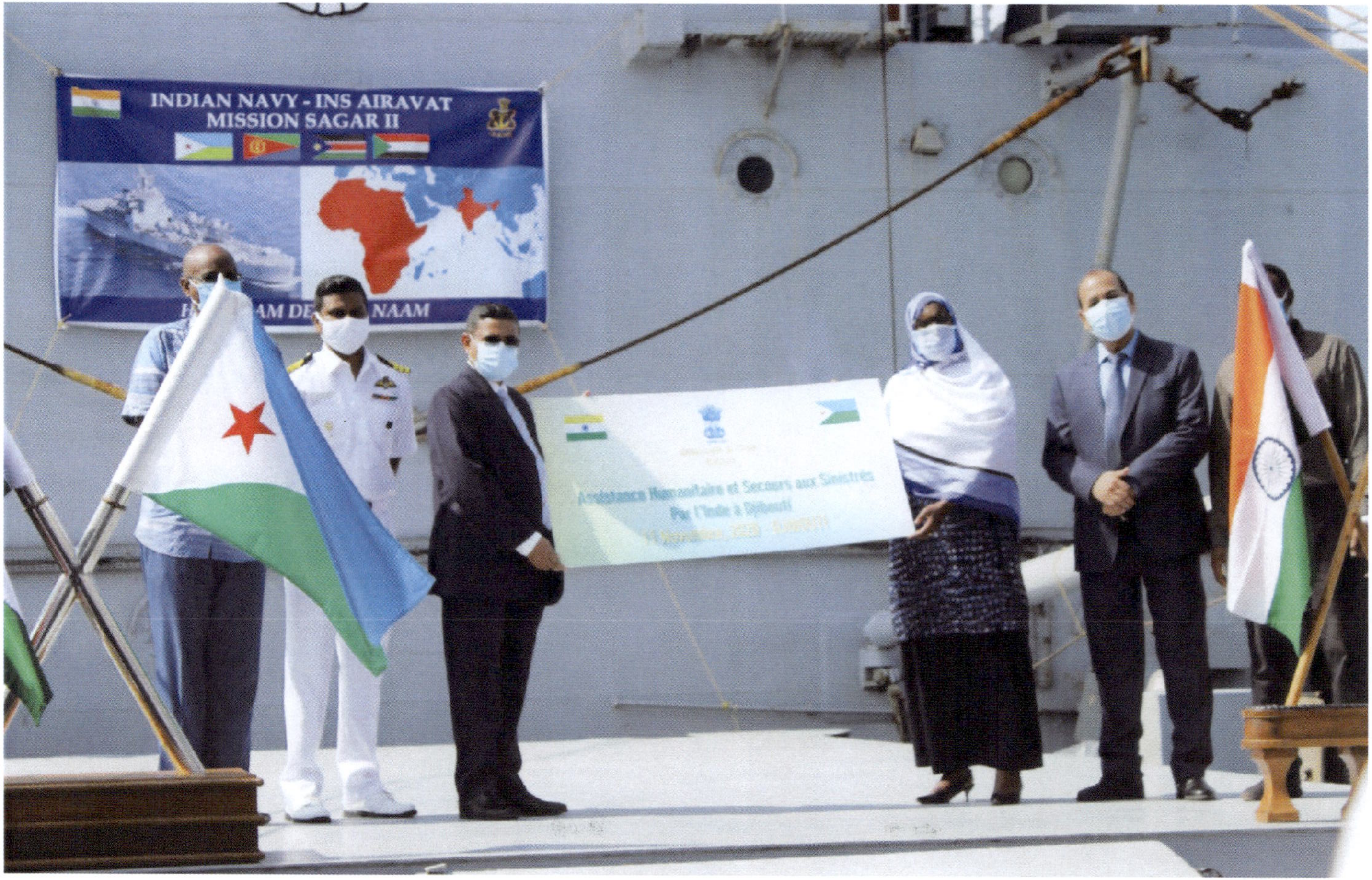
INDIAN NAVY - INS AIRAVAT
MISSION SAGAR II
Assistance Humanitaire et Secours aux Sinistres
Par l'Inde à Djibouti

A gift of 50 metric tonne of food items to Djibouti as part of humanitarian assistance and disaster relief delivered by INS AIRAVAT

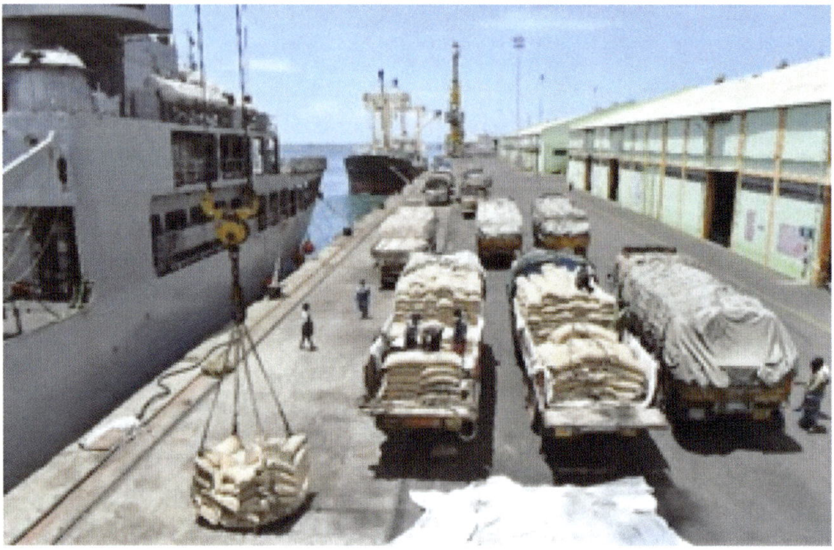

INS Kesari departs for Maldives, Mauritius, Comoros, Seychelles and Madagascar with food, COVID related Medicines including HCQ Tablets & Special Ayurvedic Medicines with Medical Assistance (not vaccines) from India

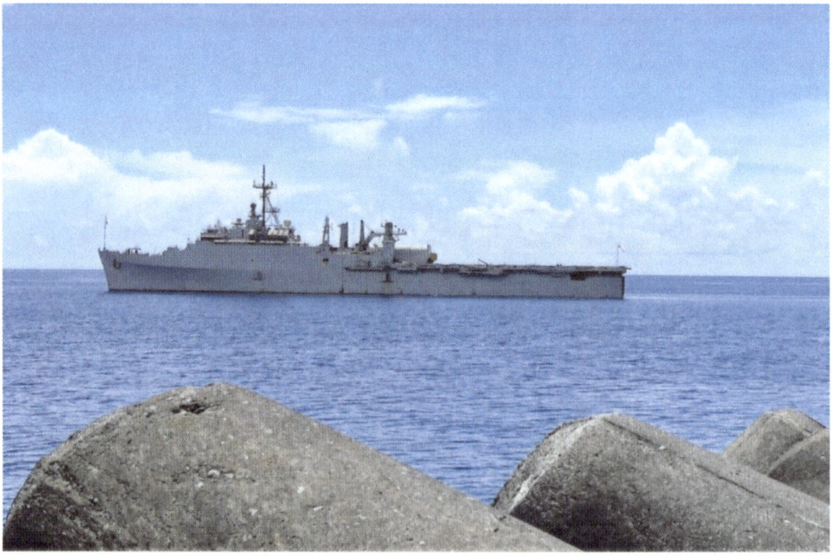

The arrival of Indian navy ship Jalashwa with a 1000 metric tonne of rice from India to Comoros fulfilling Prime Minister Narendra Modi's vision of SAGAR (Security and Growth for all in the Indian Ocean Region)

4

HUMANITARIAN ASSISTANCE AND DISASTER RELIEF

INTRODUCTION

India has an established reputation as a first responder and a responsible Humanitarian Assistance and Disaster Relief (HADR) provider. It also has an established reputation as a major centre of healthcare capacities. There was a global demand for some of these capacities during the first wave of the pandemic. Many of our partners, from both developing and developed countries, requested Indian produced medicines, pharmaceutical products, testing kits, and COVID protection gear, as well as medical expertise during this period.

This required a policy and operational response from the Ministry of External Affairs that incorporated the views and requirements of multiple stakeholders within the country. It also required the Ministry to work on balancing the need for domestic requirements, which had priority, with the requirement of protecting and preserving diplomatic and strategic equities. These had taken decades of patient hard work and perseverance to build. The top-most leadership appreciated the importance of a forward-looking agenda that made India's capacities available for the international community. India is determined to be a force for good and a responsible international citizen.

The Ministry's efforts in this arena were along four verticals. The first was the demand for certain specific products in which India's domestic pharmaceutical industry had become the centre of global attention due to its production capacity for generics as well as high-end life-saving antibiotics. These included Paracetamol, Hydroxychloroquine and Azithromycin. Second, the Ministry coordinated a massive operational exercise in which it dispatched large quantities of such medicines as humanitarian grants to developing partner countries and as commercial exports to others. Third, the Ministry worked with the Indian Navy and the Armed Forces in another vertical to make Indian medical expertise and supplies available to countries in its extended neighbourhood. These were done through a number of seaborne and airborne operations that deployed Rapid Response Teams in a number of countries and delivered expertise and supplies through Mission SAGAR and Operation Sanjeevani. Fourth, India worked to make advanced healthcare products such as vaccines available through Vaccine Maitri. This was a part of a larger effort to work with countries in our immediate and extended neighbourhood as well as through partners such as G20 to come up with a coordinated response to the pandemic. The Co-Win digital platform conclave was one such effort in this vertical.

India also responded to the requirements of countries in the neighborhood and G20 through platforms such as SAARC and G20.

India has also offered its CoWIN platform as a digital public good to the world to aid the global fight against the pandemic.

SUPPLY OF MEDICINES AND MEDICAL EQUIPMENT

It became clear during the early stages of the pandemic that global healthcare systems which were being overwhelmed by the pandemic were unable to cope with the management of other challenges. Lockdowns, and restrictions on cross-border movements of humans and goods across borders affected healthcare systems in developing countries which relied on import of drugs and medical equipment to provide regular healthcare services.

India was no different, and despite our large pharmaceutical sector, on 31 January 2020, Directorate General of Foreign Trade (DGFT) issued a notification which restricted export of around 12 medicines for which Active Pharmaceutical Ingredients (API) was being sourced from China. The apprehension was that the supply of these APIs, manufactured in the Hubei province of China, if disrupted due to COVID, could undermine manufacturing of these medicines in India.

Meanwhile, a small trial by Chinese researchers revealed that Hydroxychloroquine appeared to ease the symptoms in moderately ill patients. At the same time, former US President Donald Trump also tweeted that Hydroxychloroquine may be useful in the prophylaxis of COVID infection. This suddenly generated interest in Hydroxychloroquine, which was predominantly being used for the treatment of arthritis. India is the biggest manufacturer of the API of this medicine. Demand for Hydroxychloroquine, on commercial terms and also as humanitarian supplies, expanded dramatically. This happened at a time when trade restrictions and lockdowns were being imposed across the world. Under these circumstances, given the increase in demand of this medicine, and the possible domestic requirements, DGFT issued a notification on 4 April 2020 prohibiting export of Hydroxychloroquine. This naturally resulted in several countries seeking exemptions from export restrictions. The demand for Hydroxychloroquine was accompanied by a rise in the demand for Paracetamol.

Several nations including some major partners took this matter up with Indian leadership at the top-most levels. Indian Heads of Mission across the world received requests from host governments for supplies of Hydroxychloroquine and Paracetamol.

A major policy intervention through the inter-Ministerial process was required to deal with this issue. The issue had to be examined from multiple angles. First, India is one of the major exporters of medicine formulations; in fact, it is called 'the pharmacy of the world'. This brand equity needed to be protected and preserved. Second, exporters were being adversely affected. They faced pressures due to decrease in production following labor shortages during the lockdown. They were also under pressure due to their inability to respect the contracts that they had already entered into. These imperatives had to be reconciled with the prevailing situation and the uncertainties associated with it.

The Ministry engaged closely with the Department of Pharmaceuticals, Ministry of Health, DGFT and other stakeholders to put in place a mechanism to allow exports without compromising on domestic obligations. With the help of various Government of India agencies, COVID Cell and Development Partnership (DPA) II Division computed the export surplus by directly contacting domestic manufacturers of these medicines and made stock assessments as well as our dependency on API imports. The information was tabulated and shared with the Department of Pharmaceuticals which in turn made a presentation to the Committee of Secretaries in April 2020. Exports and donations were cleared on the basis of real-time information on domestic demand and surpluses.

Based on the stock assessment, export restrictions on medicines were gradually lifted, after mandating domestic manufacturers to meet some targets for domestic use. A mechanism was put in place for allowing purchases by foreign entities on a case-by-case basis through the 'Empowered Committee on Ensuring Availability of Essential Medical Export Production, Procurement, Import and Distribution'. The COVID Cell also liaised with various foreign Missions and projected their requirement to the Department of Pharmaceuticals for seeking approval of the Empowered Committee to allow exports to specific countries. The COVID Cell also liaised with DGFT to get specific instructions issued to the Customs Authorities to permit export of medicines. Subsequently, all export restrictions on Hydroxychloroquine, including for formulations and APIs, were lifted on 18 June through DGFT notification(s) at ***Annexure 3a.***

In April 2020, the government also banned the exports of Paracetamol, Azithromycin along with Hydroxychloroquine which had then started being used in the treatment of COVID, as also for protective gear, N-95 masks and sanitizers, etc., which were in short supply. In the early days of the pandemic, before the ban on exports, the Ministry of External Affairs had, through DPA-II division and in coordination with its territorial divisions, dispatched N-95 masks, gloves, PPE kits and medical equipment to China, Italy, Israel and Iran. This was achieved by undertaking the Ministry's own tendering processes for identifying private suppliers/vendors and obtaining country specific approvals/ exceptions for donations as needed, of these items as Humanitarian aid.

Domestic production of these essential medical supplies was ramped up, as Indian industry rose to meet the challenge. This placed India in a situation where it was able to supply surplus production of these items to other countries.

Indian pharma responded to global demands for commercial supply of drugs like Paracetamol, Hydroxychloroquine and Azithromycin. The Ministry then launched a major logistical operation to dispatch these items across the world. This highly complex operation involving multiple agencies and partners in India and destinations across the world was executed in the midst of a global lockdown. India dispatched large quantities of medicines to our developing partner countries in the neighbourhood, Indian Ocean region, Africa and Latin America and Caribbean regions as humanitarian grants. Between April and August 2020, at the height of the global pandemic, 800 tonnes of essential drugs, antibiotics and PPE kits (worth around INR 100 crore) were delivered to 80 developing partner countries in these regions. These included 10 million tablets of Hydroxychloroquine and 5.5 million tablets of Azithromycin.

Procurement was centralised in Ministry's DPA-II Division. It worked in partnership with HLL Ltd, a Government of India undertaking. HLL Ltd had long experience in working with central and state governments. An enabling MoU between the Ministry of External Affairs and the Ministry of Health and Family Welfare allowed HLL Ltd to float procurement tenders on behalf of the Ministry for a fee. This was, however, a time when both the Ministry of Health and HLL Ltd were under considerable pressure due to domestic procurement priorities. HLL Ltd initially declined requests for processing external donations, and only did so after intervention by the Ministry of Health and Family Welfare due to the importance of fulfilling international commitments.

DPA-II division, working with the territorial divisions in the Ministry (ESA, CWA, WANA, LAC) formulated a comprehensive yet rationalised package of essential medicines, life-saving antibiotics and COVID-protection gear. Developing partner countries who had sought Indian assistance were offered this package as grants-in-aid through our Missions. This package was rationalised in both quantity and content. It met the requirements of the recipient country while taking into account the domestic supply situation.

The procurement cycle also had to be adapted to the compressed time frames. The Ministry worked with HLL Ltd, Department of Pharmaceuticals and Bureau of Pharma PSUs of India (BPPI) to generate solutions. The mechanism of lateral transfer (drugs procured by BPPI for its stocks, and transferred at same prices to HLL so that HLL needn't go through a lengthy price-discovery process) was used in order to obtain stocks within 30 days. DPA-II Division was able to coordinate with Indian pharma companies to obtain zero-cost consignments of valuable drugs like Azithromycin as donations.

Procurement of products from within the country had to contend with a complicated maze of logistics and clearances. Each individual shipment then had to be transported through a global logistics system that had virtually come to a standstill. Organising transportation and delivery of such supplies in response to medical emergencies, is in normal circumstances, a comparatively simple affair. It typically involves delivery to a single country through established production, supply and logistics chains. The pandemic disrupted these well-established mechanisms. The Ministry had to navigate these disruptions and improvise and innovate to ship supplies to 80 nations in a very short period of time. Supplies were delivered to 27 counties in South America, 25 counties in Africa, and multiple countries in the neighbourhood, Indian Ocean Region and in Central Asia within emergency time frames.

This required intensive planning to work out the time frames and bottlenecks at each step of the logistic chain in an atmosphere of extreme uncertainty. The established practice of mounting an Air India flight or Ministry of Defence vessel or aircraft was available only for the neighbourhood and few other cases. Air India had expressed its inability to mount chartered flights or freighters to execute deliveries in Africa or Latin America. Similarly, individual airline carriers also had expressed their inability to provide load capacity as commercial carriers had suspended scheduled operations. Even chartered operations were seriously affected due to lockdown rules at hub airports.

DPA-II division of the Ministry then approached the Logistics Division of Department of Commerce for advice. It suggested that given the size and scale of the Ministry's requirement, the only feasible technical solution was to engage express couriers. A coordination mechanism was thereafter created by DPA-II Division which included HLL Ltd, Drug Controller of India, BPPI, Air India, express couriers representatives and other stakeholders. This mechanism was able to develop a plan that linked supplies and procurement to a tentative delivery plan.

HLL Lifecare Ltd was able to work out, after an intense effort, a delivery solution with express couriers for all recipients (25 countries in LAC, 27 countries in Africa, plus a few other destinations). This involved among other things, splitting consignments, often into 10-14 parts. These could be moved easily particularly to small island countries, using small-capacity aircraft. This was particularly true for Caribbean and Latin American countries. While this arrangement solved logistics hurdles at lockdown affected hubs across the world and resolved problems created by sluggish production and packaging within the country, it increased the workload for the Ministry and its Missions. Multiple import permissions and destination clearances were required. HLL Ltd and the couriers operated a dedicated caller-helpline facility, where one operation manager from courier tracked each Airway bill and informed designated nodal officer in Missions at two mandatory points—once before airlift in Delhi and once within 24-hr of expected arrival. All consignment-wise shipping documents were made available to the Missions as soon as they were generated at port-of dispatch. DPA-II division ensured real-time liaison with customs and drug control authorities at New Delhi airport so that there were no unanticipated blockages at cargo terminals.

The final step in the process was to ensure the delivery to the recipient governments. Apart from ensuring regulatory compliances, Missions also had to overcome logistic problems in ensuring delivery from airport to designated warehouses. Organising delivery by Mission destinations where they only had concurrent accreditation proved to be a problem. Many of them had suspended cross-border transportation due to COVID restrictions. This required another set of innovative solutions, often at a distance and working through local contacts.

Attention to detail was critical. Mistakes were more likely to happen in the chaos caused by the lockdown. HLL Ltd's ability to "work the system" was severely impacted. They also had no experience of conducting an operation of such scale or complexity. Ministry worked closely with HLL Ltd on measures such as ensuring that the names of countries correctly printed on labels, boxes or airway bills; ensuring local police permissions to move trucks from warehouses in India to airport; ensuring timely manual data-entry at customs (when ICT systems went down); mobilising labour for loading aircraft. A similar operation had to be conducted on the other side. Particular care was given to making sure that all instructions given to procurement and logistic agencies were clear, precise, technically accurate and given in writing, so that there was no occasion for confusion or ambiguity.

It was largely due to these efforts that within a short span between April and August 2020, at the height of the global pandemic, 800 tonnes of essential drugs, antibiotics and PPE kits (worth around INR 100 crore) were delivered to 80 developing partner countries. The Ministry was able to organise centralised procurement at scale and speed, through better inter-Ministerial and intra-Ministerial coordination.

In all, India provided medical assistance to more than 150 countries in the form of medicines and medical equipment. This includes both grant assistance as well as facilitation of commercial exports of Paracetamol (96 countries) and Hydroxychloroquine (83 countries).

This generated considerable goodwill for India in the form of diplomatic equity. It also enhanced India's standing as a reliable component of global healthcare supply chains in difficult times. Prime Minister received more than 50 messages of appreciation from world leaders (Annexure 3b).

It also established a global footprint for Indian HADR capacities.

RAPID RESPONSE TEAMS

India also shared its medical expertise by dispatching Rapid Response Teams to Kuwait and Maldives.

Maldives

A composite COVID Rapid Response medical relief team went to the Maldives in March 2020. The team was tasked with assisting Maldives in setting up testing systems, and train local medical professionals.

Kuwait

During bilateral discussions at the highest political levels, that of Prime Minister and EAM, in the early days of the pandemic, Kuwait underscored the need to augment the medical resources of Kuwait Defence Forces. Government of India responded swiftly to the request from the Kuwaiti leadership by dispatching a Rapid Response medical team with a mandate of assisting in COVID testing and capacity building on 11 April 2020, for a period of two weeks.

A considerable amount of goodwill was generated with the leadership, the government and the senior officials, especially from the Ministries of Defence and Health, acknowledging the timely assistance from India. Positive press coverage ensured amplification of the goodwill and further strengthening Brand India in Kuwait, as a reliable partner.

Mission SAGAR

Launched in May 2020, Mission SAGAR was India's initiative to deliver HADR and COVID related assistance to the countries in the Indian Ocean region, over three phases. Mission SAGAR is a major milestone in our engagement with the countries in the Indian Ocean Region, in line with Prime Minister's vision of 'SAGAR- Security and Growth for All in the Region'. Mission SAGAR saw the deployment of Indian Naval Ship (INS) Kesari to deliver assistance to our maritime neighbours: Maldives, Mauritius, Madagascar, Comoros and Seychelles.

Mission Sagar II was launched in November 2020. As part of Mission Sagar II, INS Airavat delivered food aid to Sudan, South Sudan, Djibouti and Eritrea. Following this, India carried out Mission Sagar III wherein INS Kiltan offered HADR assistance to flood affected people in Vietnam and Cambodia.

Maldives

INS Kesari entered the port of Male, Maldives on 12 May 2020. Maldives was the first destination of INS Kesari during Mission Sagar. INS Kesari delivered 580 tonnes of food provisions supporting food security during the pandemic for India's important neighbour. The food provisions included 200,000 kg of parboiled rice; 140,000 kg of wheat flour; 80,000 kg of sugar; 120,000 kg of yellow dal; 26,000 kg of onions and 14,000 kg of potatoes. In view of the COVID pandemic in the region and social distance norms, an online handing over ceremony was held on 12 May 2020. The ceremony was attended by Maldives' Foreign Minister Abdulla Shahid and the Defence Minister Mariya Ahmed Didi. The Indian side was represented by the High Commissioner. President Solih thanked India for being a "true friend" to Maldives. Foreign Minister Shahid appreciated the assistance provided by India.

Comoros

In response to a request for medical assistance from the Comorian side during a telephonic conversation between the Foreign Minister of Comoros and EAM in April, 2020, a 14-member Medical Assistance Team visited from India onboard INS Kesari from 31 May 2020 to 18 June 2020. They provided assistance to Comoros in its fight against spread of COVID and Dengue. The medical team visited three islands of Comoros, viz., Anjouan, Moheli and Grand Comore and held camps along with Comorian health authorities. A consignment of medicines which included Hydroxychloroquine was also donated by India to Comoros.

Madagascar

INS Kesari visited the port of Antsiranana from 26-28 May 2020 to deliver a consignment of medicines meant for treatment of COVID. From 22-25 March 2021 INS Jalashwa visited the port of Ehoala to deliver a donation of 1000 MT of rice and 100,000 tablets of Hydroxychloroquine to the people of southern Madagascar.

Seychelles

Government of India donated two consignments of essential medicine supplies to Seychelles on 15 April 2020 and 6 June 2020 respectively. These shipments had a variety of essential medication, including 50,000 tablets of Hydroxychloroquine. A 3.4 tonnes consignment of urgent medical supplies was also airlifted by a chartered Air India aircraft and delivered on 15 April 2020. It was received by Secretary of State for Foreign Affairs for Seychelles, Amb. Barry Faure, on behalf of the

Government of Seychelles. Subsequently, INS Kesari, when it reached Seychelles on 6 June, as part of Mission SAGAR, was jointly received by Secretary of State for Health, Amb. Marie-Pierre Lloyd, and Secretary of State for Foreign Affairs, Amb. Barry Faure.

Djibouti

India provided 50 MT of food aid to Djibouti that was delivered by INS Airavat on 11 November 2020. A 5.9 tonnes consignment of medicines was gifted to the Government of Djibouti on 12 April 2021.

Sudan

On 2 November 2020, 100 MT of food aid, consisting of wheat flour and sugar was handed over to the Government of Sudan in a ceremony held at Port Sudan on board the visiting Indian Naval Ship Airavat, under Mission SAGAR—for the flood and pandemic affected population of Sudan. The first batch of 8,28,000 doses of AstraZeneca COVID Made in India vaccines under WHO's COVAX Facility, and in collaboration with UNICEF, arrived at Khartoum on 3 March 2021. On a request by the Federal Ministry of Health of Sudan for the supply of essential medicines related to the pandemic, an air consignment of 5.9 tonnes of life saving and essential medicines was gifted by Government of India to Sudan on 19 April 2021.

Others

Indian initiatives such as Vaccine Maitri and CoWIN also have a presence in the pandemic related HADR activities. Separate sections have been included about Vaccine Maitri and CoWIN in Chapters on Vaccines.

PROCUREMENT PHASE I

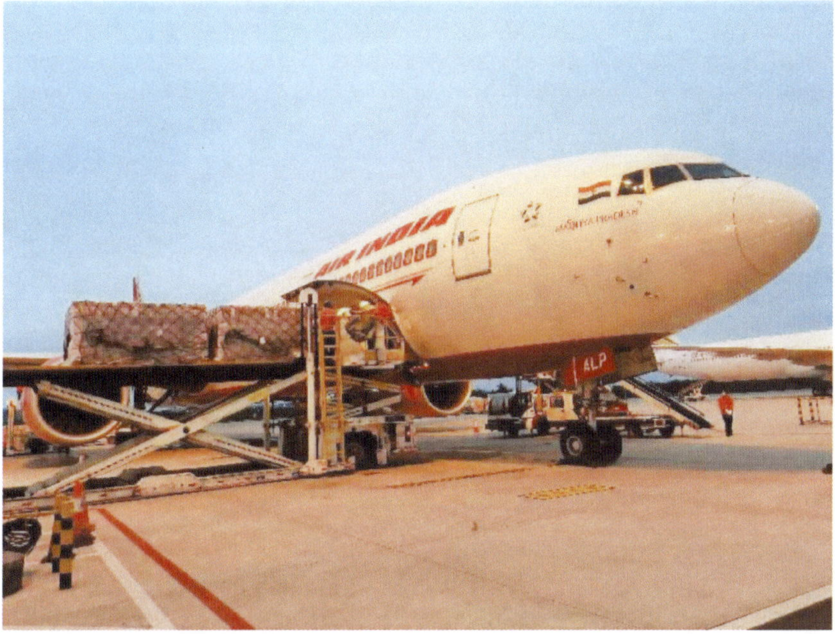

Air India flights bringing in 78 tonnes cargo to India as part of 1 million PPE kits acquired through a Singapore-based company

5

PROCUREMENT PHASE I

The COVID pandemic has gone through several "waves". The waves caused spikes in the case load and on the demand for medical services and medical products. The demand for medical services, such as medical and nursing services, was met without recourse to imports. The country however confronted acute and often, crippling, shortages of medical products and essential medical supplies. Procurement of medical products and essential medical supplies thus became one of the greatest challenges faced by the Government of India in responding to the pandemic.

Healthcare is a highly globalised industry and medical products, and supplies are produced by global supply chains. Sourcing such products and supplies during a pandemic therefore was, by necessity, a global effort.

The Ministry worked with the Department of Pharmaceuticals and Ministry of Health and Family Welfare in facilitating procurement of essential medical equipment required to overcome domestic shortages. Its network of Missions and Posts around the world were the global arm of this extraordinary procurement. During the first wave, they coordinated and executed a global sourcing operation to tide over the situation. This was parallel to and also supported the process of scaling up of domestic manufacturing capacity to meet demand and supplement the health infrastructure.

Missions in China, South Korea and Singapore were initially the major hubs of this procurement and supply operation.

Prior to the constitution of the Empowered Group system, Ministry of Health and Family Welfare had requested the Ministry to facilitate procurement of the following medical items from China: (i) PPE kits—1 million (ii) Ventilators—10,000 (iii) N95 masks—4 million and (iv) 3-ply surgical masks—10 million. Further, Ministry of Health and Family Welfare had also requested procurement of 10,00,000 PPE kits from Singapore and 20,00,000 PPE from South Korea. These orders would have helped India meet its growing demands for medical devices and masks.

The Indian Embassies in Beijing, Seoul and the High Commission in Singapore reached out to multiple entities and organisations to identify potential suppliers of the equipment. The Ministry, through its Embassy in Beijing, also approached the Chinese Ministry of Foreign Affairs and Ministry of Commerce to enlist their help.

EMPOWERED GROUPS

Ministry of Home Affairs, Government of India constituted 11 Empowered Groups (EG) on 29th March 2020 on different aspects of COVID management in the country to take informed decisions on issues ranging from containment plans and guidelines on a wide range of subjects related to travel, behavioural & psycho-social health, surveillance, laboratory support, hospital infrastructure, clinical management, rational use of PPE, etc. The 11 Empowered Groups (EG) were:

1. Medical emergency management plan,
2. Availability of hospitals, isolation and quarantine facility, disease surveillance & testing and critical care training,
3. Ensuring availability of essential medical equipment, production, procurement, import and distribution,
4. Augmenting human resource and capacity building,
5. Facilitating supply chain and logistics management,
6. Coordination with private sector, NGOs, and international organisations for response related activities,
7. Economic and welfare measures,
8. Information, communications and public awareness,
9. Technology and data management,
10. Public grievance and suggestions, and
11. Strategic issues related to lockdown.

In the absence of domestic manufacturing and the huge projected demand for essential medical equipment the EG devised an import strategy to address immediate needs. A combination of procurement through Indian Missions and Invest India and corporate donations was employed in this phase. Indian Missions helped to identify global suppliers in a highly competitive seller's market in order to augment procurement and ensure regular supplies. In addition to scaling up domestic manufacturing, a product-wise strategy was implemented to secure essential medical equipment such as PPE kits, masks, testing kits, ventilators, hand sanitizers, etc.

The Ministry was represented in Empowered Groups. From the Ministry, Joint Secretary (EA) was part of the Empowered Group-3 which was constituted for ensuring availability of essential medical equipment such as PPE, Masks, Gloves & Ventilators; Production, Procurement, Import & Distribution.

In May 2020, Chairman of the EG-3 on Ensuring Availability of Essential Medical Equipment, Production, Procurement, Import and Distribution presented a brief overview on the production and procurement of medical supplies, in the country's fight against COVID. The key points of the presentation were:

- Against a total demand for 75,000 ventilators, close to 20,000 were available and additional orders were placed for more than 60,000. The demand for ventilators was met through handholding and facilitation, and assistance via training and installation.
- More than 4 lakh oxygen cylinders were available, orders for more than 1 lakh oxygen cylinders were placed, and industrial oxygen too was converted into medical oxygen.
- Against projected demand of around 2 crore PPEs, orders were placed for more than 2.2 crore PPEs. Also, orders for 1.4 crore PPEs from 111 indigenous manufacturers were placed.
- 9 new labs for PPE testing were added including Institute of Nuclear Medicine and Allied Sciences, Delhi; Aerial Delivery Research and Development Establishment, Agra and 6 labs of Ordinance Factory Board. DRDO developed 3 types of new PU coated nylon and transferred the technology to domestic manufacturers.
- From a production capacity of around 3,300 COVID PPEs per day in March end, capacity was augmented to 1.8 lakh PPEs per day.
- For N-95 and N-99 masks, orders were placed for 2.5 crore, out of which 1.5 crore were from domestic manufacturers.

- Against a demand for 35 lakh combined RT-PCR kits, ICMR ordered more than 21 lakh kits. The Government of India has decided to handhold states in purchasing VTMs and RNA extraction kits.
- Production of Hydroxychloroquine was augmented from 12.23 crore tablets to 30 crore. Also, 9 crore tablets were supplied as against the requirement of 2.5 crore.

PROCUREMENT OPERATIONS

Through its Missions and Posts, the Ministry was able to reach out to companies and organisations across the globe to identify potential suppliers of essential medical equipment. They were also asked to forward proposals.

Orders were subsequently placed for Ventilators, PPE kits, N-95 masks, 3-ply surgical masks and testing kits. These orders partly helped India meet its demand for medical devices and masks, especially when domestic manufacturing of these items had not picked up scale.

It may be noted that this was during a time of global shortages and a supplier's market in which vendors dictated the terms of supply including advance payments without any guarantees.

To overcome this challenge and ensure that orders could be placed in a timely manner, Department of Expenditure (DoE) issued appropriate instructions to allow EG to decide to waive off the conditions of consultation of financial advisors for full advance payment, obtaining bank guarantees from suppliers for making advance payment and performance security on the recommendations of Indian heads of mission. DoE further stipulated that the specifications, price and quantity of medical equipment and essential supplies would be fixed in the manner prescribed by the EG.

TESTING KITS AND VENTILATORS

Diagnostic kits were secured through imports and by supporting procurement material for domestic manufacturers. Through the months of April and May 2020, as more was learnt about the virus, the ways to test for it also changed repeatedly. The changing testing strategy and lack of clarity on rapid testing kits, combined with insufficient laboratory infrastructure and the lack of availability of testing support materials in bulk such as swabs and Viral Transport Medium (VTM), etc., were significant challenges in meeting the demand for testing. EG-3 launched an effort to acquire RNA extraction kits and such materials that were already in short supply. It streamlined the procurement procedure and issued tenders according to the requirements projected by EG-1. Testing kits and polymer swabs were sourced primarily from Italy, Germany, China, and the United States to conduct COVID tests.

In order to cater to the urgent domestic requirement for Ventilators, orders were placed with M/s Sinopharm International Corporation for 1,000 units through the Ministry making advance payment to the supplier. Carefully evaluated proposals were forwarded to the Technical Committee on Ventilators, constituted by the EG-3 and approved ventilators were procured at rates fixed by the EG, based on the recommendation of the committee.

Based on the outreach by Indian Missions following orders were finally placed after approval of EG for procurement from other countries:

China

Following an EG-3 decision, Embassy of India, Beijing, acting on behalf of HLL Lifecare procured 1000 VG70 model ventilators from China Sinopharm International Corporation. Delivery was completed in August 2020.

The Embassy also procured large volumes of PPE for health care professionals on behalf of HLL Lifecare. The orders that were placed included: (a) Supply of 1 million protective goggles by M/s Beijing Convisto/Riccino on 8 April; (b) Supply of 1 million each of protective gowns, N-95 masks, gloves of two sizes and goggles with M/s Chinabidders/VFLO on 8 April; (c) supply for a further 6 million PPE kits of the type already contracted on 8 April with M/s Chinabidders/VFLO on 15 April,. However, due to delays in delivery, with the approval of EG-3, the last two contracts were revised to supply the following items: 2 million protective gowns, 3 million goggles, 4 million pairs of gloves and 7.8 million masks.

All these consignments were airlifted by three Indian aviation companies, namely Air India, Blue Dart and SpiceJet in 97 Flights from 22 April 2020 to 2 August 2020. These flights operated from Shanghai, Guangzhou, and Dalian. Flight clearances, requisite permission for carrying dangerous goods, mobilisation of consignments at various airports at the right time and right quantity, their storage, and completion of customs clearance processes in time had to be worked out on a daily basis by the Embassy with the Ministry of Civil Aviation, three Indian aviation companies, HLL Lifecare and Chinese suppliers.

Singapore

During the initial phase of the pandemic, in April 2020, the close partnership between the two countries helped NITI Aayog purchase 30,000 test kits from Singapore through the good offices of Temasek Foundation. Temasek Foundation donated an additional 100,000 PCR testing Kits in April 2020.

1 million PPE kits and 6.77 million KN95 masks were acquired on behalf of HLL Lifecare and Ministry of Health and Family Welfare through a Singapore based company. A consignment of high-tech components acquired through Bharat Electronics Limited for local manufacturing of ventilators and patient monitoring systems in India, was shipped on 2 May 2020.

After the Ministry had placed the orders, in some cases there were contract modifications and a few contract terminations including in some of the above-mentioned cases. The Ministry also requested concerned Missions to get specific medical supplies from China tested and inspected by third parties, approved by technical agencies in India.

The Ministry worked in close coordination with several other ministries thereafter. In addition to procuring essential equipment, the Ministry facilitated requests from different Ministries and Departments to expedite supply and shipment of medical products, machinery, and components. For instance, it supported import of components for ventilators being produced by BEL and AMTZ, testing inputs such as RNA Extraction Kits, Roche Cobas testing machines, and testing kits from US, Germany, China, Switzerland, and Singapore.

In some cases, orders placed by ICMR for COVID testing with Indian suppliers were facilitated by Missions abroad by pursuing with their original suppliers in various countries.

PROCUREMENT PHASE II

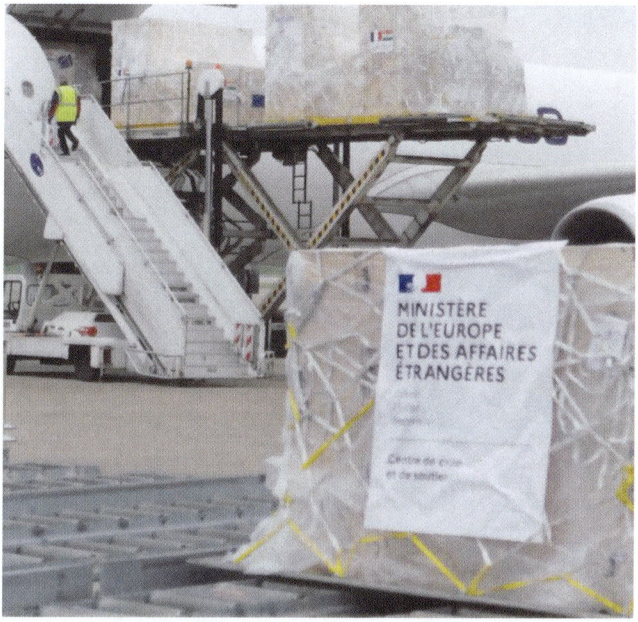

Oxygen Supplies delivered by France to India

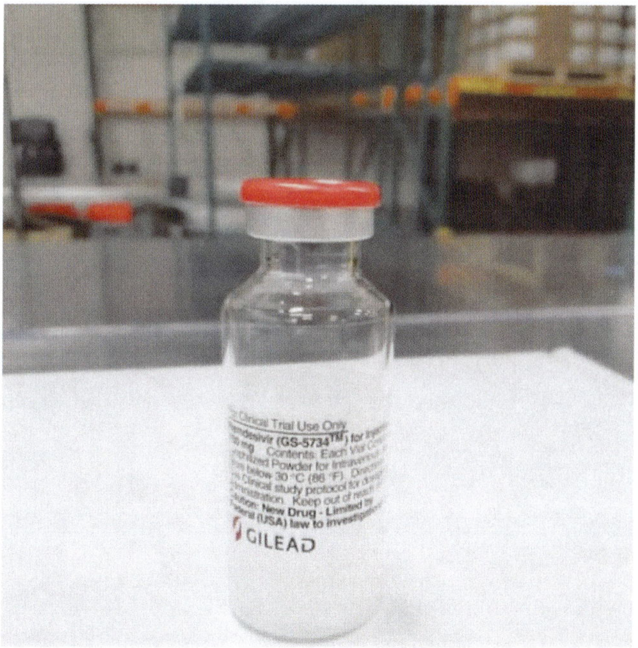

Remdesivir doses donated by Gilead Sciences, USA to India

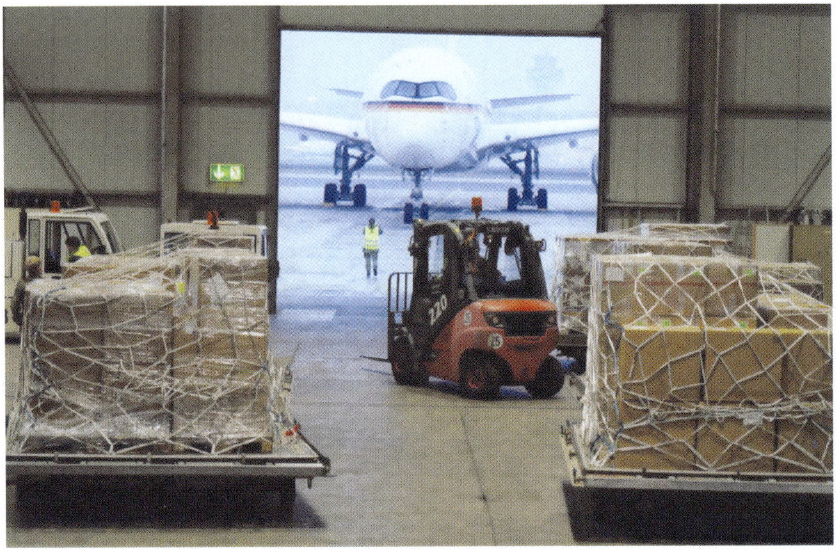

German Air Force AirBus with 120 Oxygen respirators en route New Delhi

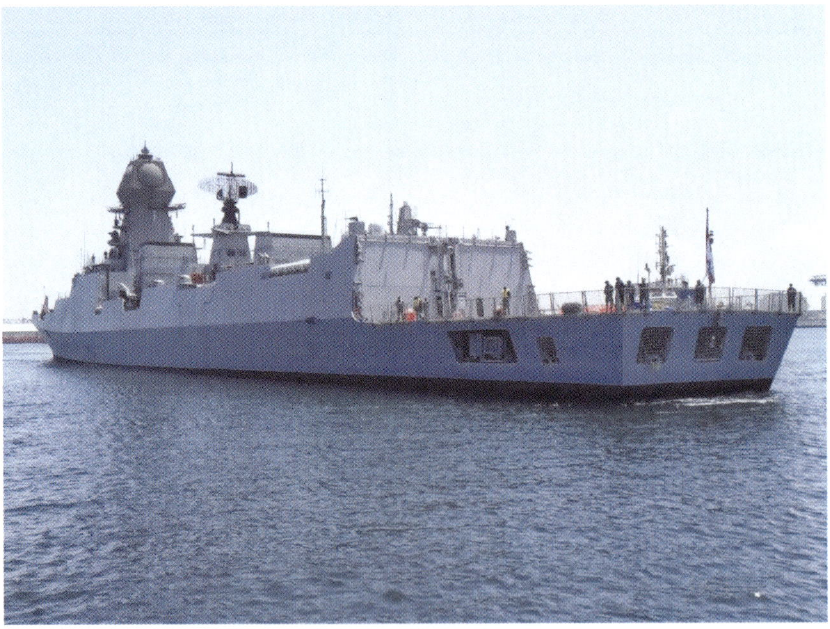

INS KOLKATA arriving at Shuwaikh Port, Kuwait for the shipment of ISO cryogenic tanks of LMO gifted by the Government of State of Kuwait

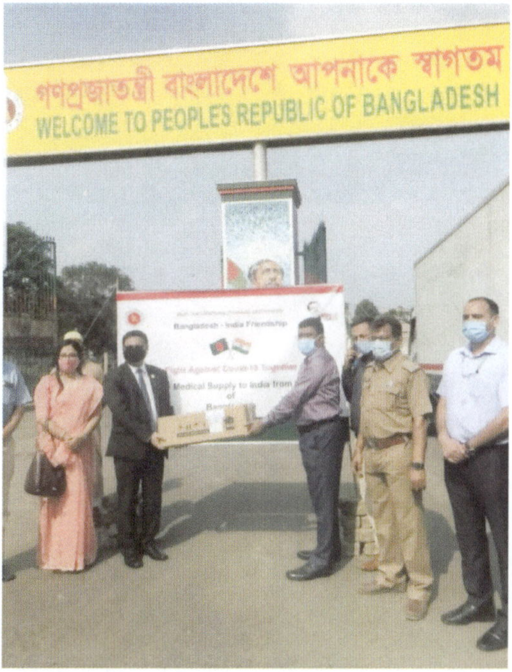

10,000 Vials of Remdesivir Injections handed over by Bangladesh to India

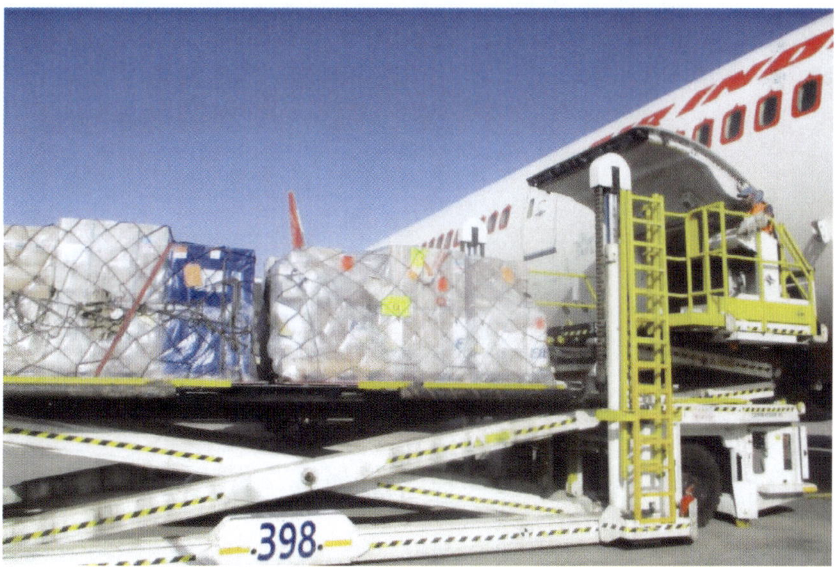

Oxygen cylinders and generators donated by Israeli Company Elbit Systems arriving in India

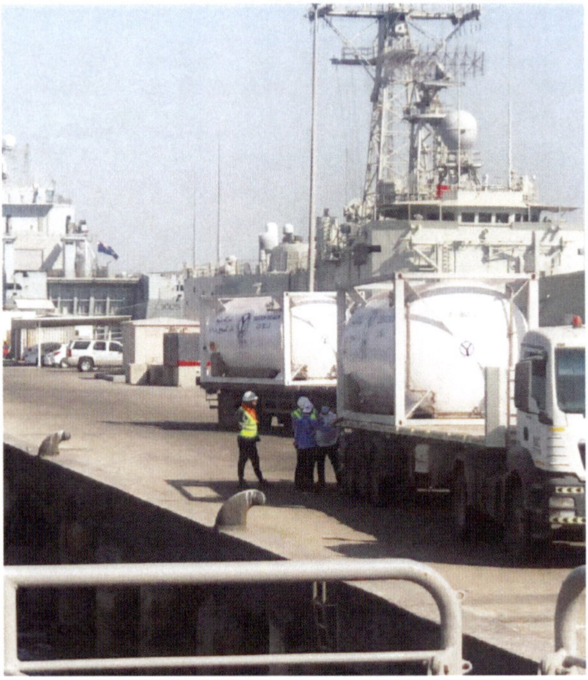

Operation Samudra Setu-II: Indian Naval Ships at the port of Manama, Bahrain for embarking and transporting LMO to Mumbai

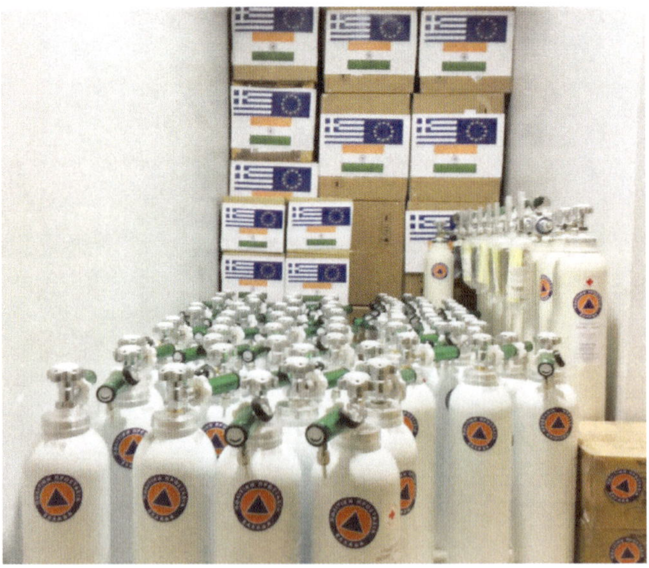

Greece offers oxygen cylinders and medical supplies to India

6

PROCUREMENT PHASE II

While the peak of the first wave was in September 2020, the peak of the second wave was in April and May 2021. The second wave caused enormous stresses. The shortage of critical medical supplies such as oxygen had catastrophic consequences. A global effort to source these critical supplies had to be mounted literally overnight. The procurement effort was accompanied by logistical efforts, unprecedented in its size and complexity, to get the supplies to locations across India. It was a whole of society effort that added a civil society and private sector contribution to a whole of government effort.

Procurement and logistics during the second wave proved to be much more daunting than the first. The numbers of infections, critically ill patients, and deaths were much higher. The quantities involved were accordingly larger. The wave also spiked very rapidly. This meant that the supplies and products were required at very short notice, i.e., on an emergency basis. The entire operation was mounted without the benefit of any previous experience of a similar undertaking on a similar scale or involving similar volumes.

India has impressive disaster management capacities. The policy stance previously had been to focus on domestic disaster response and take international assistance where required. This policy had to be rapidly discarded. It was decided to accept international assistance. A policy and operational framework had to be created to accept supplies that came in from all over the world. An enormous amount of goodwill obviously existed and was translated into material support. The challenge was to get the right kind of support to the right place at the right time. A logistical system also had to be created to bring these supplies in, match supply with demand, and channel the supplies to where they were needed.

Separate mechanisms were created for LMO supplies and non-LMO donations.

LIQUID MEDICAL OXYGEN (LMO)

The most pressing shortage was that of LMO. Demand for LMO spiked rapidly from 3,842 MT per day on 12 April 2021 to 8,400 MT per day by 25 April, and further up to 11,000 MT per day by the beginning of May—before gradually reducing as the number of fresh cases declined. The existing supply chains were stressed and disrupted.

The procurement and sourcing effort had a number of components that operated in parallel. LMO had to be sourced, LMO production capacity had to be increased substantially and LMO transportation capacity had to be similarly enhanced.

While a major effort was made to re-engineer and re-purpose existing domestic LMO supply chains, a simultaneous international effort was underway at a global level. This international effort operated along multiple axes. Government attempted to procure the necessary supplies from international locations either from governmental or private/non-governmental sources.

On 7 April 2021, Empowered Group-2 (EG-2) had directed that alternate source for import of liquid oxygen in Asia and Oceania region may be explored (note: a similar exercise was done in early December 2020). A short-term tender issued by HLL (16 April 2021) for procurement of 50,000 MT of liquid oxygen was circulated through our Missions to prospective suppliers. Several responses received through our Missions were shared with HLL and EG-2 members. It became apparent during this process that no single company would be able to meet such a large amount. Besides constraints in supply of liquid oxygen there was also an acute shortage of cryogenic tanks to transport them from other countries to India (note: The shipment is only through ships not air as it is classified as dangerous goods).

On 23 April, after the approval of EG-2, Ministry of Health Family Welfare approved procurement of LMO from (i) Gulf Industrial Gases (UAE) for 1800 MT; and (ii) Sing Swee Bee (SSB Singapore) for 200 MT. In both cases the companies had indicated that they could help lease cryogenic tanks for shipment. The supply time was indicated to be about 30 days. However, it emerged that the ISO tankers that SSB were to lease were bought by Tatas and brought to India to help with the shortage of tankers for inland LMO transportation. Gulf Industrial

Gases too, later, expressed inability to arrange 10 tankers and instead offered only 3 tankers that would do round trips, which would have delayed the overall delivery period. Therefore, these orders were not pursued any further.

On 27 April, HLL issued an amendment to the original Short Term Global Tender. The amendment lowered the minimum quantity that a single supplier could quote for and relaxed some provisions in the original tender. This was circulated to all Missions and Posts. However, this tender did not result in any bids.

The main constraint for import of LMO was availability of ISO tankers for transportation. Due to non-availability of cryogenic tankers in general, the majority of companies conveyed they could only supply liquid oxygen only on 'ex-works' basis, and the Government of India would have to arrange for ISO containers for transportation.

A related issue was that of losses due to shipping distances and long travel times. Most companies invoiced for oxygen at loading point and would not undertake responsibility for losses in shipment. Several companies, especially in Europe, also mentioned local requirements due to COVID situation in their region and expressed inability to cater to external demand.

The constraints notwithstanding, a combination of outreach by the Ministry and by Missions and Posts, and due to the tremendous goodwill that India enjoys, supplies of LMO as well as ISO Cryogenic Tanks from several countries in the form of donations and gifts could be secured. These include Bahrain (40 MT to Karnataka and 2 ISO tanks); Kuwait (approx. 2400 MT in total through 7 ISO Tanks and 3 Trailers); of this amount 425 MT has already reached India (Karnataka and Kerala); UAE (DP World–140 MT to Delhi and 7 ISO Tanks ; Abu Dhabi National Oil Company (ADNOC)—60 MT and 3 ISO tanks for 6 months); France/Qatar/Air Liquide (total of 600 MT; Maharashtra); Thailand (300 MT to Andhra Pradesh/Tamil Nadu) (Annexure 6a).

In addition, Indian Oil Corporation Ltd and GAIL also negotiated commercial contracts for procurement of LMO from suppliers in the Middle East as well as in Southeast Asia. For most of these contracts, transportation was worked out by a coordination team consisting of officers from the Ministry, DPIIT, Indian Navy, Indian Air Force, HLL and IOCL.

The timely supply of LMO through these arrangements was crucial in alleviating the difficult situation caused due to oxygen shortage in the country due to sudden rise in demand.

Simultaneously, capacity for production and supply/transportation of LMO within the country was also ramped up.

The Ministry and Missions were able to identify and subsequently facilitate procurement and long-term lease of cryogenic ISO containers. ISO containers were obtained *inter alia* from ADNOC, Kingdom of Bahrain, DBS Singapore, Linde, etc. This helped address the major bottleneck for domestic LMO supply and distribution. Several ISO containers were also received as donations, or as free lease for 2-6 months.

The logistics of LMO import and transport was coordinated with the Armed Forces. Naval Ships brought in LMO supplies and empty tanks were transported back for refilling by the Air Force. IAF Special flights also flew in leased/hired tanks to India from various foreign sources ranging from Southeast Asia to Europe

In view of the constraints on supply and transportation of LMO, other technological solutions like oxygen concentrators and oxygen generators were also considered. Several commercial offers were received. A large number of offers were received at that time for donations/gifts of oxygen generating plants as well as concentrators, as Government-to-Government (G2G) and Private-to-Government (P2G) donations. These offers were compiled, tabulated, and shared with Ministry of Health and Family Welfare and EG-2 for assessment.

The technical committee opined, on consideration, that procurement of Oxygen Generator plants through imports would not be feasible for several reasons including. A problem that frequently arose during this period related to the technical specifications of equipment. The offers of supplies for oxygen generating plants, for example, had to weigh against the following factors:

(i) the numbers were small—most offers are in single digits.
(ii) transportation and installation would be time consuming.
(iii) they might also require provision of diesel generating sets which are not usually part of the offer.

Oxygen Concentrators (which are portable units), needed to:

(i) provide a flow of at least 10 Litres per Minute (LPM) of Oxygen (i.e., 10 LPM or more).

(ii) have battery backup.

(iii) be compatible with 220 V, 50 Hz AC supply in India; and

(iv) have provisions for after-sales service as Concentrators require servicing regularly depending upon usage.

Coordination with government, quasi-governmental and private sector bodies which were involved in the procurement of oxygen concentrators, generators, and cylinders such as ONGC, TPCI, and NMDC was conducted on a real-time basis.

France

This Mission, in the first wave, largely carried out the coordination and research for various medical devices and products required to fight COVID. Mission reached out to a number of companies, including Arkema, Air Liquide, Gaz Systemes, Novair, Mil's, Linde, Scaleo Medical, Boemedical, Cryolor, SOS Azote, Wika, Eurotainer, Azote Services, Cryo Diffusion, Posaconazole, etc. to identify availability of products, quotations and delivery schedules for various equipment/items. The Mission also worked towards having Air Liquide and Rashtriya Ispat Nigam Ltd case on Vishakhapatnam plant resolved in order to channelise oxygen supplies for medical purposes. However, given stringent export restrictions from France no direct procurements were made.

Starting May/June 2020, Mission's research/information dissemination and coordination got eventually translated into delivery from France to India of:

- More than 70 oxygen generating plants
- 200 tons of high-grademolecular sieves
- Thousands of oxygen concentrator ordered by various French and Indian businesses, associations and governments.
- 600 metric tonnes of crucial high-grade zeolite absorbers—a key component in oxygen generating plants were finalised for supply from French company Arkema.
- The Mission followed up on Bharat Biotech's order with French company Biowest for supply of 2.5 million litres of "Dulbecco's

Modified Eagle Medium" (DMEM)—a crucial component in vaccine production. In response Biowest was able to ramp up its production to be able to fulfil all requirement from India at the rate of 400,000 litres per month.

- The Mission closely followed up on order of 4 tonnes of Betadex—a crucial raw material for the production of Remdesivir, ordered by Zydus Cadila from the French company Zach Systems. Zach systems was able to augment its production capacities to fulfil this order timely.
- The Mission facilitated direct contact between oxygen plant generating companies and the Indian Armed Forces. The Air Force was able to order and airlift five oxygen generating plants and close to 200 concentrators in its C17 flight from Bordeaux.
- The Mission facilitated coordination and transportation of 20 oxygen generating plants for use by the Delhi government ordered from the French company Novair.
- Given the close strategic ties between India and France and large presence of French companies in India, French Government mobilised about 60 French companies which contributed in different capacities to deliver 8 Oxygen Generation Plant, 18 OSIRIS Transport Respirators, 5 Liquid Oxygen Container, 200 Electric Syringe Pumps and many Respirators for Intensive Care.

Zeolites

DRDO and CSIR had sought the Ministry's assistance in ensuring assured supply of specific adsorbents (zeolites) for molecular sieves required in the manufacture of PSA Oxygen Generators. These included Lithium-based, Calcium-based and Sodium-based Zeolites. A parallel operation involving Missions/Consulates around the world was launched to source and transport Zeolites. COVID cell mobilised the network of Missions/ Consulates and responses were tabulated and shared with CSIR and DRDO for technical evaluation based on specifications required for their PSA Oxygen generator plant technology.

The sourcing of zeolites by the Tatas and some other private industrial partners of CSIR from abroad and their transportation through EG-2 logistics arrangements through the Air Force was facilitated.

CSIR had also sought the Ministry's help to secure long-term Zeolite supplies from France and the United States. Missions were requested to urgently liaise with concerned companies (Arkema, France; and UOP, United States). Arrangements were worked out and the supplies were assured till September. Missions in Moscow and Beijing, as well as Consulates in Guangzhou and Shanghai, were directly approached by DRDO and CSIR for zeolites. They provided necessary assistance to ensure the supply of zeolites of required specifications.

This was primarily only for commercial procurement through imports. In case of gifts from foreign governments, separate lists of priority items along with their technical specifications were sent by the Ministry of Health and Family Welfare from time to time.

Non-LMO

A large number of governments from across the world offered supplies and assistance. Supplies reached India through commercial agreements and as donations/gifts and sometimes as both. Civil society and the private sector, both in India and abroad, were involved. The present chapter provides a detailed analysis of procurement initiatives put in place by the Government of India and the Ministry to address the second wave of COVID pandemic

INTER-MINISTERIAL GROUP/ MINISTRY OF EXTERNAL AFFAIRS COVID TASK FORCE

Policies and mechanisms for receiving, allocating and distributing the medical aid received by India had to be created to ensure their effective utilisation. The medical relief supplies from abroad also had to be as per Indian requirements. This process needed extensive inter-ministerial discussions and coordination. An Inter-Ministerial Group (MG) was created on 26 April 2021, to address these issues. It had senior officers to represent:

- Ministry of External Affairs
- Ministry of Health and Family Welfare
- Ministry of Home Affairs
- Ministry of Civil Aviation
- NITI Aayog

- HLL Lifecare Ltd
- Indian Red Cross Society

Within the Ministry, Foreign Secretary constituted the COVID Task Force. It was led by OSD (COVID) and had 2 Joint Secretaries (Anurag Bhushan and Jayant Khobragade) and 8 IFS officers who had earlier worked on the Vande Bharat Mission. A special control room was set up in the South Block which functioned 24/7.

The Inter-ministerial Group and Ministry of External Affairs COVID Task Force (CTF) met regularly for smooth and effective coordination. IMG met virtually at 9.30 am every morning including weekends to plan the receipt of the incoming donations and to sort out all pending issues. Till the next day's meeting, it closely coordinated and monitored the relief supplies on WhatsApp group.

IMG worked on the following specific areas:

(i) framing policies on the receipt of donations including, identifying priority equipment and drugs as per the requirement, determining the threshold technical specifications, etc.;

(ii) deciding on the equipment and drugs which did not meet the threshold;

(iii) obtaining permission from Drug Controller General of India (DCGI) on the medical drugs received including Remdesivir and other lifesaving drugs;

(iv) coordinating on logistics of the medical aid from the time of its arrival in India till its distribution to the intended entities including hospitals, institutions, States, UTs;

(v) resolving issues related to the Indian regulatory framework, compatibility of equipment with the Indian standards and infrastructure, etc.

NON-LMO PRIORITY LIST

Items and supplies that were critical in responding to the second wave were identified and publicised into priority lists. The priority list underwent changes as per the requirements of the changing epidemiological situation. The initial priority list comprised of following items and drugs:

- Oxygen Cylinders with 10 litres and 45 litres LMO capacity;
- Oxygen Concentrators;

- Ventilators/BIPAP;
- Remdesivir;
- Tocilizumab.

Subsequently, the priority list was revised to:
- ECMO machines,
- Oxygen Cylinders,
- PSA,
- Oxygen Generation Plants,
- Tocilizumab,
- Amphotericin,
- Isavuconazole.

There was a period of overlap and transition during which shipments from both the priority lists were processed simultaneously.

NON-LMO DONATION POLICY

Non-LMO donations were divided into two categories: Government-to-Government (G2G) and Private-to-Government (P2G). The latter included all entities other than the government such as Indian Associations, NGOs, private companies, private individuals, etc. Thus, any aid coming to the Government of India was dealt with by this group. All the decisions on the donations have been taken in line with the Government of India's foreign policy. Donations were restricted only to in-kind donations.

NITI Aayog coordinated all private donations (i.e. donations other than the government donations). NITI Aayog created a separate platform called COVAID and processed all the offers of donations through the portal (http://niti.gov.in/covaid). The Ministry was actively engaged in this process. OSD (COVID) was a part of the group chaired by CEO NITI Aayog on P2G donations. Initial coordination including the vetting of the credentials of the private donor/entity, assessment of the donated items was conducted by the Ministry.

MINISTRY'S ROLE

Incoming supplies were organised into a "pipeline." IMG and CTF served as the central node in this pipeline that coordinated the policy and operational aspects of the entire operation. The Ministry participated in this central coordination process. The "pipeline", however, had a number of Ministry-specific roles that were performed by the Ministry and Missions /Posts abroad. These included:

- It became the starting point for considering the donations and channelling them from foreign partner countries, Indian associations, private companies, individual donors, etc.
- A number of policy guidelines/SOPs were formulated to guide Missions/Posts. The Ministry issued SOPs became the standard reference and were applicable across the board. SOPs were dynamic in nature, as the pandemic produced rising and, often, fresh challenges, with changing demand and requirements, SOPs were issued to create frameworks for issues as and when they emerged.
- Upon the receipt of donation/grant offers from foreign governments and private entities/associations abroad, Indian Missions/Consulates would then forward the medical assistance offers to CTF. CTF carefully vetted the offers in accordance with the Ministry of Health and Family Welfare priority list and threshold technical specifications. Offers which qualified for the minimum threshold limit and technical specifications were cleared by CTF under intimation to the Ministry of Health and Family Welfare. Others were forwarded to the Ministry of Health and Family Welfare for clearance.
- On receipt of the Ministry of Health and Family Welfare and CTF clearances, Missions/Consulates liaised with the donor for the shipment. The shipment details were then shared with the IMG and to ensure smooth processing at the receiving airport.

Incoming supplies as per list generated by CTF and IMG were distributed as per the Ministry of Health and Family Welfare's decision. These decisions were conveyed in advance to HLL Lifecare Ltd which was entrusted with the operational responsibility for arranging the onward logistics for distribution and delivery of the items.

Coordination with Customs through IMG and directly ensured fast track clearance of incoming supplies.

The Ministry also provided inputs for decisions relating to waiver of customs duties, health cess on goods classified as priority items by the Ministry of Health and Family Welfare, and GST waiver for these priority items. Subsequently, the actual waiver was effected on the basis of an MoU/Agreement between external donors and Indian Red Cross Society which was made the consignee for all incoming donations. Ministry's territorial divisions were actively involved in finalizing the texts of such MoUs and Agreements. Upon the receipt of all necessary documents for the incoming donation, IRCS issued the necessary certificates immediately to HLL for processing customs and regulatory clearances at Airports/Seaports/Land ports. IRCS also ensured liaison with the Ministry of Health and Family Welfare and HLL so that delivery of relief supplies was quick without delay.

CTF and IMG made enormous efforts to ensure that every piece of medical aid received from abroad has been accounted for and put to good use. More than 300 consignments were received over a period of 9 weeks. Reconciliation of data relating to receipt, distribution of data and transparency were made a major priority. Individual data sets and records maintained by individual Ministries/Departments were reconciled by an IMG sub-group that located missing items and ensured 100 per cent transparency in distribution.

The Ministry also liaised with resident foreign Missions in Delhi who naturally had queries about the distribution and utilisation of the aid coming from the respective countries. Interaction with these Missions took place through territorial divisions, with COVID Cell directly, and through joint the Ministry of Health and Family Welfare-Ministry of External Affairs briefings.

SOPS FOR DONATIONS

Once it was decided to accept donations from friendly countries, the first order of business was to ensure that the right materials reached India. This was done by informing Missions and Posts across the world about priority items and how they were to be processed. SOPs had to be generated at short notice and the first set of instructions were issued on 27 April 2021 (Annexure 6b).

SOPs and guidelines were subsequently issued about:

- Conditions on arrival of crew, other passengers and cargo on 29 April. RT PCR testing for crews of flights coming from Middle

East, Europe and UK, who did not have layover in foreign stations, crew of international relief flights (with clearance from the Ministry) and of cargo airlines (including all type of relief flights), which are playing a significant role in transportation of medical cargo (Annexure 6c).

- Ad hoc blanket exemption on 4 May of customs, IGST, No Objection Certificates etc. in order to streamline and expedite the receipt of donations coming from abroad directly to States/ UTs and to entities, relief agencies or statutory bodies, specified by States/ UTs (Annexure 6d).
- Clarifications on procurement by and donations to States/UTs to Missions that asking them to facilitate consignments being sent directly to States/ UTs, and to guide private donors to avail air cargo facility extended gratis by some airlines/agencies such as Qatar Airways, Emirates, Fedex, Maersk, etc. for delivery up to its "ultimate destination" (Annexure 6e).
- States and other stakeholders were informed about medical equipment and drugs available for procurement in 15 countries, viz., Australia, Canada, France, Hungary, Israel, Netherlands, New Zealand, Serbia, South Korea, Sweden, Russia, Taiwan, Thailand, Turkey and Greece.
- Providing publicity to foreign donations assigning responsibilities to the Ministry's territorial Divisions to liaise with IRCS and HLL Lifecare Ltd for receiving relief consignments, to coordinate with foreign heads of mission and resident Missions in New Delhi on such consignments and to keep XP Division informed (Annexure 6f).
- Efficient handling of donations of medical assistance coming from abroad through civilian and military aircraft, in consultation with Ministry of Defence (Annexure 6g). Ministry's territorial divisions and Indian Missions/Posts were asked to facilitate clearance by forwarding load manifests of incoming civilian and military aircraft to the Ministry of Defence. Details of dealing with the crew, handing of the cargo, etc., were clarified.
- Free transportation/facilitation of donations by private entities (nodal authority NITI Aayog) including P2G, P2IRCS, P2States, P2PSUs and P2P donations.

PROCUREMENT OF FINISHED ESSENTIAL DRUGS AND RAW MATERIALS

Substantially increasing availability of Remdesivir and Tocilizumab in India was a very high priority during the second wave. This entailed:

- immediate procurement from abroad
- simultaneous multi-fold increase in domestic production of the medicines.

Remdesivir, developed by Gilead Life Sciences, USA, was manufactured domestically by 7 Indian licensees (Mylan, Cipla, Dr. Reddy's Laboratories, Biocon, Zydus Cadila, Hetero Drugs and Jubilant Lifesciences).

Tocilizumab was supplied solely by Roche, Switzerland through the Indian company, Cipla and was not being manufactured in India.

The Ministry mobilised Missions and Posts abroad to scout for sources of the two medicines for immediate supply.

Remdesivir

Within two days, Missions were able to get immediate positive response from as many as 23 suppliers in 13 countries for supply of Remdesivir, either as donation or for commercial purchase.

Offers of commercial purchase (total quantity of these commercial offers were in the excess of 16 lakh vials, with 4 lakh vials from licensed suppliers and 12 lakh from unlicensed suppliers) were shared with Ministry of Health and Family Welfare. After examination, Missions were directed to seek quotations and delivery schedules from 13 suppliers in 9 countries, namely United States, Bangladesh, Germany, Uzbekistan, Egypt, United Arab Emirates, China, Lebanon, and Russia.

The quotations were submitted to EG-2 which approved procurement of 3,00,000 vials from Gilead-licensee Eva Pharma in Egypt. The Embassy of India in Cairo thereafter placed an order for 3,00,000 vials of Remdesivir with this Egyptian company.

Gilead Life Sciences, USA offered the largest single donation of 450,000 doses of Remdesivir, which were received in subsequent weeks in multiple consignments.

REMDESIVIR—SUPPORT FOR DOMESTIC MANUFACTURING

Subsequent to Government of India's call to ramp up production to 1 crore doses a month, Indian manufacturers sought Ministry's help in sourcing critical raw materials from countries abroad, mainly from China, United States and Europe. Missions and Posts reached out to the suppliers and also sought support from foreign governments. A sustained effort was made to speed up delivery schedules. This showed results. Specific instances of successful interventions by Indian Missions abroad include:

Hungary

- M/s Cyclolab which committed to supply Betadex SBECD, a critical raw material, to Indian manufacturers and indicated its readiness to expand capacity, and transfer technology to any Indian company willing to produce Betadex SBECD. The offer of technology transfer, in particular to M/s Anthem Biosciences Bangalore, was forwarded to Department of Pharmaceuticals for onward transmission to Drug Controller General of India and to other potential manufacturers.

Portugal

- M/s Hovione committed to 24×7 production of another Remdesivir ingredient, viz, Captisol (ingredient for Remdesivir) and expedited shipments to Indian companies Mylan, Zydus and Hetero. Its customer, M/s Ligand Pharmaceuticals/Cydex in the US, also worked to expand supply to the Indian market.

France

- M/s Zach Systems confirmed that it would supply half of the requested quantity of Betadex SBECD to Cadila Healthcare at a time of low production and very high demand.

Germany

- M/s Sartorius, a German company, expeditiously supplying 128 micro-filters to M/s Mylan, which placed further orders of 500 such filters. The same German company delivered 16 pieces of sterile midicap to the Indian manufacturer Jubilant Generics and committed to deliver the 38 pieces in two weeks. Merck Life Sciences from Germany also expedited supplies of orders of filters placed by M/s Lupin's, which were arranged to be dispatched phase wise.

United States

- TM/s Ligand, which owns Cydex Pharmaceuticals-the main supplier of Betadex SBECD, confirmed that it was working over time to accelerate all deliveries to the Indian manufacturers-Mylan, Cadila Healthcare and Jubilant Generics. Several American companies such as M/s Pall Corporation and M/s Thermofisher Scientific, which supply Bioreactor bags/Mixer bags, assured full support in expediting deliveries. M/s Gilead Life Sciences also offered full support in asking its subsidiaries to ramp up production of BCD to India. M/s West Pharmaceutical assured expedited delivery of Rubber stoppers to Dr. Reddy's Laboratories and Hetero Biopharma. US-India Business Council (USIBC) assisted the Embassy in identifying Telefax-USA, which manufactured filters and this information was shared with the Indian Pharmaceutical Association, which had shared a list of items required for production of medicines, including Remdesivir.

China

- Constant contact was maintained with the suppliers of BCD in China, specifically Shandong Binzhou Zhiyuan Biotechnology Ltd., and Xi'an Deli Biochemical Industry Co., Ltd to ensure that the orders were delivered as per schedule.

Italy

- The Mission in Rome liaised with M/s Datwyle Pharma Packaging for supplies of Rubber and Aluminium vials to M/s Mylan, the licensed Indian manufacturer of Remdesivir.

A direct line of communication was also established between the Indian manufacturers and our Missions abroad to ensure smooth and timely flow of information so that specific issues related to supplies are tackled at the earliest. The work by Missions to speed up delivery schedules of critical raw materials to licensed Indian manufacturers of Remdesivir, contributed to increasing the availability of the medicine within a period of few weeks during the peak of the second wave of the pandemic.

Tocilizumab

The Mission in Berne engaged with the top management of M/s Roche to increase and expedite allocation of Tocilizumab to M/s Cipla India the sole Indian importer for the Indian market. Allocation was significantly expanded following this intervention. M/s Roche immediately supplied 50,000 vials to India, promised to ship another 50,000 vials in subsequent weeks, expanded production and doubled delivery. It also worked with external manufacturers on transferring technologies to further increase global Actemra (Tocilizumab) supply as quickly as possible.

M/s Roche was also requested to consider temporarily granting voluntary licenses for manufacturing Tocilizumab in India. As a result of sustained efforts, M/s Roche agreed not to assert any patents against the use of Actemra to treat COVID in India during the current pandemic.

Missions across the world reached out to alternate suppliers and could secure assurances of some donations including 1000 infusion vials of Tocilizumab 400 mg from Oman.

Others

Upon approval of an antibody cocktail (Casirivimab/ Imdevimab) in India, Germany donated 20,000 vials of monoclonal antibodies Casirivimab/ Imdevimab.

LIPOSOMAL AMPHOTERECIN-B

During the pandemic, it emerged that a new disease, Mucormycosis was being increasingly seen amongst those who had recovered from COVID. Liposomal Amphotericin-B was recommended for the treatment of the disease and accordingly, its supplies had to be ramped up by both increasing its domestic production and getting immediate supplies from abroad.

Missions were once again mobilised to scout for suppliers of the drug abroad as well as for alternative drugs. Based on Ministry of Health and Family Welfare's recommendations, Ministry asked concerned Missions and Posts to approach various identified sources and seek firm quotations. Several sources expressed inability to supply due to various reasons such as i) inability to participate in procurement process due to a coordinated global response by their partner to secure shipments to India, ii) lack of authorisation from the original manufacturer to market outside country of jurisdiction, ii) do not manufacture Liposomal Amphotericin B but other drugs, iv) limited supply, and v) labelling issues. All these updates were regularly shared with the Ministry of Health and Family Welfare. Alternative sources for drugs such as Conventional Amphotericin B, Amphotericin B Lipid Complex, Posaconazole and Isavuconazole identified by Missions were also shared with the Ministry of Health and Family Welfare.

The Ministry presented firm quotations received for the desired drugs to EG-2 for consideration. EG-2 approved proposals for procurement of 10,688 and 1,200 vials of Liposomal Amphotericin B from Mexico and Taiwan respectively because of the larger volumes and lower cost implications. The Mission in Mexico placed an order for supply of 10,688 vials of Amphotericin-B Liposomal from the Mexican company. The Taiwanese company conveyed their inability to meet CDSCO's minimum regulatory requirements i.r.o. provision of certain information in English on product pack and vial.

Ministry also requested the Mission in Washington DC to reach out to M/s Gilead at an appropriately high level and request them to expedite allocation of Liposomal Amphotericin B to M/s Mylan Pharma, which imported the drug for supply in the Indian market. M/s Gilead committed to expediting supply of up to 1 million doses to India through M/s Mylan and withdrew stocks from third countries for supply to India.

Several Indian manufacturers of Liposomal Amphotericin-B also approached the Ministry for expeditious supply of key excipients DSPG and HSPC, required in the production of the drug. Eight Indian companies, Bharat Serums and Vaccines (BSV), BDR Pharmaceuticals, Lifecare innovations, Cipla, Dr. Reddy's laboratories, Alembic, Emcure and Mylan, had placed orders for supply of the two key excipient from

M/s Lipoid, Germany. The Mission in Berlin approached M/s Lipoid for expeditious supply of these two excipients. M/s Lipoid conveyed that it would be able to supply small quantities of the excipient on a monthly basis, despite nearly the entire production of DSPG-Na being earmarked for the Pfizer vaccine. M/s Lipoid decided to increase emergency production and supply of HSPC and DSPG, to India and identified an Indian company Lifecare Innovation that had the know-how to produce an anti-fungal drug using a lipid that is different from DSPG which was available in larger quantities. The Mission in Berlin worked with M/s Lipoid to expediting delivery schedule, on exemptions (with Department of Pharmaceuticals) on Indian labelling.

In an effort to identify alternate sources for the key excipients, the Mission in Tokyo reached out to NOF Corporation, Japan, which confirmed the availability of the key excipient HSPC. This information was used by Indian manufacturer Bharat Serums and Vaccines (BSV) who decided to place an order with the Japanese company.

Cipla India approached the Ministry for facilitation of supplies of key excipient DSPG from M/s Corden, Switzerland. The Mission in Berne reached out to M/s Corden which agreed to increase supply to India after diverting it from a US based client which was taken into confidence.

ISAVUCONAZOLE

A source in Argentina had stocks but was not authorised by its Swiss manufacturer of the drug to export to India. The Mission in Berne, on Ministry's request, reached out to the Swiss company M/s Basilea Farmaceutica to obtain a quotation. The company, and its authorised partner in India M/s Pfizer, then granted this third company a one-time right to sell directly to the Indian government.

VACCINES

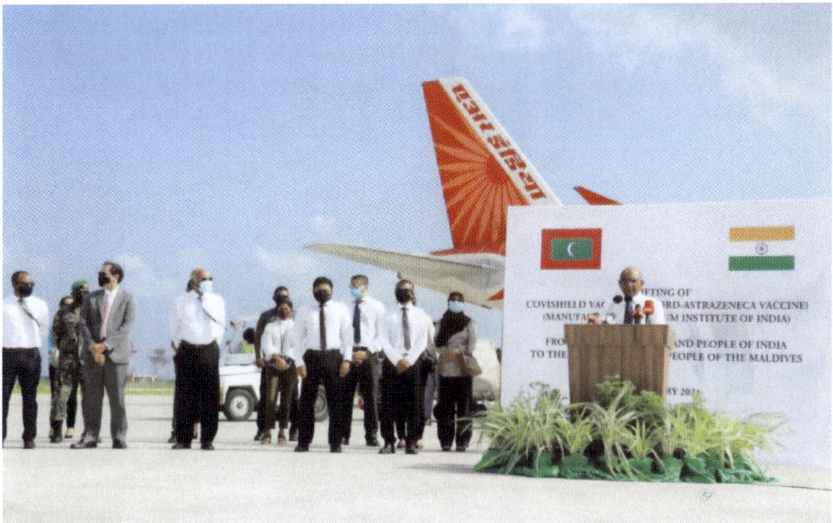

100,000 doses of Covishield vaccine donation by India to Maldives

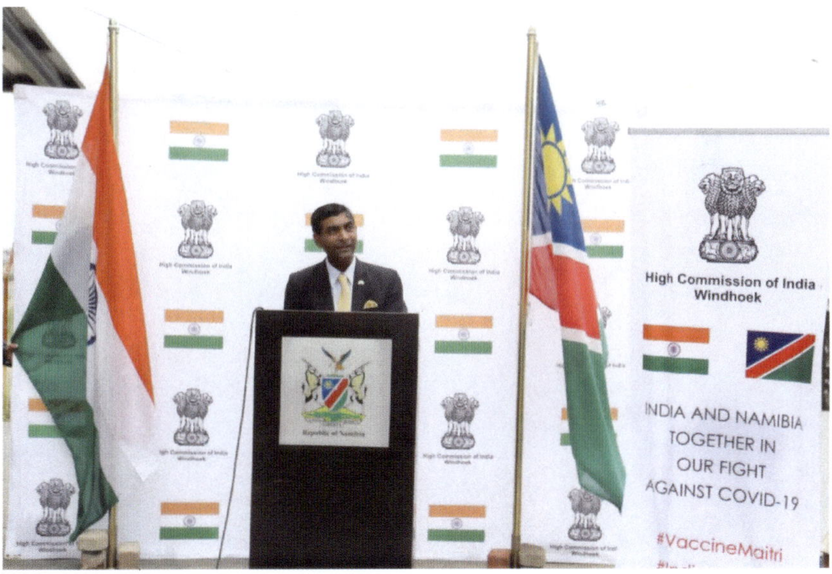

30,000 doses Covishield vaccine donation by India to Namibia

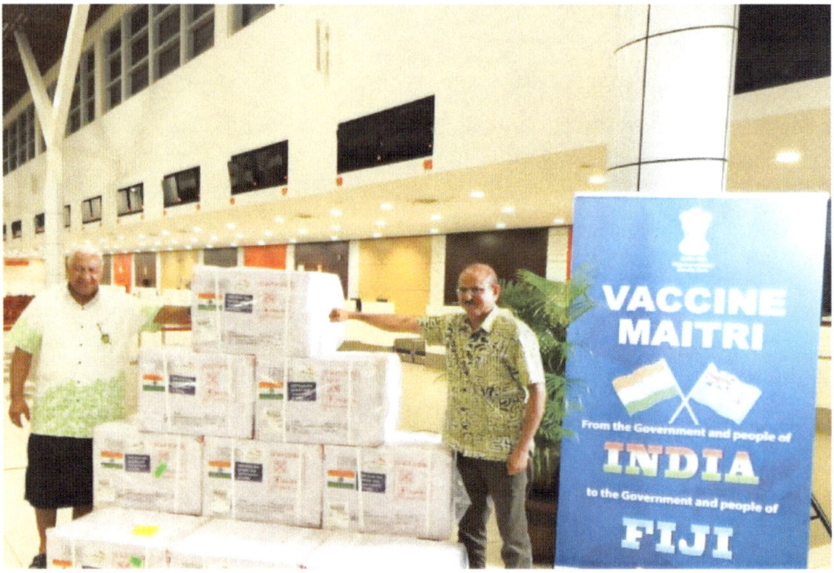

100,000 doses of Covishield vaccine donation by India to Fiji

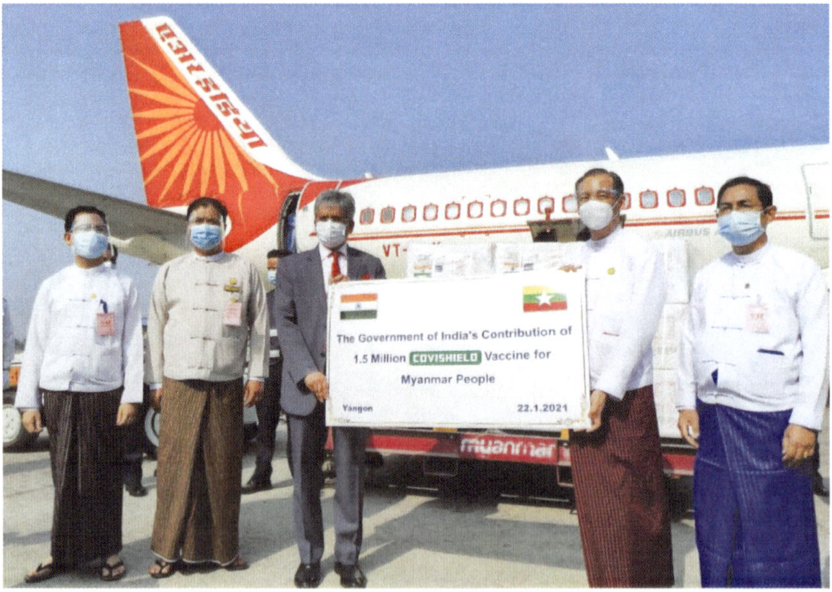

Act East Policy in action: Indian vaccines arrive in Myanmar to contribute to Myanmar's inoculation efforts

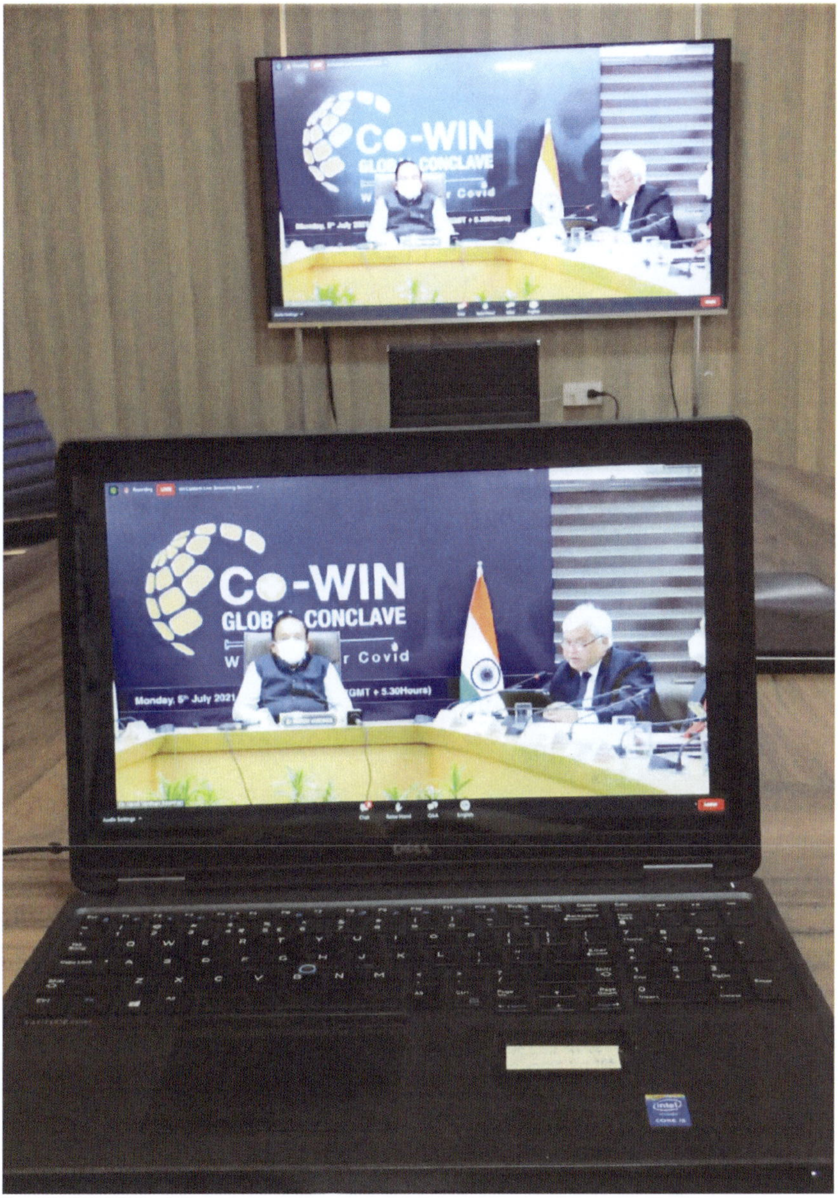

Over 140 countries participated in Global Co-WIN Conclave addressed by Prime Minister Modi and Health Minister of India besides health ministers from several countries, to share expertise in to joint fight against COVID.

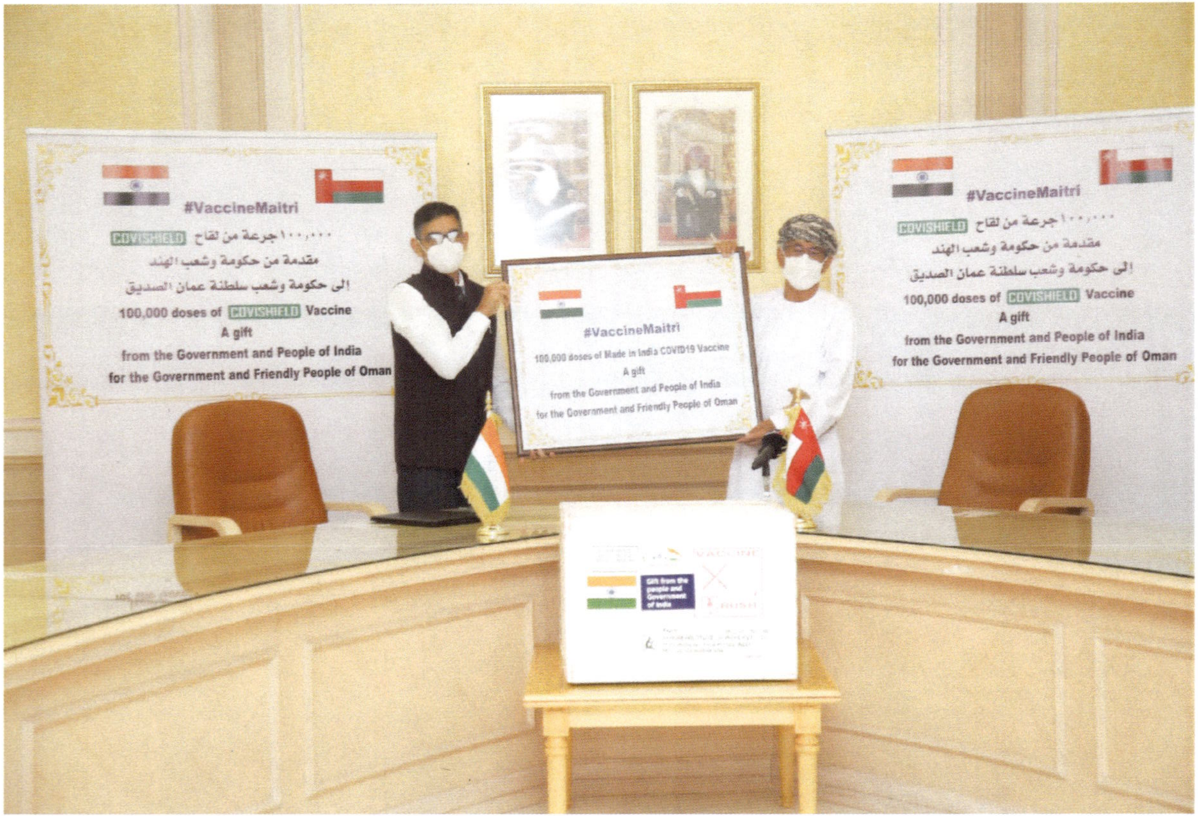

100,000 doses of Covishield vaccine donation by India to Oman

7

VACCINES

Vaccines have been one of the most important elements of the pandemic response. There was no vaccine available at the outset of the pandemic. It was recognised that vaccination would be the optimal course of action and an unprecedented effort was made to rapidly develop vaccines and deploy them around the world. India, because of the size and capacity of its indigenous vaccine industry, and with the vulnerabilities associated with its large population, played a role in many strands of the vaccine story as it unfolded.

The Ministry, with its network of Missions and Posts, played both inward and outward facing roles. In its inward facing role it facilitated access to vaccines, vaccine technology and vaccine raw material for Indian entities. In its outward facing role, it worked on expanding the global relevance of India's vaccine capacity by linking Indian manufacturing and research and development capacities with markets and global institutions.

TASKFORCE ON COVID VACCINE / NEGVAC

The Government of India created a number of vaccine-focussed structures. The two principal structures were the Taskforce on COVID Vaccine and the National Expert Group on Vaccine Administration for COVID (**NEGVAC**). Among the specific tasks assigned to NEGVAC were:

- The selection of COVID vaccine candidates for the country.
- Procurement of vaccines.
- Leveraging domestic vaccine manufacturing capacity for meeting national and international need for COVID vaccines.
- Engaging with international teams under the aegis of the Ministry to address the concerns and requirements regarding COVID vaccinations of neighbouring and friendly countries.

All of the above had a major international component and involved the Ministry and its network of Missions and Posts. AS (IO) in the Ministry (V. Doraiswami, and later Vinay Kumar) was designated as the focal point for vaccine related matters. This focal point was scaled up as and when required by making the capacities of other officers and units were deployed as and when required. For example, Joint Secretary (Administration) was the nodal point for logistics during Vaccine Maitri. Joint Secretary (Americas) was a focal point in Ministry for obtaining critical raw material from the United States and for the Quad Vaccine initiative.

ROLE OF SUB-GROUP OF NEGVAC IN VACCINE MAITRI

National Expert Group on Vaccine Administration of COVID (NEGVAC) consisted of senior officials from the Ministry of External Affairs, Department of Pharmaceuticals, Ministry of Health and Family Welfare, and Department of Expenditure. This subgroup was formed before the first external supplies were undertaken on 20 January 2021. All matters relating to vaccine supplies were dealt with by an Additional Secretary rank Officer [AS (IO & Summits)] who is also a member of NEGVAC from the Ministry. The sub-group, co-led by Foreign Secretary and convened by Secretary (Pharma), met frequently to assess the availability of vaccine supplies, based on domestic production and requirements of the phased roll out of national vaccination programme and, after ensuring adequate quantities of vaccines for domestic needs, approved the proposals made by the Ministry for supply to various countries.

Continuous requests received from territorial divisions and our Missions abroad were processed and prioritised and, proposals of priority countries, along with number of doses of vaccines for each country, were put up for approval by the sub-group of NEGVAC. After approval, DPA-II placed purchase orders for the Ministry grant supplies to Serum Institute of India and later on with Bharat Biotech also, as the case may be.

To work out the complex logistics and smooth supply of vaccines, an inter-ministerial team of senior officers was formed. JS (AD) led the logistics team from the Ministry of External Affairs, along with senior officials from Ministry of Civil Aviation and Department of Customs, among others. The team closely liaised with the officials of Serum Institute of India and later on with that of Bharat Biotech to ensure fast and smooth transportation of Made in India vaccines to various countries around the world in the form of Grant, commercial sales by manufacturers and through GAVI's COVAX facility. Approval for movement plan of every consignment of vaccine was taken from the sub-group was taken by JS (AD). This entire process, including that in the preceding para, which started from mid-January, continues till date.

PROCUREMENT OF FOREIGN VACCINES AND EXPLORING JOINT VENTURES FOR VACCINES PRODUCTION IN INDIA

A 5-member team of Officers was constituted under the chairmanship of Member (Health), NITI Aayog to deal with issues related to procurement of COVID vaccines from foreign manufacturers. AS (IO & Summits)] and JS (L&T)] represented Ministry of External Affairs Other members of the team were Secretary, Ministry of Health and Family Welfare and Secretary, Department of Legal Affairs.

FOREIGN VACCINES INTO INDIA

Ministry worked with the Russian Direct Investment Fund (RDIF) on the introduction of the Russian vaccine Sputnik V in India. The Ministry's role in this may broadly be categorised as follows:

Working with RDIF and other stakeholders in India and Russia, including regulatory authorities and commercial entities on the clinical trials in India that were a condition for approval for emergency use. Clinical trials were undertaken in collaboration with Dr. Reddy's Laboratories and based on the results of the same, Drug Controller General of India approved restricted emergency use in April 2021.

Making 3 million people doses available in May and June 2021 and obtaining RDIF assurance for 18 million doses of the finished product of Sputnik V vaccine by July. Our constant interventions ensured that even in May and June, we were able to receive more than 3 million doses. As a symbolic gesture, 1.5 lakh doses were received on 1 May and another 1.5 lakh doses arrived subsequently.

RDIF gave the complete marketing and selling rights in India only to Dr. Reddy's Laboratories. Ministry worked with RDIF and Dr. Reddy's Labs on bulk imports from Russia, which would be bottled and finished in India. Delivery schedules were drawn up and flow of supplies was managed with RDIF and Dr. Reddy's Laboratories.

Indian companies—Gland Pharma, Hetero Drugs, Panacea Biotech, Stelis and Virchow were selected by RDIF for contract manufacturing. Two other candidates were subsequently added. The capacity to manufacture Sputnik V in India was to be the largest outside Russia. The two-dose Sputnik V vaccine uses different technologies for the first and second doses. Technology was transferred for both. While Indian companies were able to absorb the technology transfer for the first dose, producing the second proved to be difficult. The Ministry worked on troubleshooting these problems by facilitating dialogue between Indian entities and RDIF.

A team of RDIF scientists visited the Indian manufacturers to provide support for absorption of technology transfer for the second dose. RDIF offered another vaccine, Sputnik Light, which has already received regulatory approval in Russia. The Ministry is working on issues relating to Sputnik Light's possible entry into India, after the necessary regulatory approvals.

USA / PFIZER, MODERNA AND JANSSEN VACCINES

Towards accelerating US-India vaccine partnership, the Ambassador regularly engaged with key interlocutors including Surgeon General Dr. Vivek Murthy, National Institute of Allergy and Infectious Diseases Director Dr. Fauci, Centers for Disease Contol and Prevention Director Dr. Walensky and United States vaccine manufacturers. The vast network of institutional engagements brought scientific communities of the two countries together to jointly respond to COVID research and its management.

Indian vaccine companies have collaborated with United States based agencies to develop and produce vaccine against COVID. At least seven vaccine candidates have been developed through bilateral engagement including one vaccine being developed using mRNA platform.

With a view to expand the basket of COVID vaccines in India, Ministry and the Mission in Washington, facilitated discussions with the top leadership of US based vaccine manufacturers, namely Pfizer, Moderna and Johnson & Johnson.

Pfizer agreed to supply several million doses of Pfizer vaccines but insisted on an indemnity agreement to waive liability of the company, and the requirements of sovereign jurisdiction and arbitration.

Discussions with Moderna revealed that they would be in a position to supply vaccines only in 2022 as their orders were fully booked for 2021. Moderna's leadership also demonstrated interest in exploring production of Moderna vaccines in India in the next few years.

Johnson & Johnson top management was engaged and agreed to further discuss supply of several million doses to India, along with the technical and legal requirements on the same.

The production of United States vaccines in India by Indian companies was discussed in the meetings held with the leaderships of United States based vaccine manufacturers.

EXERCISE TO DETERMINE LIABILITY CLAUSES IN AGREEMENTS BETWEEN PFIZER AND VARIOUS COUNTRIES

The offers for supply from United States based vaccine manufacturers were: Over 70 million doses by Johnson & Johnson (commercial procurement); nearly 50 million doses by Pfizer (commercial procurement); and nearly 7 million doses of Moderna (through COVAX by the United States Government).

Conditions put forth by United States based vaccine manufacturers for supply of vaccines to India were discussed by the team led by Member (Health), NITI Aayog. During the process, Missions were requested to obtain agreements between Pfizer and other countries for supplies of vaccines to understand the liability and other clauses/conditions agreed to by other countries. It was found out that other countries had indeed agreed to such conditions. Keeping all the issues in mind, several rounds of discussions were held with the representatives of Pfizer, Moderna and Johnson & Johnson on the conditions for import of vaccines from these companies. The details of requirements from the United States companies are as below:

Requirements	Vaccine Manufacturers which have these requirements
1. Indemnity and Liability agreement	All United States manufactures—Johnson & Johnson, Moderna, Pfizer
2. Legal/administrative regime for the patients/vaccine recipients who may have adverse impact and may put claims	All three
3. Creation of No Fault Compensation Fund—to meet the claims from vaccine recipients whose claims are held valid under the above mentioned legal/administrative regime	All three
4. Waiver of sovereign immunity—to meet the eventuality in which the government is not able to meet the claims of the beneficiaries through the above mentioned No Fault Compensation Fund and a court orders the manufacturer to meet the claims	Pfizer
5. Creation of a Reserve Fund—a limited amount in an escrow fund to meet any claim which a court adjudicates against the manufacturer	Moderna (*This fund was our proposal in lieu of a full waiver of sovereign immunity; Moderna agreed to our proposal.*)

India does not have a legal framework for indemnification of domestic vaccine manufacturers. Due to these requirements having financial, legal, sovereign and precedent setting implications, India has not yet procured vaccines from United States based vaccine manufacturers.

RAW MATERIAL FOR VACCINES

Manufacturing of COVID vaccines requires import of at least 75 critical items from various companies based in the United States and several countries of Europe. The Indian vaccine manufacturers- Serum Institute of India, Bharat Biotech and later on Biological-E and those manufacturing Sputnik V, namely Virchow, Shilpa Biotech, Gland Pharma, Stelis Pharma and Hetero Drugs had a long list of requirements of numerous critical raw materials to be sourced from companies in the United States and Europe.

Several meetings with Indian vaccine manufacturers were organised to understand their needs and the bottlenecks in the supply of raw materials. While there was a general global supply constraint, the United States Defence Production Act (DPA) made it mandatory for suppliers in the United States US to supply to its domestic vaccine manufacturing companies, thereby adversely impacting supplies of critical raw materials to Indian vaccine manufacturers.

All Indian vaccine manufacturers were asked to give a list of their monthly, quarterly, and long-term requirements along with details of their orders placed with the suppliers. Regular meetings and communication about orders and delays ensured that the necessary matters were being taken up appropriately with suppliers as well as with the United States Government. Simultaneously, Indian Missions in Germany, France, Denmark, Singapore, Poland, Sweden, Netherlands, Ireland, and Japan engaged with suppliers located in these countries for enhanced and expedited supplies of critical raw materials to Indian vaccine manufacturers. The issue of supply constraint was also raised and discussed in the Quad vaccine Experts' group meetings.

The issue of supplies from the United States was further taken up at multiple levels, including at the ministerial level. EAM spoke to his counterpart Secretary Blinken and forwarded the requirements of Indian vaccine manufacturers at meetings in London and in Washington in early and late May respectively. Foreign Secretary also spoke to his counterpart in the United States on the issue. The issue was also taken up with the United States Embassy in New Delhi as well as in Washington by our mission, which constantly engaged with the United States Government authorities.

After the visit of EAM to Washington in late May 2021, United States Government announced removal of Defence Production Act priority ratings on AstraZeneca, Novavax and Sanofi vaccines, allowing

United States companies to decide on their own priority on the supplies to vaccine manufacturers. This decision of the United States Government directly benefited Serum Institute of India.

TAKING INDIAN VACCINES GLOBAL

Regulatory Support

Even before the vaccination programme started, the Ministry was facilitating the approval process for the indigenously developed vaccine Covishield. The Mission in London engaged with the United Kingdom Medicines and Healthcare products Regulatory Authority (MHRA) for collaboration with the Central Drugs Standards Control Organisation (CDSCO) of India. A MoU on cooperation in the field of Medical Products Regulation was finalised between CDSCO and MHRA. The Drug Controller General of India also observed the proceedings of MHRA's study and analysis of the data of trial of the vaccine.

Promotion of COVAXIN Abroad

Missions were tasked to promote indigenously developed COVID vaccine (COVAXIN of Bharat Biotech) in their respective countries. Regular supply of updated documentation was ensured to Missions. The Ministry, through its Missions abroad, facilitated the regulatory approval process of COVAXIN by drug regulators in various countries. Meetings and presentations by Bharat Biotech with regulatory authorities of various countries were facilitated. This coordination and support played a role in emergency use authorisation for COVAXIN in 12 countries. Missions continue to facilitate the approval process in several other countries by reaching out to the host government at various levels and sharing various technical data as provided by Bharat Biotech. Foreign Secretary held a meeting with the leadership of Bharat Biotech and assured full support of the Ministry of External Affairs in its application process for WHO Emergency Use Listing (EUL) of COVAXIN.

To enhance the recognition of COVAXIN abroad, especially in the neighbourhood, a proposal was mooted for its trials in Bangladesh. Towards this end, the Ministry facilitated the visit of a team of officials from Department of Biotechnology and Bharat Biotech to Dhaka to discuss the proposal with Bangladeshi officials. It also obtained approval for funding the clinical trials in Bangladesh.

For increasing vaccine availability in India and also globally, India offered joint production of COVAXIN through transfer of technology in interested countries. Missions in several countries worked on determining interest and identified potential partners. This was shared with the Department of Biotechnology for further action, in consultation with Bharat Biotech.

Promotion of India's Vaccination Portal Co-WIN

India's experience of its indigenously developed digital platform Co-WIN that provided the software backbone for India's mass vaccination campaign has been made available to the international community. The Ministry, through its Missions, offered the Co-WIN platform as open-source software free of cost to interested countries. They also mobilised interest and participation of healthcare authorities, administrators, and IT specialists of their host governments in a well-attended Co-WIN virtual global conclave organised by National Health Authority.

Vaccine Maitri

Vaccine Maitri is an initiative of Government of India to supply Made-in-India COVID vaccines to various countries across the world, while keeping in view the domestic production capacity and the requirement of the national vaccination programme. The initiative is in line with the commitment made by the Prime Minister during his speech at the United Nations General Assembly in September 2020 that "India's vaccine production and delivery capacity will be used to help all humanity in fighting this crisis."

The planning for external supplies of vaccines had been on-going for several months in anticipation of indigenous vaccine development and production. Missions were asked to give data on expected vaccine requirements of each country, based on parameters such as population, percentage of healthcare and frontline workers and other vulnerable groups as also regulatory frameworks and requirements for emergency use authorisation for vaccines. Based on the data provided by Missions, a list was drawn up for possible supply of vaccines, once the national regulator

(CDSCO) approved the restricted use of two COVID vaccines in early January 2021.

To facilitate the external supplies of COVID vaccines under Vaccine Maitri initiative, an inter-ministerial subgroup of National Expert Group on Vaccine Administration of COVID19 (NEGVAC) was formed, consisting of senior officials from the Ministry of External Affairs, Department of Pharmaceuticals, Ministry of Health and Family Welfare, Department of Expenditure and Ministry of Commerce. In November 2020, a comprehensive briefing on India's vaccine development programme was given to Heads of Missions resident in Delhi by senior officials such as Chairman of NEGVAC, Principal Scientific Advisor to Prime Minister, Foreign Secretary, Health Secretary, Secretary of Department of Biotechnology and Secretary, Department of S&T. Subsequently in December 2020, foreign envoys were taken for a visit to vaccine manufacturing facilities in Hyderabad.

The first external supplies were undertaken on 20 January 2021. All matters relating to vaccine supplies were dealt with by the Additional Secretary (International Organisations) who represented the Ministry in NEGVAC. The NEGVAC inter-ministerial sub-group, co-led by Foreign Secretary and convened by Secretary (Pharma), met frequently to assess the availability of vaccine supplies, based on domestic production and requirements of the phased roll out of national vaccination programme and, after ensuring adequate quantities of vaccines for domestic needs, approved the proposals made by Ministry for supply to various countries.

Continuous requests received from territorial divisions and Missions abroad were processed and prioritised and, proposals of priority countries, along with number of doses of vaccines for each country, were put up for approval by the sub-group of NEGVAC. After approval, DPA-II placed purchase orders for grant supplies to Serum Institute of India and later on with Bharat Biotech also, as the case may be.

To work out the complex logistics and smooth supply of vaccines, an inter-ministerial team of senior officers was formed. Joint Secretary (AD) represented Ministry in this team which included senior Ministry of Civil Aviation and Customs officials among others. The team closely liaised with the officials of Serum Institute of India and Bharat Biotech to ensure fast and smooth transportation of Made in India vaccines to various countries around the world in the form of Grants, Commercial Sales by manufacturers and through GAVI's COVAX facility. Approval for movement of every consignment of vaccines was taken from the sub-group by taken by Joint Secretary (AD). Total supplies by end May 2021 amount to 663.698 lakh doses for 95 countries, UN Peace keepers and UN Health workers.

Other avenues such as research and development of vaccines, possibility of joint manufacturing, cooperation between regulatory bodies of India and other countries were also explored and meetings between experts, including drug regulators, of various countries and of India were facilitated. The most prominent cooperation came out in the form of the Working Group on Vaccines under the Quad framework, which continues to work together, and includes members from Ministry of External Affairs, Ministry of Health and Family Welfare, Department of Pharmaceuticals, Department of Biotechnology and CDSCO.

Under the PACT Initiative (Partnerships for Accelerating Clinical Trials), the Department of Biotechnology offered training programmes for several countries, especially from our neighbourhood, Africa and Gulf nations to enhance and build capacity in those countries for vaccine development, trial and even covering administration and operational aspects of vaccine distribution and delivery. In the first session of the training programme, 771 participants from 7 countries participated. The second session, which started in February 2021 under PACT initiative, saw participation of more than 100 participants from 9 countries, including from Africa and Gulf nations. In the training session conducted on 19-20 January 2021 covering operational and administrative aspects of vaccination, more than 150 participants from 13 countries participated. A workshop on 'COVID Management: Experience, Good Practices and Way Forward' with 10 neighbouring countries was organised on 18 February 2021, in which health secretaries and technical experts shared their experiences in tackling COVID pandemic.

Data regarding supply of vaccines was maintained on a daily basis and was uploaded on the Ministry's website twice daily. XP Division and the Missions were tasked to give wide publicity to India's Vaccine Maitri initiative.

India's initiative of supplying COVID vaccines to the world despite its huge domestic requirements has been widely appreciated, including by the UN Secretary General, WHO, Heads of State/Heads of Government of several countries, Foreign Ministers and even by the public at large around the world.

Overall, Vaccine Maitri initiative has been a big diplomatic success for India and has helped raise our stature in the comity of nations, including establishing India as the 'Pharmacy of the World'. A presentation by the Foreign Secretary at the concluding meeting of the Parliamentary Standing Committee on External Affairs (2020-21) on "COVID Pandemic: Global Response, India's Contribution and Way Forward" delivered on 10 March 2021 (Annexure 7a).

DIPLOMATIC INITIATIVES

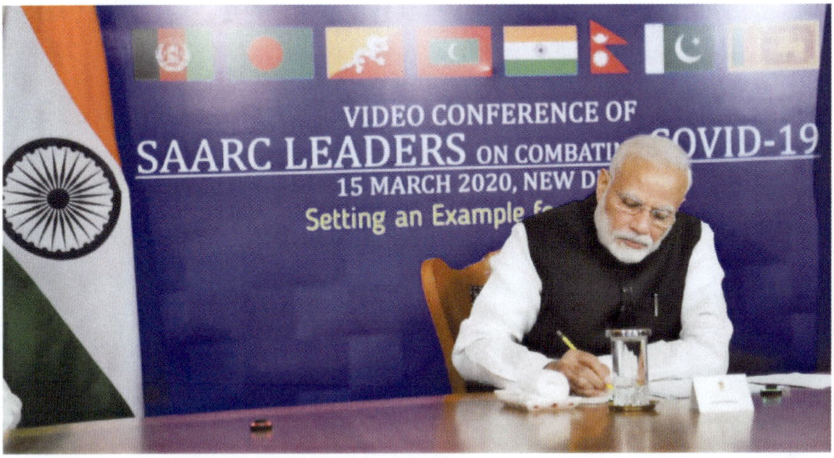
VIDEO CONFERENCE OF
SAARC LEADERS ON COMBATI COVID-19
15 MARCH 2020, NEW D
Setting an Example

SAARC: Prime Minister Narendra Modi shared the real meaning of the message 'Vasudhaiva Kutumbakam' at the video conference of SAARC leaders to collectively fight the global pandemic and improve relations between the nations.

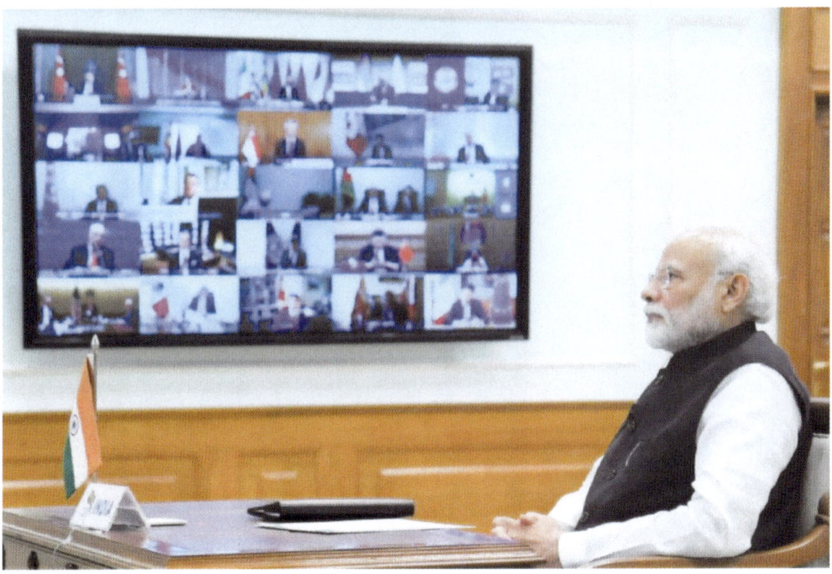

G20: Prime Minister Narendra Modi joined other G20 Leaders at the G20 Virtual Summit to advance a coordinated global response to the COVID pandemic and its human and economic implications

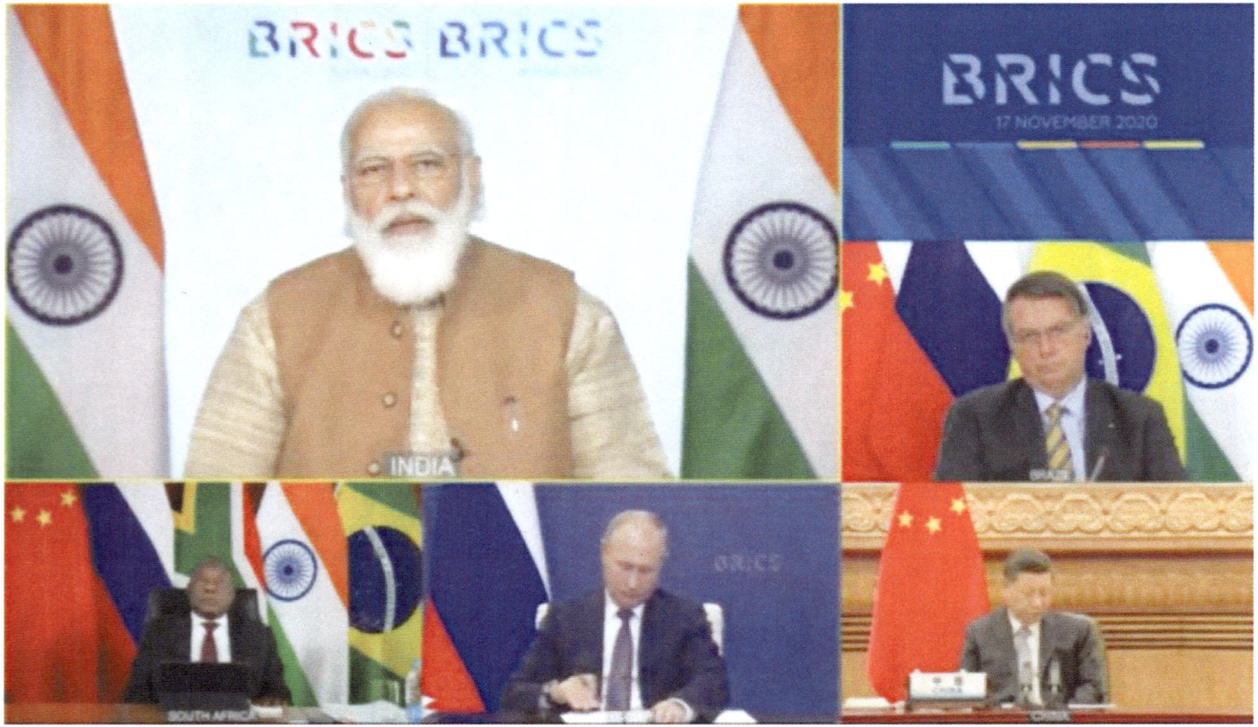

BRICS: Prime Minister Narendra Modi addresses the 2020 BRICS summit held in a virtual format

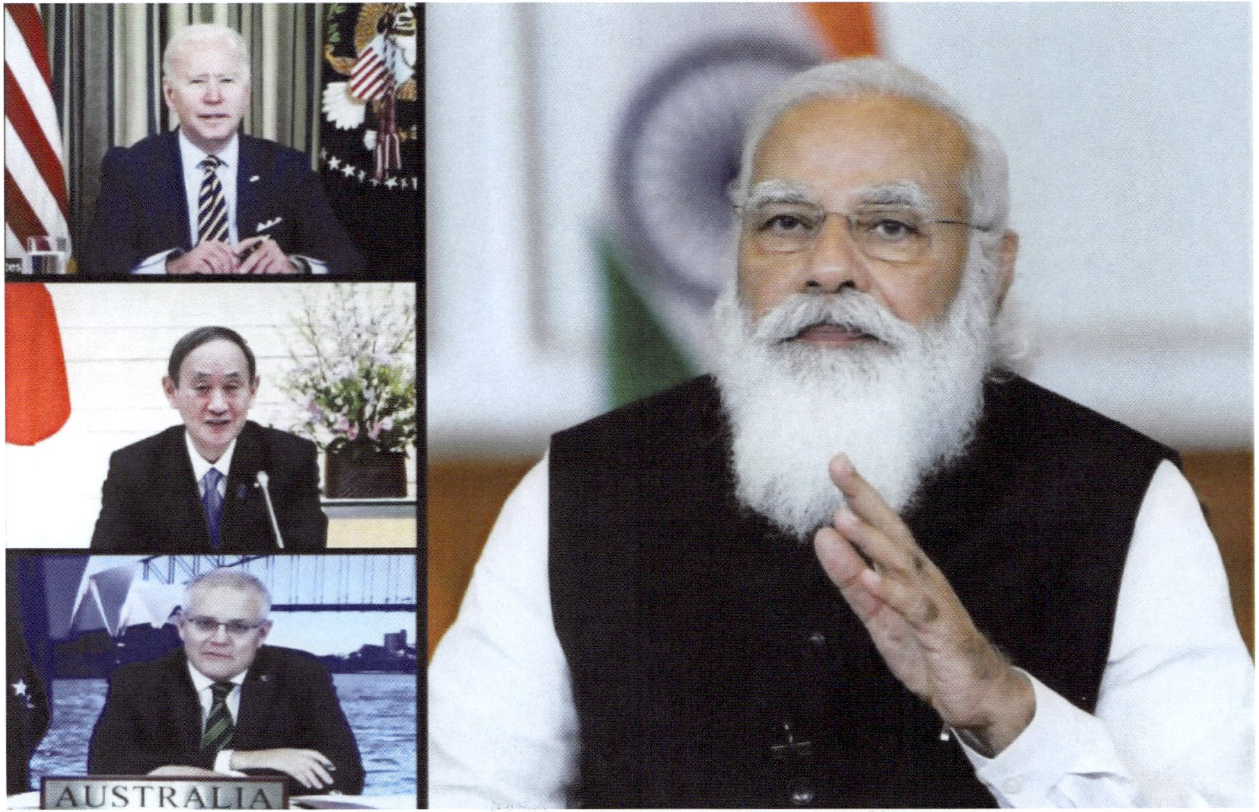

Quad Virtual Summit

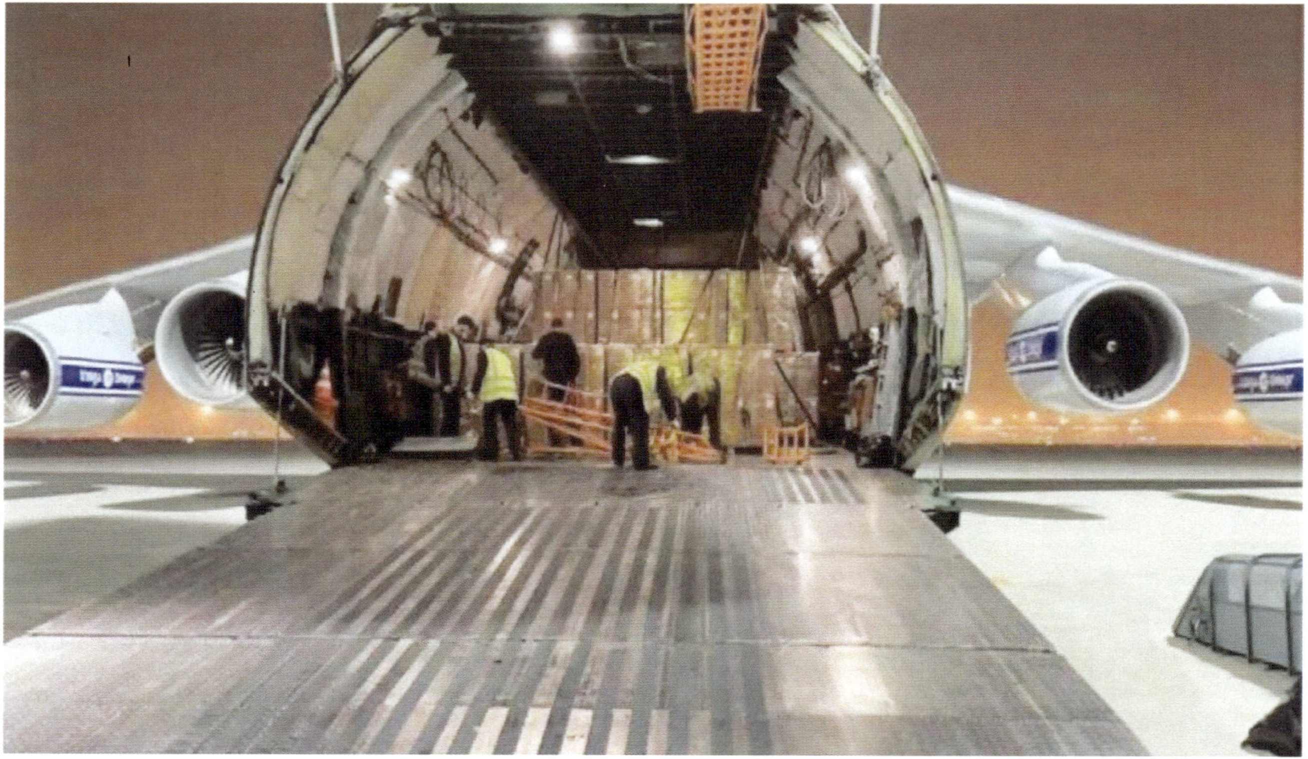

WHO: WHO chartered flights to supply medical supplies, hospital beds and additional critical equipment to India during COVID surge in May 2021

8

DIPLOMATIC INITIATIVES

The pandemic was not just a healthcare and economic shock. It is a significant geopolitical event. Amongst other things, it established that crises of this nature require more international cooperation, and not less. Existing mechanisms of intergovernmental cooperation in this area were subject to heavy stresses and not all were satisfied with their functioning. India took a number of initiatives that placed it at the forefront of global efforts to combat COVID. India joined and catalysed a number of diplomatic initiatives that dealt with various aspects of the pandemic. This included multilateral and plurilateral platforms such as SAARC, G20, WHO and WTO. The Quad undertook a number of pandemic related activities as did BRICS. India also supported organisations such as GAVI.

Through these initiatives India stressed the importance of international cooperation. It also stressed that it was willing to contribute more than its fair share in cooperative efforts to combat the pandemic. India believes in being a global force for good and is interested in generating solutions and assisting countries that seeks its help. India has also been working on shaping international regimes by seeking a TRIPS waiver for vaccines and related products.

ENGAGEMENT WITH SAARC

1. At the initiative of Prime Minister of India, a Video Conference of SAARC Leaders was held on 15 March 2020 to discuss regional response to combat COVID pandemic. The Presidents of Afghanistan, Maldives and Sri Lanka; the Prime Ministers of Bangladesh, Nepal and Bhutan, the Minister of State for Health of Pakistan, and the Secretary-General of SAARC attended the conference.

2. India announced several initiatives including the setting up of a COVID Emergency Response Fund to meet the immediate costs of combating the pandemic. India took lead in pledging a voluntary contribution of USD 10 million to the Fund followed by other SAARC members: Sri Lanka (USD 5 million), Bangladesh (USD 1.5 million), Nepal (USD 1 million), Afghanistan (USD 1 million), Maldives (USD 200,000) and Bhutan (USD 100,000). Pakistan has pledged USD 3 million subject to the condition that it be administered by the SAARC Secretariat in accordance with the SAARC Charter.
3. Responding to the requests of the countries in the region, India immediately operationalised the Fund with supply of essential drugs, medical consumables, COVID protection and testing kits, and other equipment worth INR 30.09 crore (approximately USD 4.05 million), the details of which are given below:

S. No.	Country	Aid provided under COVID ERF – Medical supplies	Amount in INR
1.	Afghanistan	Medical supplies consisting of essential medicines and equipment	2.58 crores
2.	Nepal	Medical supplies consisting of test kits and essential medicines	15.9 crores
3.	Bhutan	Medical supplies consisting of test kits and essential medicines	2.15 crores
4.	Bangladesh	Medical supplies consisting of test kits and essential medical equipment	4.01 crores
5.	Sri Lanka	Medical supplies consisting of test kits and essential medicines and equipment	1.55 crores
6.	Maldives	Medical supplies consisting of essential medicines and other supplies	3.9 crores
Total (approximately USD 4.05 million)			**30.09 crores**

4. Further, India launched a COVID Information Exchange platform 'COINEX' (on 9 May 2020) with an expenditure of INR 41.75 lakh to facilitate exchange of specialised information among designated health professionals of SAARC countries covering topics such

as disease surveillance, contact tracing, travel restrictions and evacuation, risk assessment, diagnostics, isolation and quarantine methods and facilities, clinical management of patients, treatment options and protocols and safety of health care providers. This was complemented by a website developed by SAARC Disaster Management Centre Interim Unit with an expenditure of INR 4.8 lakh, to provide reliable information and updates on the evolving situation. The total expenditure on the development of COVID specific websites was INR 46.55 lakh (approximately USD 63,826). Thus, the total expenditure on medical supplies and development of websites as India's response to fight the pandemic in the region was INR 30.56 crore (approximately USD 4.19 million).

5. In addition, since the emergence of the pandemic,
   - (i) India hosted a video conference of health professionals representing all SAARC countries at the level of Director General of Health Services (DGHS) on 26 March 2020 to share information and best practices among member states;
   - (ii) India hosted a video conference of trade officials of SAARC countries to discuss the impact of travel restrictions and the larger COVID situation on intra-regional trade including the need for simplified import procedures on 8 April 2020;
   - (iii) India participated in the virtual meeting of the SAARC Health Ministers to discuss COVID pandemic on 23 April 2020. India was represented by Directorate General of Health Services, AIIMS and Ministry of Health and Family Welfare;
   - (iv) India supplied 2000 MT of rice to Bhutan in May 2020—the first ever transaction under SAARC Food Bank mechanism;
   - (v) Under the SAARC currency swap framework for 2019-2022, India extended USD 150 million foreign currency swap support to Maldives to address short term liquidity requirements and the financial impact of COVID. India has also extended currency swap support of USD 200 million to Bhutan and USD 400 million to Sri Lanka during 2020;

(vi) Premium Indian institutes organised webinars and e-ITEC courses for practising medical professionals in the SAARC countries to share experiences on management of COVID, testing strategies, infection control measures and bio-medical waste management. The details are given below:

S. No.	Date	Event
1.	04, 06 and 08 May 2020	Webinars for practising medical professionals in the SAARC countries by AIIMS, New Delhi
2.	11-15 May 2020	e-ITEC course on Managing COVID Pandemic – Experience and Best Practices of India organised for health-care professionals by PGI Chandigarh
3.	12 – 13 May 2020	e-ITEC course on COVID Management (in Bengali language) for Bangladesh Healthcare professionals/administrators organised by AIIMS Bhubaneshwar
4.	18 May 2020	e-ITEC Capacity Building Programme on COVID organised by PGI Chandigarh for Health Care Administrators

G20

Prime Minister participated in the Extraordinary Virtual G20 Leaders' Summit on 26 March, 2020 during the Saudi Presidency. Prime Minister thanked the King of Saudi Arabia for convening this extraordinary session of G20.

In his remarks, Prime Minister noted the alarming social and economic cost of the pandemic. He added that 90 per cent of the COVID cases and 88 per cent of deaths were in G20 countries even as they share 80 per cent of world GDP and 60 per cent of the world's population. He called on the G20 to come out with a concrete action plan to fight the global pandemic.

Prime Minister underscored the need to put human beings at the centre of our vision of global prosperity and cooperation, and freely and openly share the benefits of medical research and development. He also stressed on the need to develop adaptive, responsive and humane health care systems, promote new crisis management protocols and procedures for an interconnected global village, strengthen and reform intergovernmental organisations like WHO and work together to reduce economic hardships resulting from COVID particularly for the economically weak.

Prime Minister called on the Leaders to help usher in a new globalisation, for the collective well-being of humankind and have multilateral fora focus on promoting the shared interests of humanity.

Prime Minister participated in the 15th G20 Summit convened by Saudi Arabia, on 21-22 November, 2020. At this summit meeting, Prime Minister termed the COVID pandemic as an important turning point in the history of humanity and the biggest challenge the world is facing since World War II. He called for decisive action by the G20, not limited to economic recovery, jobs, and trade, but to focus on preserving planet earth, noting that all of us are trustees of humanity's future.

Prime Minister called for a new Global Index for the post-COVID world that comprises four key elements—creation of a vast talent pool; ensuring that technology reaches all segments of the society; transparency in systems of governance; and dealing with mother earth with a spirit of trusteeship. Based on this, the G20 can lay the foundation of a new world.

Noting that 'Work from Anywhere' is a new normal in the post COVID world, Prime Minister also suggested the creation of a G20 Virtual Secretariat as a follow up and documentation repository.

G20 Ministerial meetings and that of senior officials also discussed COVID related issues.

G7

Prime Minister participated in several sessions of the G7 Summit on 12-13 June 2021. Speaking at the session, titled 'Building Back Stronger—Health', focused on global recovery from the COVID pandemic and on strengthening resilience against future pandemics, Prime Minister expressed appreciation for the support extended by the G7 and other guest countries during the recent wave of COVID infections in India. He highlighted India's 'whole of society' approach in fighting the pandemic, synergising the efforts of all levels of the government, industry, and civil society. He also explained India's successful use of open-source digital tools for contact tracing and vaccine management, and conveyed India's willingness to share its experience and expertise with other developing countries.

Prime Minister committed India's support for collective endeavours to improve global health governance. He sought the G7's support for the proposal moved at the WTO by India and South Africa, for a TRIPS waiver on COVID related technologies.

Prime Minister said that G7 meetings should send out a message of "One Earth One Health" for the whole world. Calling for global unity, leadership, and solidarity to prevent future pandemics, Prime Minister emphasised the special responsibility of democratic and transparent societies in this regard.

UNITED NATIONS

Prime Minister virtually addressed the 75th session of United Nations General Assembly in

September 2020, wherein he emphasised on the need of reform within the United Nations. Prime Minister also assured that India, as the largest vaccine producing country, will use its vaccine production and vaccine delivery capability to take the whole humanity out of the COVID pandemic.

TRIPS WAIVER FOR VACCINES AND RELATED PRODUCTS

In view of the global health crisis and the need to combat the COVID pandemic, India and South Africa, on 2 October 2020, proposed a relaxation in the norms of the agreement on TRIPS at WTO, to ensure quick and affordable access to vaccines and medicines for developing countries. As a result of the proactive outreach by India and other like-minded countries, the proposal received support of more than 120 countries.

The waiver is more than just a legal mechanism; it is a statement of intent by all countries that they accord highest value to protecting human lives rather than protecting private profits. The TRIPS Waiver Proposal is an enabler and will be invoked to ensure that intellectual property barriers do not come in the way of scaling up of manufacturing capacity. It will complement and serve to off-set some of the challenges faced by these various mechanisms in responding adequately, effectively and timely to this global health emergency.

INDIA AND WORLD HEALTH ORGANISATION (WHO)

India actively engaged in the negotiations and discussions that transpired during the 73rd World Health Assembly in the immediate aftermath of the outbreak of the pandemic and led to the adoption of the COVID Response Resolution in May 2020. India substantially contributed in the discussions that led to the comprehensive, independent and impartial evaluation of the WHO's response to the pandemic. India also contributed to the discussions that led to the call for study of the origins of the SARS-CoV2 virus.

Consequently, inter-alia, WHO established an Independent Panel for Pandemic Preparedness and Response with which India engaged actively, including at the level of the Health Minister for sharing our national experiences and lessons learnt during the pandemic.

Permanent Mission of India in Geneva, in coordination with the Ministry and Ministry of Health and Family Welfare, also formalised India's approach paper on WHO reforms which was shared with all stakeholders, including the Independent Panel for Pandemic Preparedness and Response. Based on this Approach paper the Mission actively engaged with the 74th World Health Assembly to present India's position particularly on issues of our prime concern like TRIPS waiver for vaccine manufacturing and the Nagoya Protocol on Access and Benefit sharing and the leveraging of digital technologies.

SUPPORT EXTENDED BY WHO TO INDIA DURING THE COVID PANDEMIC

By mid-May 2021 several States and Union Territories across India had begun receiving consignments of oxygen concentrators and tents for temporary health facilities brought by WHO to support India's COVID surge response. Chandigarh, Haryana, Punjab, Rajasthan, Uttarakhand, and Uttar Pradesh are among the states that received oxygen concentrators on 17 May 2021. A large consignment for the Northeast states left the warehouse on the same day.

WHO extended support to fill critical gaps in the availability of oxygen, testing kits, and hospital beds. It has provided 1.2 million respirator masks (KN95), 4000 oxygen concentrators, 128 tents for auxiliary health facilities, 1.2 million reagents and 400,000 PCR test and swab kits.

WHO has a network of over 2600 technical officers supporting the government in elimination of tuberculosis and Neglected Tropical Diseases, Routine Immunisation and Non Communicable Diseases programmes covering all States and Union Territories. These teams were repurposed last year to support the pandemic response at the grassroot level. In the recent surge, they are redeployed again to support State governments in responding to the second wave.

WHO continued to bring out a weekly India Situation Report on Coronavirus Disease. Last such report was published on 16 June 2021.

Quad

Prime Minister participated in the Quad Leaders Meeting convened by the President of the United States on 12 March 2021. The Quad Leaders' Joint Statement: "The Spirit of the Quad" had references to "the global devastation wrought by COVID" and pledged "to respond to the economic and health impacts of COVID". It spoke of joining forces to "expand safe, affordable, and effective vaccine production and equitable access, to speed economic recovery and benefit global health. With steadfast commitment to the health and safety of our own people, we also recognise that none of us can be safe as long as the pandemic continues to spread. We will, therefore, collaborate to strengthen equitable vaccine access for the Indo-Pacific, with close coordination with multilateral organisations including the World Health Organisation and COVAX. We call for transparent and results-oriented reform at the World Health Organisation." It said that Quad would combine "medical, scientific, financing, manufacturing and delivery, and development capabilities and establish a vaccine expert working group to implement our path-breaking commitment to safe and effective vaccine distribution".

The Quad Vaccine Partnership was created wherein it was stated that "Quad" partners will launch a landmark partnership to further accelerate the end of the COVID pandemic. Together, Quad leaders are taking shared action necessary to expand safe and effective COVID vaccine manufacturing in 2021 and will work together to strengthen and assist countries in the Indo-Pacific with vaccination, in close coordination with the existing relevant multilateral mechanisms including WHO and COVAX.

Quad Foreign Ministers also met in October 2020 and February 2021. The 3rd Quad Ministerial Meeting on 18 February 2021 noted that "the Ministers discussed ongoing efforts to combat the COVID pandemic, including vaccination programmes. They expressed their commitment to cooperate in addressing this challenge, enhancing access to affordable vaccines, medicines and medical equipment. India's efforts at providing vaccines to 74 countries was recognised and appreciated."

Quad senior officials at the level of Foreign Secretary held a number of meetings during the early days of the pandemic. This created a mechanism for coordination, information-sharing and exchange of views on issues relating to managing the pandemic and its fallout.

BRICS AND COVID

India assumed the rotational Chair of BRICS on 1 January 2021, for the calendar year 2021, and has utilised this platform to augment cooperation on combating COVID.

Under the 10th BRICS Health Ministers meeting theme on *"Era of COVID -19: Global BRICS Solidarity for Health Safety"*, in 2020, the Health Ministers agreed to deliver decisive, coordinated and inclusive multilateral efforts to fight against the COVID pandemic, while maintaining the spirit of trust and partnership amongst the BRICS countries even in the post-COVID era.

BRICS cooperation in health has been strengthened in the context of combatting the COVID pandemic. It is likely to remain an important area for BRICS cooperation even in the post COVID world. The strength of BRICS on Health lies in presenting fresh and inclusive approaches to global health through robust intra-BRICS engagement and based on genuine developmental partnership and South-South cooperation models among others and in reshaping the Global Health architecture and mechanisms.

At the 12th BRICS Leaders' Summit on 17 November 2020, Prime Minister in his remarks stated that India would focus on consolidation of intra-BRICS cooperation including in the fields of Traditional Medicines and Digital Health, people to people ties and cultural exchanges and would work towards boosting BRICS collaboration in these fields.

GLOBAL VACCINE SUMMIT 2020

At the Global Vaccine Summit hosted by the Prime Minister of the United Kingdom and held on 4 June 2020, India pledged USD 15 million to GAVI.

In his address, Prime Minister pledged that the world can "count on India's support" in the critical mission of vaccination against infectious diseases, highlighting India's role as the world's fourth-largest producer of vaccines. He highlighted that during this pandemic, India shared its stock of medicines with over 120 countries by forging a common response strategy in its immediate neighborhood and by providing specific support to countries that sought it, while also protecting India's own vast population.

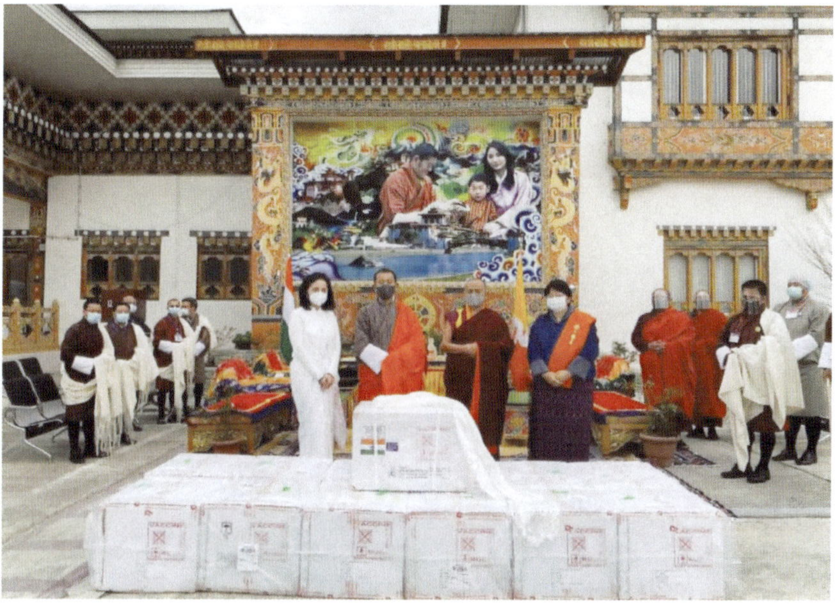

An AN 32 aircraft of Indian Air Force delivered 150,000 doses of Covishield vaccines from India, making Bhutan the first country to receive the gift, just four days after India's own massive roll out of the vaccine

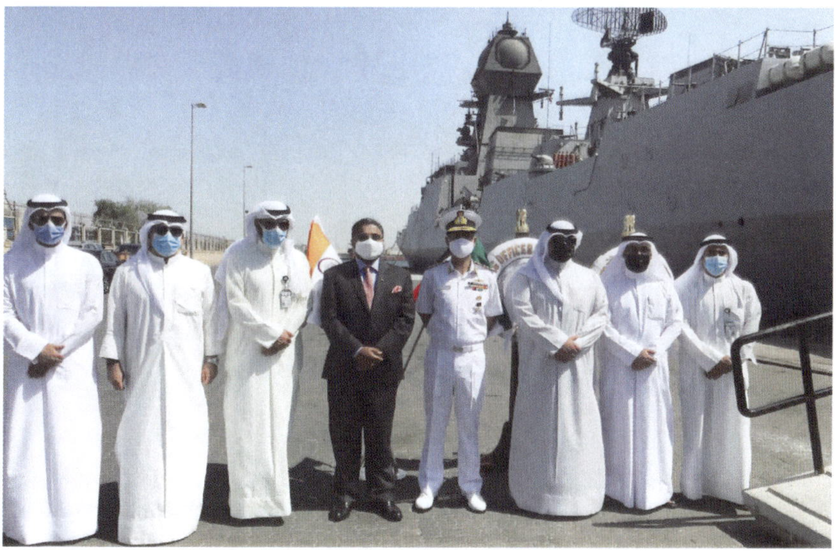

INS KOLKATA at Shuwaikh Port, Kuwait for shipment of ISO cryogenic tanks of liquid medical oxygen (40 MT) gifted by Government of State of Kuwait and 500 Oxygen cylinders & 4 Oxygen concentrators arranged by the Indian Community in the collective fight against COVID

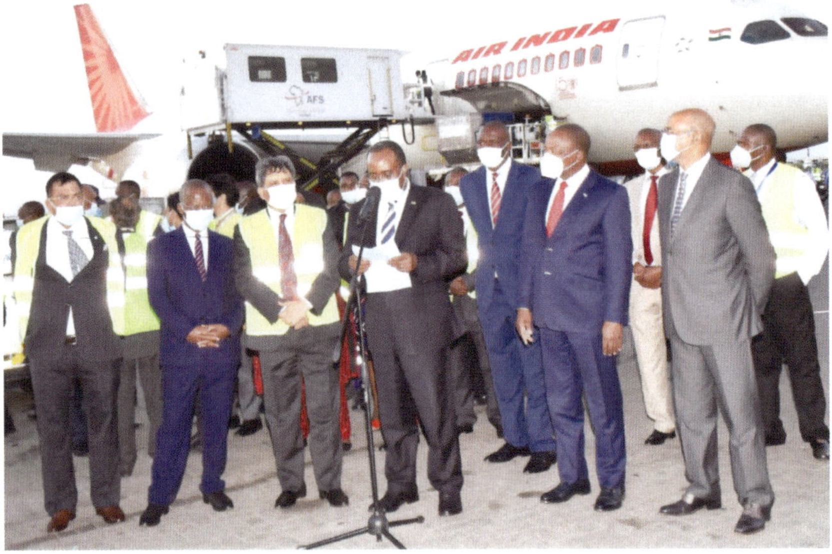

100,000 doses of Covishield vaccines donated by the Government of India received by Kenya's Health CS Mutahi Kagwe and Foreign Affairs officials

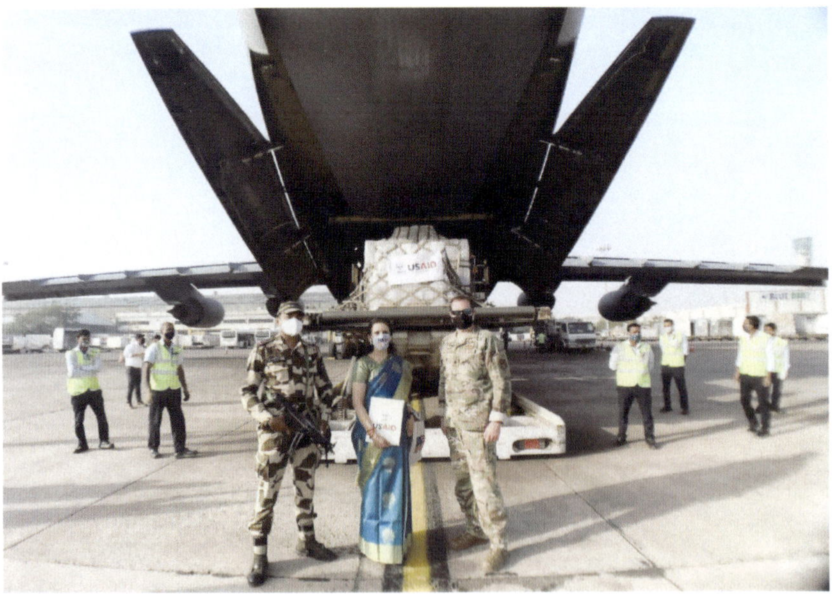

Emergency shipment from US to India carrying 500+ oxygen concentrators to help hospitals create oxygen from air & 100,000+ N95 masks

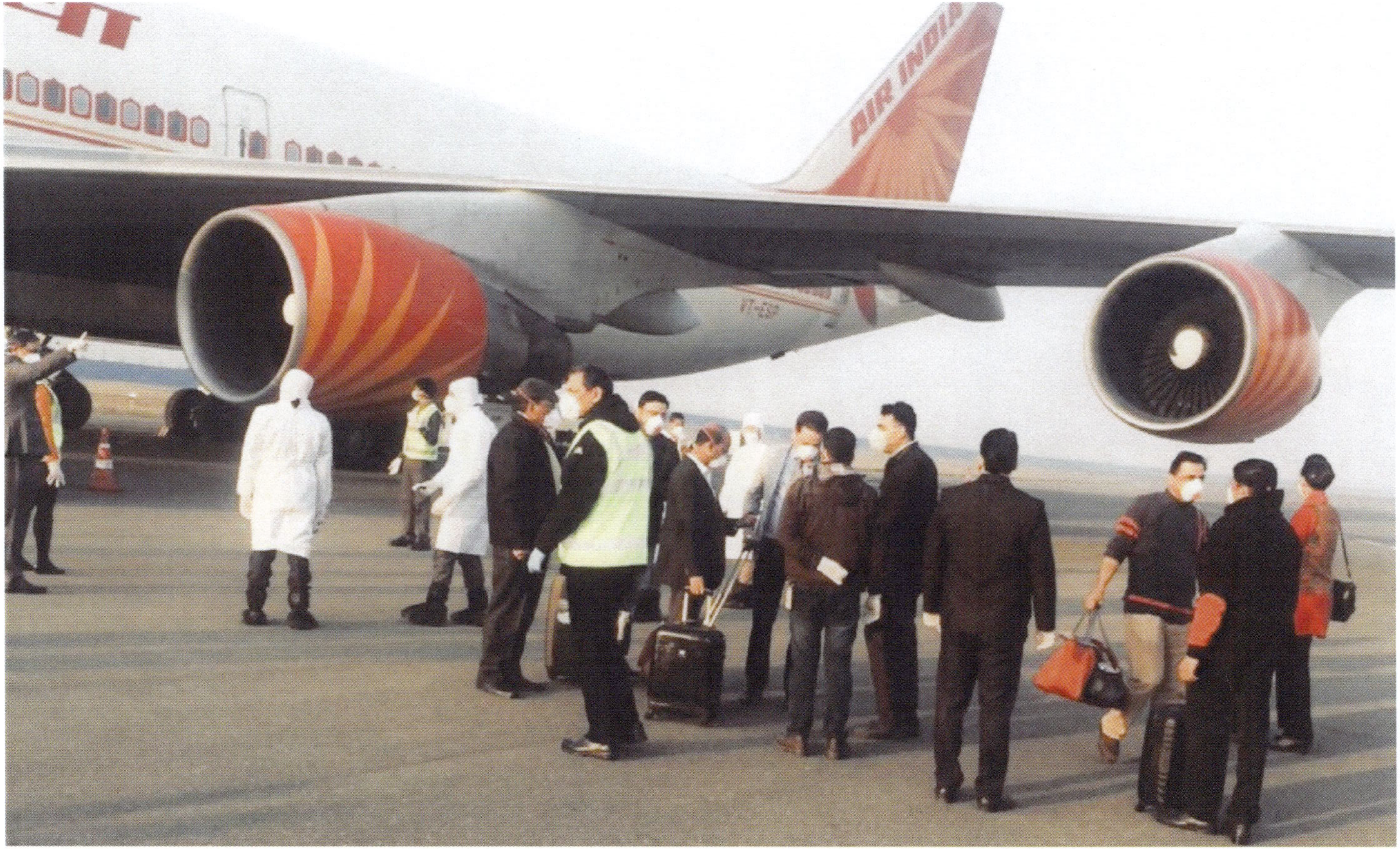

Air India flight carrying 324 Indian nationals from Hubei Province of China took off from Wuhan in the early hours of 1 February 2020. Majority of the passengers were Indian students

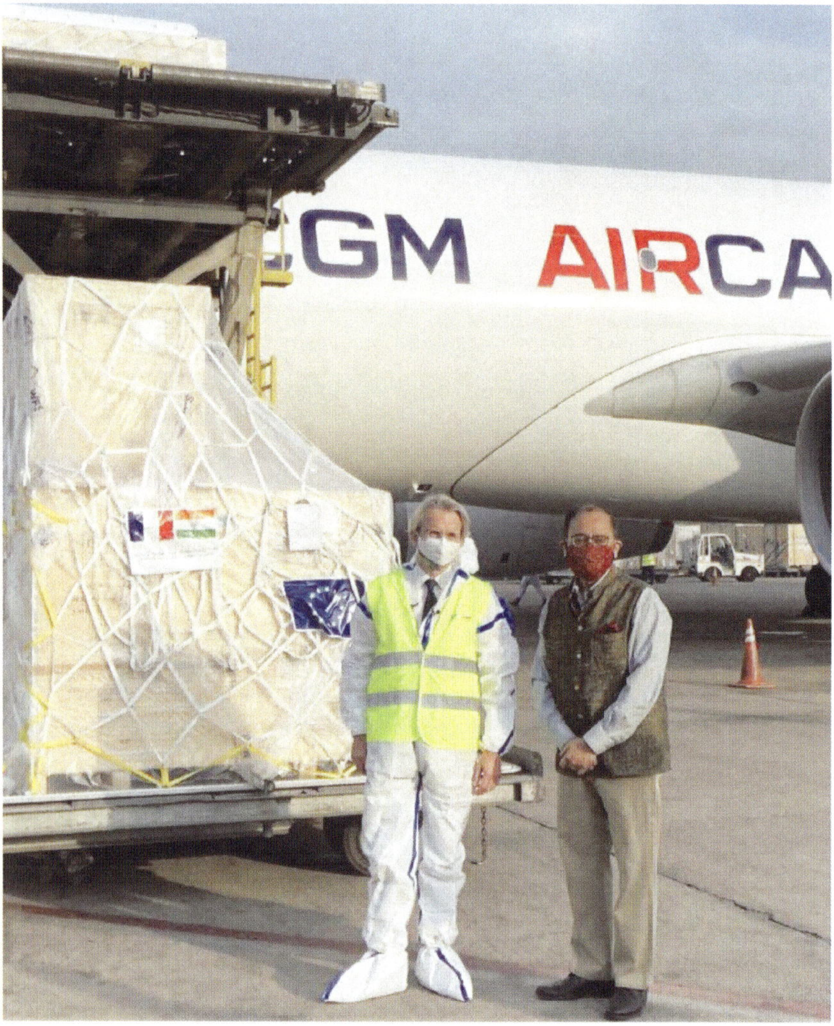

28 tonnes of medical equipment including 8 hospital-level oxygen generators and other medical supplies arrive from France

9

ROLE OF MISSIONS

INTRODUCTION

The Ministry of External Affairs operates a network of Missions and Posts abroad. This is a system with a worldwide presence and reach. This network was mobilised to meet the varied and constantly changing requirements of the international aspects of the response to the pandemic and its impacts.

An overview of operations by this network of Missions and Posts reveals that activities took place along a series of well-defined verticals. The first of these was the worldwide mission to help Indians stranded in various parts of the world. The second vertical worked on repatriation of Indians to India. This was done through a combination of Vande Bharat Missions, charter flights and land and sea voyages. The third vertical was related to procurement. The first wave of the pandemic produced a demand for PPEs and essential medical supplies. In the second wave, Missions and Posts around the world worked as a part of the network that delivered essential supplies from various parts of the world to destinations in India. The fourth vertical was outward looking and coordinated Indian outbound HADR. Essential medical supplies were delivered to 150 countries, rapid response teams were inserted, and Mission Sagar was launched. The fifth vertical dealt with vaccines. A number of vaccines were involved in Vaccine Maitri and in India's vaccine diplomacy to safeguard critical vaccine supply chains, reach out to vaccine manufacturers across the world, regulatory approvals and in efforts to obtain TRIPS waivers. A sixth vertical was concerned with outreach and to the more "normal" aspects of diplomatic functioning that persisted through the disruptions. The seventh and last vertical coped with the stresses and strains of maintaining this worldwide network in this time of disruptions. Officers and staff had to continue to operate across time zones and differing degrees of restrictions. Like many such organisations, the Ministry struggled to keep its systems "running" with the exception that it had to deal a massive geographical spread. Officers and staff abroad often worked in very difficult circumstances. Many were exposed to the virus in the line of duty. Some fell seriously ill. A few died.

These required a major coordination effort between headquarters and Missions, between and amongst Missions and Posts, and between Missions and Posts with other agencies in the Government of India and Indian States. Missions coped using modern communication and technology. The existing networks and channels of communication within the Ministry and amongst officers across the world proved resilient. Information and requirements from headquarters could be disseminated rapidly. Feedback loops also worked well, and Missions were able to find solutions and problems.

The Ministry and its network in other words remained a coherent organisational unit with rapid communication, swift execution of decisions and good reflexes.

Missions were also constantly updated about the developing situation in India.

Broadly speaking, main line of efforts by Missions and Posts may be classified into the following lines of operation:

Stranded Indians

- Lockdowns and restrictions on physical movements meant that Indians were stranded in various locations.
- Some in isolated areas that were difficult to reach
- Indian Community Welfare Fund operations

Returning Indians/Vande Bharat Missions

- Assessment of population to be repatriated—linked to REPAT portal Logistics of Vande Bharat Mission
- Liaison with local authorities
- Charter flights
- Prioritising those who wished to return
- Land and sea journeys

Inbound Procurement

- First Wave
- Second Wave

Outbound HADR

- Essential medical supplies
- Requests from world
- Rapid Response Teams
- Mission Sagar

Vaccines

- Vaccine Maitri
- Vaccine diplomacy
- Safeguard vaccine supply chains
- Outreach to manufacturers
- Regulatory approvals
- TRIPS waivers

Outreach

- Prime Minister's meeting with HoMs
- EAMs coordination meetings
- Foreign Secretary's coordination meetings
- Logistics
- Keep channels of communication open; keep the India story alive

DIGITAL/VIRTUAL DIPLOMACY

Stranded Indians

India's Missions abroad extended all possible assistance to the stranded Indians after COVID related restrictions were imposed. The assistance varied based on the needs of the people. Missions set-up 24×7 COVID emergency helplines for all kinds of assistance to Indian nationals in need. In some countries, Indian nationals were provided with masks and sanitizers, food kits, preliminary medical consultation, along with aid, boarding and lodging, and even tickets in the most deserving cases.

These initiatives were conducted by the Missions through the Indian Community Welfare Fund as well as through close cooperation with the local Indian community and their local associations. Some Missions sought the help of local Gurdwaras and community centres for providing lodging and boarding or created innovative makeshift arrangements for the same.

In consultation with host governments, Missions also helped in timely dissemination of local government guidelines on health, preventive measures, and provided medical facilities, facilitated travel logistics. Missions also assisted in testing for symptoms and other facilitation at the airports at the time of an individual's departure to India.

Missions played an important role in arranging chartered flights in cooperation with local Indian communities and companies to repatriate their workers.

Even though the critical phase of repatriation of stranded Indians was mostly over by December 2020, Missions continued to oversee the smooth functioning and forwarding of the manifests of chartered flights, air bubble flights and other flights under Vande Bharat Mission, as per the extant guidelines of the Government of India.

OUTREACH OF INDIAN MISSIONS ABROAD

Once the Standard Operating Procedures were put in place on receipt donations/gifts from abroad, many of Indian Missions abroad actively pursued the matter with the host countries. The steps taken by Missions included:

(i) Writing to the Prime Minister of the country and the Head of the Regional governments informing them about the priority requirements of Government of India;

(ii) Consul Generals following up with the regions/provinces under them;

(iii) Interacting with the Indian Associations, private companies and individuals;

(iv) Interacting with the private companies on getting technical specifications and quotations for commercial procurement;

(v) Informing all the stakeholders in India including Government of India entities, State governments and Union Territories, NGOs, businesses, chambers and associations, in some cases entities from foreign countries such as Singapore and the USA, in response to various offers of assistance for India on the range of products, including oxygen generators, molecular sieves and ingredients for life saving medicines. Such kind of information has resulted in timely procurement of equipment and drugs;

(vi) The Missions also conveyed requirements of the Indian companies in terms of ingredients and raw materials including for the vaccines;
(vii) Establishing sea-bridges and air-bridges for the transportation of Liquid Medical Oxygen;
(viii) Organising public display of solidarity with India in the host country;
(ix) Leveraging host countries manufacturing capabilities, strong trade and supply chain networks in the region to help source the oxygen-related supplies and transport them to India.

While aid has been received from 53 countries, as an illustration of action taken by Missions abroad, experience shared by some of the Missions is enclosed herewith.

MISSIONS MOBILISED TO PROVIDE UPDATES ON INDIAN EFFORTS TO COMBAT COVID

Prime Minister held a video conference with the Heads of all of India's Embassies and High Commissions worldwide on 30 March 2020 to discuss responses to the global COVID pandemic and give guidance.

Reporting

Assessments of the pandemic and its consequences were sought from Missions across the world. This was collated into a comprehensive scenario-building and projection exercise.

Mission Inputs

Inputs from a representative sample of Indian Missions and Posts have been collated. They are from all major geographies. Some of the Missions are large in size. Others are small. Some were involved in the whole spectrum of COVID related operations. Several Missions operated in some, or many, parts of the spectrum. The accounts of their activities have been broadly arranged according to region.

THE NEIGHBOURHOOD

Embassy of India, Thimphu

With the outbreak of pandemic, and in keeping with India's unique and special ties with Bhutan as well as the Ministry's Neighbourhood

First policy, the Embassy of India, Thimphu responded proactively to all challenges faced by the Royal Government as well as Indian nationals residing in Bhutan.

Vaccine Maitri: Bhutan was the first country to receive vaccines under the Ministry's Vaccine Maitri Initiative. Under Phase I of Vaccine Maitri, Bhutan received 150,000 doses of Covishield vaccines on 20 January, 2021 and under Phase II, Bhutan received 400,000 doses of Covishield on 22 March, 2021. The total number of 550,000 doses of Covishield were given to Bhutan on a grant basis. In addition to the two consignments of vaccines, Government of India delivered 11 medical consignments to Bhutan containing essential medicines including Paracetamol, Cetrizine, Hydroxychloroquine and medical equipment including PPE kits, N95 masks, RT-PCR test kits and 7 portable digital x-ray machines.

Vaccine Maitri involved coordination with the Ministry as well as liaising with the local authorities in Bhutan—both the Ministry of Foreign Affairs and the Ministry of Health. Coordination with the media was also a part of the Mission's digital diplomacy strategy to ensure appropriate publicity to India's gesture to gift vaccines to its longstanding partner and friend, Bhutan. India's vaccine donation enabled Bhutan to administer the first dose of the vaccine to its entire eligible population.

Repatriation of Indians from Bhutan: The Embassy organised the repatriation of approximately 12,000 Indian nationals across Bhutan. The repatriation was arranged via the land border route of Phuentsholing-Jaigaon, Gelephu-Dadgiri-Samdrup Jongkhar and also through Druk Air flights under the air bubble arrangement. Around 385 buses and taxis were hired to ferry Indians from Thimphu to the border points. This exercise involved coordination with the Royal Government for a special single window check point for hassle-free immigration clearances. This exercise involved coordination with the Royal Government of Bhutan—National COVID Task Force, Immigration authorities, Dzongdag (district) authorities and the Department of Immigration.

Inbound procurement (2nd wave): With the onset of the second wave of the pandemic in India and the surge in the number of positive cases, attention turned to one of the most critical life saving commodities in the fight against the pandemic-medical oxygen. In April 2021, the Health

Minister of Bhutan and the Chief Minister of Assam had requested the Ministry to explore the possibility of importing liquid oxygen from the Royal Kingdom. Within an hour of receiving the Ambassador's request, all necessary approvals were obtained from Bhutan's top leadership for setting up SD Cryogenics Gases Pvt. Ltd in Motanga Industrial Estate in the eastern district of Samdrup Jongkhar bordering Assam. The plant will supply close to 10,000 cylinders of oxygen per day to Assam and Manipur.

Mitigate disruption in the movement of goods between India and Bhutan: In 2020, India opened five new trade routes: Ahllay, Nagarkata, Agartala, Pandu and Jogighopa to step up connectivity between the two neighbours and to allow the movement of goods between the two countries despite the pandemic.

Consulate General of India, Birgunj, Nepal

The following consular services were rendered during the pandemic to the Indians as well as Nepali nationals residing in the jurisdiction of the Consulate which includes eight Terai districts viz. Parsa, Bara, Rautahat, Sarlahi, Mahottari, Dhanusha, Makwanpur and Chitwan:

(i) Issuance of Registration Cards to Indian nationals, issuance of Ordinary/Jumbo, Official and Diplomatic Passports to Indian nationals, attestation of documents, issuance of birth and death certificates;
(ii) Issuance of Certificates of Transfer of Residence to Indian nationals registered with this Post or with the Embassy of India, Kathmandu at time of their final departure from Nepal to India;
(iii) Issuance of Note Verbales to the Nepalese Ministry of Foreign Affairs for addressing the grievances/complaints of Indian nationals;
(iv) Issuance of letters to various Indian authorities for addressing the grievances/complaints of Nepali citizens;
(v) Issuance of courtesy letters based on the recommendations of Ministry of Foreign Affairs for Nepali nationals as well as Indian nationals residing in Nepal for treatment in Indian hospitals on priority basis; and
(vi) Issuance of courtesy letter/recommendation for transportation of mortal remains of Indian nationals to their home towns in India.

Land-Border Repatriation

Apart from usual consular services, the Post undertook the following:

(i) 24,563 stranded Indians including migrant workers were repatriated via Land Border route through ICP Birgunj-Raxaul during the pandemic in 2020.

(ii) 2000 distressed stranded Indians were extended assistance from the Indian Community Welfare Fund budget during evacuation and repatriation through land-border of ICP Birgunj-Raxaul. An expenditure of INR 1,29,821.02 (NPRs 2,06,00.00) was incurred by the Post from Indian Community Welfare Fund.

(iii) The Post also coordinated with local district authorities, Mayor of Birgunj and organisations like 'NGO Green City' and 'Rotary Club, Birgunj' for boarding and lodging of stranded Indians in distress during the process of land border repatriation.

SOUTH-EAST ASIA AND EAST ASIA

Embassy of India, Beijing

The Embassies inputs about its work in organising evacuations from Wuhan and procurement during the first wave has been listed under the Chapters on Vande Bharat Mission and Procurement Phase I.

Embassy of India, Manila

The Philippines imposed a complete lockdown in affected areas on 17 March 2020, which was repeatedly extended. Several Indians, especially students pursuing higher education and temporary visitors/tourists were therefore stranded in the country. After the first lockdown was imposed, the Embassy coordinated with local authorities to provide hotel accommodation to Indian tourists stranded in different islands of the Philippines. In case of Indians who were short of resources and money, arrangements were made in Gurudwaras with the help of the local community. In close co-ordination with the colleges and universities, the Embassy also arranged for distribution of face masks, sanitisers, food and essential supplies to the Indian students.

Under the Vande Bharat Mission, from 7 May 2020 till 30 September 2020, the Embassy repatriated 9477 Indians, in a total of 49 flights operated by Air India and SpiceJet.

In August-September 2020, in face of strict quarantine measures and travel restrictions on the domestic sector in both the countries, arrangements were made for the convenience of Indians located in different cities of the Philippines and those intending to travel to different parts of India. Vande Bharat Mission flights were arranged from two cities in the Philippines—Manila and Cebu. Similarly, feeder flights were arranged for passengers intending to travel from one Indian city to the other.

Under its public outreach efforts, the Embassy extensively used social media and local community WhatsApp and Viber groups to publicise related advisories. A dedicated email id and a hotline number for Vande Bharat Mission related communications was made available.

Apart from repatriation of Indian nationals, facilitation of travel of Filipino children to India for urgent liver transplants on the Vande Bharat Mission flights got visible media traction.

High Commission of India, Singapore

The High Commission's inputs about its work on procurement during the first wave have been listed under the chapter on Procurement Phase I.

During the second wave, High Commission worked with, HLL Lifecare, ONGC, GAIL, state governments, as well as corporates such as Tatas, Adani, and Reliance to identify sources for crucial items such as oxygen cryogenic tankers, concentrators, cylinders, and liquid oxygen. Although Singapore doesn't manufacture many of the required products in sufficient numbers, the High Commission was able to leverage Singapore's strong trade and supply chain networks in the region to help source the oxygen-related supplies and transport them to India via IAF planes, Indian Navy ships and commercial cargo flights. The Mission had to make arrangements for sourcing and aggregating the materials in time for the flights, ensure the requisite flight clearances, immigration and health clearances for flight and ship crews, organise ground/port handling services and also coordinate logistics arrangements for loading the materials on to the aircraft and ships. The Mission worked with a number of Ministries in the Government of India, including the Ministry of External Affairs, Ministry of Defence, Ministry of Home Affairs, Ministry of Health and Family Welfare, and the Ministry of Civil Aviation. In addition, the High Commission also liaised on a regular basis with the Indian Air Force, Indian Navy, Red Cross India, HLL Lifecare Ltd., Indian Oil Corporation Ltd. and private sector entities such as the Tata Group, Adani Group, Linde Gas and the relevant state governments.

The excellent political relationship underpinning the "Strategic Partnership" between India and Singapore is reflected in the fact that EAM and Raksha Mantri were able to reach out to their Singapore counterparts via telephone and ensure full support of the Singapore authorities for Government of India's procurement efforts. The High Commission of India liaised closely with Singapore Ministry of Foreign Affairs and Ministry of Defence to secure speedy and timely clearances for the multiple IAF sorties and Indian Navy ship visits, often at short notice and with rapidly changing schedules. Singapore Ministry of Trade and Industry, Enterprise Singapore and industry bodies and corporates worked closely with us to identify sources of key items required, in the region and beyond.

As on 29 June 2021, key items transported from Singapore to India include 121 ISO Cryogenic Tanks, 8363 Oxygen concentrators, 16616 oxygen cylinders, 51000 oxymeters, 1900 BiPAP machines, 270 ventilators, and numerous other supplies such as medicines, PPE kits, etc. These goods were transported from Singapore to India aboard twenty-six Indian Air Force sorties, three trips by INS Airavat and INS Jalashwa, and numerous commercial cargo flights. In addition, the Indian community in Singapore made its own contribution at the non-governmental level to dispatch relief supplies to India.

Donations and Fund Raising from Local Companies and Indian diaspora

The commitment of Singaporean organisations, companies and Temasek Foundation (the philantropic arm of Singapore's Sovereign Wealth Fund) is reflected in the fact that one of the earliest and largest shipments sent to India by any foreign partner was the consignment from Temasek Foundation, in partnership with a number of Singaporean companies. It consisted of over 8000 oxygen concentrators, 51000 oxymeters, over 900 BiPAP machines and 27 ventilators.

The national effort to procure relief supplies was also bolstered by the presence in Singapore of a large number of Indian professionals and other active members of the Indian community. The High Commission worked closely with the Pan-IIM Alumni Association, Pan-IIT Alumni Association, TiE (The Indus Entrepreneurs), Singapore Indian Chamber of Commerce and Industry (SICCI), Little India Shop Owners Association (LISHA) and a number of other Indian community and business organisations, to coordinate assistance for COVID mitigation efforts in India.

Embassy of India, Seoul

Republic of Korea was the first country, after China, which saw an early spike in the number of COVID cases since late January 2020. The Embassy, proactively reach out to the Indian communities through video conferences, social media and other virtual means to inform them about preventive measures and government guidelines, and more importantly to allay the initial fear and panic amongst the people which was predominant during the early days for lack of information and awareness. The Embassy distributed face masks to Indian communities as it became scarce due to higher demands in the market.

Once international flights to and from India were stopped, the Embassy played an important role in arranging Vande Bharat flights and chartered flights in close cooperation with the host government, Indian communities and the airlines, to repatriate Indians from Republic of Korea. The Embassy kept engaging the Indian community and addressed their concerns. Two Vande Bharat Flights carried 242 Indians from Republic of Korea to India, while charter flights flying with a frequency of 5-6 flights per month carried around 1420 Indians including around 70 stranded seafarers. Ten DVCs were conducted where the Ambassador or the DCM addressed queries of Indian Community members ranging from masks distribution, travel guidelines, flights information, Visa extension issues etc. Financial and medical assistance were provided to students who were in need. The Embassy has facilitated cremation and transportation of mortal remains of 16 Indian nationals since January 2020.

When COVID cases in India started rising, the Embassy reached out to reputed Korean bio-pharma companies to supply medical kits including testing kits to India. During the second wave of pandemic in India, Embassy facilitated the supply of donations in terms of oxygen cylinders, concentrators, generators, money, masks, zeolites, test kits, etc. coming from Republic of Korea Government, Local Governments like Gimhae City, companies, organisations like the Tongdosa Buddhist temple, and Indian communities. The Republic of Korea Government donated USD 4 million worth of supplies including oxygen cylinders and concentrators. Numerous companies also donated oxygen cylinders, generators, and a large amount of money during the second wave.

The Embassy reached out to major local interlocutors and media and regularly briefed them about India's efforts to address the pandemic, including the leadership shown by India at multilateral for a including the SAARC leadership summit. The Ambassador gave regular interviews and contributed articles in major media to showcase fast-paced development in India over the past one and half years. The Mission also took utmost care to ensure that officials and staff of the Indian embassy were not affected. Possibilities were explored to establish policies and practices, such as flexible work sites (work from home) and flexible work hours to increase the physical distance among employees. Local staff who use public transport were allowed to work from home. Only absolutely essential local staff attended office with reduced office timing or on rotation basis to provide indispensable services. Sufficient arrangements for masks, gloves, sanitizers, and spray were made in the Embassy for use by staff and guests. Daily temperature checks were made mandatory for all the members before entering office premises. Maximum efforts were made to conduct virtual meetings to eliminate chances of physical contact as far as possible. All the members of the Embassy arriving from India were asked to isolate themselves under home quarantine as per the stipulated time period. The Embassy cancelled all public events, cultural activities and even physical classes during COVID pandemic, and switched to online classes, including Yoga, language, music, etc.

Embassy of India, Bangkok

Thailand was the first country outside China to report COVID infection on 13 January 2020. Following the announcement of lock down in end March in India and suspension of international flights by Thailand in early April 2020, the Embassy immediately reached out to various community organisations, Indian representatives and stakeholders to take stock of the situation and affected Indian nationals. Large number of Indian tourists, students and people in transit were stranded here. The Embassy reached out to them through social media, phone calls and e-mails. 24×7 emergency COVID helpline was set up by the Mission to assist Indians in Thailand.

Indian students stranded in various provinces of Thailand were provided ration/food, accommodation through Indian Community Welfare Fund. The services of local representatives and Indian Associations were utilised. A passenger stranded at the airport was helped to enter Thailand despite the local regulations prohibiting entry of foreign national and was provided accommodation and other support until the start of Vande Bharat Mission flights between Thailand and India.

Many Indian nationals had lost their jobs and needed financial support including for treatment of COVID infection. The Mission facilitated assistance in the form of food, accommodation, jobs, financial support towards travel expenses, medical treatment, etc. to them through Indian Community associations. The Ambassador had several physical and virtual meetings with the Indian community leaders and some stranded Indian nationals.

In view of the enormous demand for COVID vaccines among the Indian Community, Mission coordinated with the Thai Government agencies and some private hospitals for vaccination of several hundred Indian nationals. Ambassador and other officers both coordinated with the concerned agencies and were present during the vaccination process.

On request of the National Security Council (under the Thai Prime Minister's Office)—the designated nodal agency for COVID management, the Ambassador also gave a detailed presentation on India's COVID management and the lessons learnt during the pandemic in a virtual meeting.

Vande Bharat Mission

During the initial phase of Vande Bharat Mission, the Mission facilitated movement of stranded Indian nationals from far-off provinces, bringing them to Bangkok and to the Airport by providing escort, arranging transportation, and reasonable transit accommodation, as travel restrictions did not allow inter-provincial travel. For the initial few Vande

Bharat Mission flights, Mission also provided packed refreshments and water for passengers in the airport terminals.

Even before the centralised database, which was communicated by the Ministry came into usage, the Mission devised its own extensive database and started registration of stranded Indian nationals. A 24-hour dedicated COVID helpline, social media platform such as Twitter, Whatsapp, Facebook were utilised to gather data and to register Indians. This database was utilised to allocate tickets to priority passengers such as pregnant ladies, the old, the infirm and those in emergency and the system was much appreciated as those in need could be prioritised as the flights were few. Within the first two months (May and June) all the priority passengers were repatriated to India by Vande Bharat Mission flights. Fifty-three Vande Bharat Mission flights in which more than 9178 Indians and 715 OCI and 53 foreign nationals were repatriated were organised. A bridge software was utilised to transfer this database to the central database.

Embassy of India, Vientiane

Lao PDR being a Least Developed Country in South East Asia is dependent on outside support to mitigate natural and other disasters. With the lockdown of Lao PDR in end March 2020 due to first wave of COVID Pandemic, the United Nations in Lao PDR, based on inputs received from WHO, requested donors and partner countries based in Vientiane to support the Government of Lao PDR in crucial preparedness and response. India favourably considered the request and dispatched a small consignment of medicines and medical supplies to help Laos. The shipment of medicines donated by India was handed over to the Lao Ministry of Health in August 2020.

In June 2020, Prime Minister spoke to the then Prime Minister of Lao PDR, Dr. Thongloun Sisoulith and the two leaders exchanged views on the health and economic challenges posed by the global COVID pandemic. The Prime Minister commended the effective measures undertaken by the Government of Lao PDR to contain spread of the pandemic in Laos.

Lao PDR is dependent on its neighbours, especially Thailand, for connectivity to outside world including India. Post-COVID outbreak, due to lockdown and travel restrictions imposed by Thailand and other neighbouring countries, travel from Laos to India became extremely challenging. Considering a small number of Indians stranded in Lao PDR, offering a Vande Bharat Mission flight to Lao PDR was also not found to be feasible on part of the Ministry due to some operational challenges and financial viability. The Mission worked with Embassy of India in Hanoi and the Embassies of Lao and Vietnam in India to operate three special chartered flights from Delhi-Hanoi-Vientiane-Delhi in the months of August 2020, November 2020 and July 2021 and evacuated 143 Indians, 3 Lao citizens and 2 Nepali citizens. The Embassy also helped some stranded Indians by providing food, accommodation and other help during lockdown.

As part of the COVAX initiative of CEPI, Gavi and WHO, 132000 Made in India Covishield AstraZeneca vaccine were supplied to Lao PDR in March 2021.

High Commission of India, Brunei Darussalam

(i) Repatriation of Indian nationals: Brunei was not covered under the Vande Bharat Mission flights during the COVID pandemic induced travel restrictions. However a large number of representations were received by the Mission from the Indian diaspora wishing to travel back to India. The Mission, therefore, in collaboration with Indian associations and local authorities, operated 13 chartered flights through Royal Brunei Airlines from Brunei to Coimbatore during the period of July 2020 to April 2021. During this period, in view of the high cost of RT-PCR test at Brunei, Mission also facilitated RT-PCR test of the diaspora community on arrival at Coimbatore airport. A total of 1808 Indian nationals were evacuated from Brunei in the 13 flights operated by the Mission. The last such flight was operated on 30 April 2021.

(ii) Humanitarian aid: The approximately 8000 members of Indian diaspora, under the patronage of the High Commission, voluntarily generated B$ 315,000.00 (INR 1.8 crore). This corpus was used to send oxygen cylinders (filled with compressed medical oxygen gas) to India in two tranches. The first consignment of 600 new and partially used cylinders of 47 liters and 50 liters capacity were sent onboard INS Jalashwa from Brunei on 12 May. The second tranche of 450 brand new oxygen cylinders of 50 liters each filled with medical oxygen gas, was sent from Singapore onboard INS Airavat on 29 May 2021.

OCEANIA

High Commission of India, Canberra

COVID Relief/Vande Bharat Mission: At the outbreak of the pandemic in Australia, there were about 2.7 lakh Indian nationals including more than 100,000 students. Mission and Posts in Australia took a series of proactive measures aimed at assisting the stranded Indian nationals in Australia, including:

- Establishment of dedicated 24×7 COVID emergency helpline and cataloging each call with a proper priority grading.
- Extensive outreach through Mission's website/social media platforms to provide critical information/guidance on real time basis in a user-friendly manner including rolling out of a 24×7 COVID *Chatbot* assistance (in collaboration with TCS).
- Outreach for registration of stranded Indian nationals desirous to return to India yielded concrete and actionable figures and aided the successful planning of repatriation flights from Australia.
- Emergency relief assistance to needy nationals in partnership with diaspora organisations to provide food, basic provisions and accommodation. More than 25,000 food parcels and grocery kits are estimated to have been distributed by Diaspora Organisations, through partial funding by Mission/ Posts from Indian Community Welfare Fund.
- Emergency medical assistance to critically ill stranded nationals through Indian Community Welfare Fund.
- Intervention with the Australian Government to facilitate visa extension/conversion to stranded Indians and liaising with Australian authorities to grant travel exemption to Indians who had compelling/compassionate reasons to travel to Australia.
- Engagement with the Australian Government and Universities/ Educational institutions to provide relief to around 100,000 Indian

students, following which a large number of Australian Universities announced plans to support international students impacted by the pandemic.

- Setting up of "Virtual Clinic" through Indian Medical Association of Australia (Queensland Chapter) to provide easy healthcare access.

As on 6 October 2021, 36,172 passengers had been successfully repatriated from Australia through 75 Vande Bharat Mission Flights (12145 pax) and 102 Chartered flights (24027 pax).

Working with Armed Forces: Four cryogenic tankers were airlifted by IAF C17 from Perth to India on 5 May 2021 (purchased by Tata group through Linde Gas/Sing Swee Bee Enterprise Pvt Ltd). One more cryogenic tanker purchased by Tata Steel was delivered by Australian Defence Force C-17A Globemaster on 6 June 2021.

Procurement/COVID support: Government of Australia delivered 3000 Non-invasive ventilators; 250 oxygen concentrators; consumables for ventilators and concentrators through five special Qantas flights on 5 May, 14 May, 22 May, 1 June and 9 June.

An Australian Pharmaceutical company MSD Australia had sent 21,600 units of their anti-fungal treatment NOXAFIL (posaconazole) to Mumbai from Australia via air freight on 30 May 2021. MSD also entered into a Voluntary Licensing Agreement with eight established Indian generic manufacturers for their oral candidate, Molnupiravir, for treatment of COVID patients in India.

Mission/Posts also facilitated donations of cash/medical equipment from individuals and diaspora organisations.

CENTRAL ASIA

Embassy of India, Ashgabat

Soon after the onset of the pandemic, Turkmenistan suspended international flights into and out of the country from 20 March, 2020. It also put in place various restrictions like closure of markets/restaurants/theatres, no inter-state movement of train/bus, ban on public events like marriage/birthday celebration etc.

Indian nationals in Turkmenistan numbered close to 250 when the pandemic began. They were mainly engaged in the construction and oil and gas sectors. Many Indians were based in Balkan province and working for foreign companies like Dragon Oil, Ilkinsaat, Al Gaama, ENI, DAMAC, etc. An Indian company, M/s. Pamposh Construction Pvt. Ltd. based in Ashgabat in the construction sector also had Indian employees. When cases of COVID increased in the country and hospitals running to full capacity, Indian workers started requesting the Mission to arrange for their return to India.

Turkmenistan was not included by the Indian Government in Vande Bharat Mission. Hence, the Mission decided to try charter flights for repatriation of Indian nationals. A notice was placed on mission's website along with registration form asking Indian nationals intending to go back to provide the details. Simultaneously, the Embassy contacted the Turkmen Government for securing permission for repatriation flight. The Turkmen Government had permitted landing and take off only from Turkmenabat, a city located 600 km from capital Ashgabat in the northern Lebap province. Embassy had to also arrange for RT-PCR test of Indian nationals and their transport from various locations inside the country to Turkmenabat. Despite the initial lack of prompt response from the host country, the Embassy was able to arrange the first repatriation flight on 18 July 2020 which carried around 60 Indians to Delhi from where they could travel to various destinations in India. Mission arranged another charter flight on 26 September 2020 and repatriated around 20 Indians successfully in a similar way. Later, on 30 January 2021, Mission assisted in repatriation of around 110 Indians through charter flights organised by the Indian company M/s. Pamposh Construction Ltd. for their workers.

During the three repatriation exercises, Mission maintained close contact with relevant authorities in India for proper liaison like COVID Cell of the Ministry, Delhi Government, Directorate General of Civil Aviation, Ministry of Health and Family Welfare, etc. All details of Indian nationals required including COVID test details were prepared in required format and uploaded on REPAT portal. Embassy officials including the Ambassador visited Turkmenabat airport to ensure hassle free repatriation and see off Indian nationals.

Embassy of India, Tashkent

As part of repatriation efforts from March to November 2020, 9 evacuation flights were operated, (8 by Uzbekistan Airways and 1 by SpiceJet) and Mission played an active role in evacuation of 934 Indian nationals including around 160 students.

On 21 March 2020, the Uzbek Airways special flight from Tashkent to Delhi which was meant to repatriate Uzbek nationals back to Uzbekistan, became the first ever foreign carrier to be permitted by the Ministry to carry Indian nationals stranded abroad to India which was so far permitted only on designated Vande Bharat Mission flights. Mission pro-actively worked towards seeking relevant permissions from the concerned authorities of Uzbekistan and India and was able to send 121 Indian nationals from Uzbekistan to India on that flight.

The Mission actively helped Indian NGOs in procurement of oxygen concentrators and sending them to the Ministry of Health and Family Welfare and other State beneficiaries in India (NGOs like Jaipur Foot USA and commercial entities in India) in an expeditious manner during the second wave of the pandemic in May 2021. Further it requested Government of Uzbekistan which was sending relief items to India on 1 May 2021 to also take on board the relief items donated by the local Indian community in Uzbekistan (oxygen concentrators). Hence, the combined shipment of relief items sent by the Government of Uzbekistan and the local Indian community was together delivered to Red Cross, New Delhi on 1 May 2021. The Mission facilitated in expediting logistical arrangements for donation of 200 Oxygen cylinders donated by Indian diaspora in Uzbekistan to Bihar Foundation, Patna, India during the second wave of the Pandemic.

Lastly, the Mission also actively tied up with JV Jurakbek Laboratories LLC in Uzbekistan for commercial export of Remdesivir injection, as sought by Ministry of Health and Family Welfare during the second wave of Pandemic.

Embassy of India, Nur-Sultan

The Embassy evacuated 1621 Indians from Kazakhstan by 11 Vande Bharat Mission flights. Around 2335 people were also evacuated from Kazakhstan by Charter flights and Indian Embassy supported the charter flight operators in obtaining Landing Permit with Ministry of Foreign Affairs, Kazakhstan.

EURASIA

Embassy of India, Ulaanbaatar

Mongolia, being a landlocked nation between China and Russia, has its own unique limitations and challenges. With the declaration of pandemic by WHO and origin of virus from its neighbouring country, on 13 February 2020, Mongolia closed its border and suspended air and land connectivity. As of October 2021, except for movement of essential goods and services, the land and air borders continued to remain closed due to COVID pandemic.

Given the strategic relationship between India and Mongolia and status of 'spiritual neighbour', India was the first country to provide 150,000 doses of AstraZeneca vaccines to counter COVID pandemic in Mongolia. The consignment was handed over to the Mongolian Government (Deputy Prime Minister) by the Ambassador on 22 February 2021 which was widely appreciated across the spectrum of the Mongolian leadership. A special letter of thanks was sent by the Mongolian Prime Minister to the Prime Minister thanking immensely for the timely support. The Mongolia Prime Minister and several other Ministers also took the first dose of Made in India vaccine.

Other important measures/assistance during Ministry's compilation are as follows:

(i) Despite Mongolia having a small population of Indian diaspora, Mission managed to arrange seats on 5 special flights operated by Mongolian Airlines for repatriation of 38 Indians in May, June, August 2020 and again in February and April 2021. No Vande Bharat Mission flights were operated on the Mongolia-India sector.

(ii) Mission also arranged transportation of engineers and other workers from India for the construction work of USD 1.2 billion Government of India funded Oil Refinery Project. Approx. 121 workers were transported and therefore, despite COVID and severe winter weather conditions, the construction work started at the ORP on 15 January 2021.

(iii) During the second wave of COVID pandemic in India, the Government of Mongolia as a special gesture donated an amount of USD 1 million to Red Cross India to supplement the COVID control efforts of Government of India. In addition, several local agencies, Indian diaspora and Friends of India collected an amount of USD 123,000 which was also donated to the Prime Minister Cares Fund/Red Cross India.

(iv) To continue its efforts in combating COVID pandemic, the Government of India granted special export permit for commercial sale of 100,000 doses of Remdesivir to Mongolia on 30 August 2021.

(v) In addition, under e-ITEC programme, online training of 3 doctors from National Centre for Communicable Diseases (NCCD), Mongolia was arranged for pandemic management protocols.

(vi) An offer of technology transfer by CSIR as well as COVID combat/ management related protocols, immunity booster medicines, etc. was extended to Mongolian Ministry of Health and was widely disseminated through a host of other Mongolian agencies like Mongolian National Chamber of Commerce and Industry, NCCD, India-Mongolia Health Cooperation Centre and Mongolia-India Business Council and pharma group MONOS.

THE GULF

Embassy of India, Kuwait

India's rapid response team to Kuwait for combating COVID Against the backdrop of COVID pandemic, early in April 2020, discussions took place at the highest political levels (Prime Minister and EAM levels), during which Kuwait underscored the need to augment the medical resources of Kuwait Defence Forces.

Government of India responded quickly to the request from the Kuwaiti leadership by dispatching a rapid response medical team with a mandate of assisting in COVID Testing and Capacity Building on 11 April 2020 for a period of two weeks. The scope included assisting in COVID testing and capacity building. Kuwait was the second country where a medical team had been sent to deal with COVID.

A considerable amount of goodwill was generated by the visit of the rapid response team with the leadership, the government and the senior Officials from the State of Kuwait especially from the Ministries of Defence and Health acknowledging the timely assistance from India. Positive press coverage ensured amplification of the goodwill and further strengthening Brand India in Kuwait as a reliable partner.

Community Support—Food, Medical

A multipronged approach was adopted by the Mission to deal with the adverse effects of the prolonged COVID crisis.

Initial phase: Treatment and quarantine of Indian nationals who were COVID affected, suspected of having COVID, and those in close contact with confirmed COVID cases at designated centres or medical hospitals was the primary concern during this phase. The Mission worked with officials of the State of Kuwait and also activated its network of Community volunteers to ensure welfare of Indian nationals at all these places. Free medical tele-consultation service was made available with cooperation from the Indian Doctors Forum in Kuwait.

Peak of the First Wave: This phase was characterised by increased restrictions imposed by rapid rise in COVID cases. Lockdowns of residential areas and restrictions on many activities meant loss of income for many Indian nationals. To ensure that Indian nationals do not face starvation, Mission formed the Indian Community Support Group, provided seed funding from the Indian Community Welfare Fund, and mobilised resources from the larger diaspora. A massive food and medicine distribution exercise was executed which saw delivery of over 6 million meals to distressed Indian nationals.

Second wave and thereafter: Mission initiated a drive to provide free lunch to all the distressed Indian nationals visiting the Embassy to address the persistent issue of COVID induced economic hardships faced by a number of diaspora members; a timely initiative which has garnered good response from the Community and the local populace as well.

Amnesty

Government of State of Kuwait announced a month long Amnesty in April 2020 during which not only penalties were waived off but travel was also arranged free of cost by the Kuwaiti side. Mission, through a specially designed mechanism, provided Emergency Certificates to thousands of those Indian nationals who did not have a valid travel document and wished to avail of the Amnesty scheme; all this at a time when COVID related travel restrictions were in place. Mission's officials were stationed at the centres of the Kuwaiti Government during the entire month to facilitate the registration process.

Further, Mission worked closely with Gulf Division, COVID cell, concerned State Governments, Civil Aviation authorities on the Indian side; and Interior Ministry officials, Health officials at the airport, Kuwaiti civil aviation and Kuwaiti Airways staff to ensure safe departure of Indian nationals under the Amnesty scheme to their respective districts and States. More than 50 flights repatriated more than 7,200 Indian nationals under this process; each of the flights were mapped according to the passengers' State/District of domicile in a massive exercise as these Indian nationals were lodged in more than 50 locations across the State of Kuwait.

Vande Bharat Mission

A specific Registration portal was designed to gather requisite information of Indian nationals wishing to travel capturing all the requisite information, including personal details and reason for travel. Each of the registered Indian nationals was provided with a unique registration number.

Categorisation of the Indian nationals was done as per the priority categories defined by the Ministry (those who lost jobs, those who needed medical treatments, students, pregnant and elderly, etc).

As of 5 October 2021, a total of 193,610 Indian nationals (20 per cent of India's diaspora in Kuwait) had registered on the platform and a large majority of these travelled to India under the temporary air services agreement.

Based on the registered numbers, demand projections on flight requirements to specific destinations were sent to the Ministry by the Mission during the various rounds of Vande Bharat Mission flight operations.

Mission, in association with Indian flight carriers, reached out to all the registered nationals on the basis of their choice of destination and prepared provisional manifests.

Mission successfully interlocuted with the Kuwaiti civil aviation authorities to get necessary per Missions for operation of Vande Bharat Mission flights. A team of Indian medical doctors were stationed at the airport during the operations to assess and assist travel of Indian nationals.

On the data/information front, Mission prepared passenger manifests as per the Ministry's template and promptly shared and uploaded them on the repatriation portal.

Medical Oxygen Supply

During the second wave of COVID pandemic in India, Kuwait Government and Indian Diaspora in Kuwait emerged as the major supplier of Liquid Medical Oxygen (LMO) to India. India had supported Kuwait in its moment of crisis in 2020 by deploying a Rapid Response Team comprising military medical professionals and also responded to Kuwait's call for assistance by supplying 200,000 doses of COVISHIELD vaccine. And when India has faced the unexpected crisis, Kuwait responded in equal measure by taking regional lead in dispatching assistance. Kuwaiti Cabinet met at an emergency session and offered immediate support.

When the crisis began, the Mission took the first step to catalogue the priority list of medical supplies needed in India, maintained a running database of all the requirements, carried out a preliminary market survey by reaching out to all the potential suppliers of the priority medical items, including Liquid Medical Oxygen, Oxygen cylinders, and Oxygen concentrators, in Kuwait and the wider region.

EAM and Kuwaiti Foreign Minister Sheikh Dr. Ahmed Nasser Al-Mohammed Al-Sabah had a telephonic conversation where Kuwait offered supply of Liquid Medical Oxygen. The possibility of a Sea-Bridge between Kuwait and India for regular flow of LMO and other medical supplies to India was also explored.

Once the sources and the volume of supplies were identified, Mission activated the Indian Community networks which in turn mobilised the financing and incremental supplies. Simultaneously, interlocution with the concerned authorities of the State of Kuwait, including the Foreign Ministry and the concerned Public Department, was initiated. Instant support for financing and mobilising supplies were secured. Regular follow-up meetings with host government interlocutors and Indian diaspora members helped in securing support and commitments. Once support commitments were secured from host government authorities and the Indian Community, all available medical supplies were reserved for supply to India. Ambassador in Kuwait visited major industrial gas plants in Kuwait and arranged the flow of tankers and semi-trailers to India.

The main bottleneck for uninterrupted supply of liquid medical oxygen was the limited availability of empty ISO cryogenic tanks and semi-trailers. A quick operational turnaround of these assets was essential for flow of oxygen from Kuwait to India. The Mission along with the Kuwaiti authorities and in close coordination with the Ministry, other line Ministries and Indian Navy and Air Force established a sea-air bridge to transport oxygen and oxygen storing assets. Consequently, Indian Naval ships were deployed to carry filled LMO tanks, semi-trailers, oxygen cylinders and oxygen concentrators from Kuwait to India. And Indian Air Force aircrafts were deployed to ferry empty assets from India to Kuwait for refilling. The cycle was repeated flawlessly a couple of times until the requirement in India waned.

The movement of ships and aircrafts were executed smoothly on the back of a well-coordinated operation. At each stage of the operation, Mission tied up the logistics in advance with all concerned authorities in Kuwait, including customs, ports, civil aviation, local foreign office and line Ministry officials to minimise the risk of disruption. To ensure a seamless connection between air and sea operations, a uniform ground handling agency was selected so that the asset flows directly from the airport to the factory for refilling and then onto the ship with an operational turnaround in a few hours.

A total of six Naval ship visits, four Aircraft sorties, one commercial ship operation and one Kuwaiti military aircraft were deployed during the current phase of supply of medical relief from Kuwait to India. The total supplies that were mobilised from Kuwait to India were: 425 Metric Tonnes of Liquid Medical Oxygen, 12,507 oxygen cylinders, 67 oxygen concentrators, 11 ventilators and tonnes of other medical equipment including PPE kits.

On 26 to 28 May the iconic Kuwait Towers lit up in the Indian Tricolour in a message of support and solidarity from Kuwait in the collective fight against COVID. The flow of Liquid Oxygen from Kuwait to India as government-to-government assistance and support from Indian diaspora to Government was the best example of what a traditional partnership of two friendly countries and the Indian diaspora can do when faced with exceptional challenges which is to help each other unconditionally in times of need. All supplies to India from Kuwait were a gift with no expenses for Government of India.

Embassy of India, Bahrain

India and Kingdom of Bahrain have excellent cooperation and collaboration in dealing with COVID. The Government of Bahrain provided food, medical and other necessary support to the Indian community in Bahrain, besides providing free COVID vaccination to all including Indian community in Bahrain. Bahrain also announced an Amnesty Scheme till 31 December 2020 to enable regularisation of stay/ facilitating travel to home country of illegal expats including Indians in Bahrain. The Mission established dedicated COVID Cell and a 24/7 helplines for COVID related queries and assistance of stranded Indians. Mission quickly formed dedicated teams for continuous communication with local government authorities, Indian community associations as well as the concerned authorities in Government of India and State governments. This enabled timely assistance to our community members in repatriation through Vande Bharat Mission/chartered flights; medical, food and other assistance; availing of Amnesty scheme by Indian community members; vaccination drive as well as smooth flow of support and assistance related to medical supplies as well as health professionals on bilateral basis.

India gifted 1 lakh doses of Covishield vaccine to the Kingdom of Bahrain generating huge positivity towards India in Bahrain. This also provided high visibility to India's central role in fighting this global pandemic. Earlier Government of India provided 1.5 million Hydroxychloroquine tablets on commercial basis and facilitated travel of nurses and medical professionals to Bahrain. Bahrain also quickly responded to the Oxygen need of India during the severe second wave of pandemic. The Indian community in Bahrain also participated voluntarily in providing relief materials such as oxygen concentrators, cylinders to India (900 Oxygen cylinders and 35 oxygen concentrators).

The INS Talwar and INS Kolkata visited Bahrain from 30 April-1 May 2021, for shipment of two cryogenic oxygen containers containing 40 MT LMO provided by Bahrain in support of India's efforts to fight the second wave of COVID pandemic. This was the catalyst for the launch of Indian Navy's Operation Samudra Setu-II. The national carrier of Bahrain, the Gulf Air, extended its support to airlift urgent medical supplies and relief material to India, free of charge, on space availability basis on all its flights to India.

India and Bahrain operationalised the air bubble agreement on 11 September 2020 and first flight under this operated on 13 September 2020. This provided a great relief for the mobility of the huge Indian community in Bahrain. In fact, Bahrain is the only country in the GCC region and perhaps in the world which did not stop flights from India even during the second severe wave of pandemic. Bahrain's National Health Regulatory Authority (NHRA) approved the emergency use of Covishield in January 2021 and Covaxin in November 2021.

Embassy of India, Muscat

Assistance Offered to Stranded Indians

The Mission established dedicated 24/7 helplines via Telephone/Email/WhatsApp for COVID related queries and assistance of stranded Indians. COVID related information and advisories were disseminated in English and multiple Indian languages through social media, website and local media. Open House was conducted regularly during the pandemic and the lockdown to reach out to Indian nationals albeit over telephone.

The Mission established a network of social workers and community organisations across Oman and coordinated food (distributed approx. 15,000 food kits) and medical assistance to needy Indian nationals using community's resources and Indian Community Welfare Fund. The Mission also established a network of Indian doctors and social workers, so that patients or suspected patients could seek advise from Indian doctors on COVID and seek prescriptions through tele-medicine. Mission established a phone helpline in coordination with Indian doctors and Oman's Ministry of Health for Indian COVID positive cases, to provide psychological help and other information in several Indian languages.

Mission continued to Issue NOCs in death cases, including during lockdown. Mission facilitate and coordinated airlifting of mortal remains (non-COVID) to India.

Mission worked on providing shelter to destitute housemaids who have no accommodation.

Mission worked closely with Board of Directors (BOD)—Indian Schools in Oman and Ministry of Education to resolve issues relating to students studying in Indian schools including deferment of fee hike, fee concession and permissions for conduct of CBSE and other competitive exams during the period.

Mission also constantly engaged with Oman's Ministries of Foreign Affairs and Health for taking up issues faced by Indian community in Oman, like extensions of visit visas, allowing movement of Indian social workers in lockdown areas, etc. In coordination with Oman's Ministry of Health, Mission worked on expansion of isolation facilities for Indian nationals.

Facilitated return of approx. 100,000 Indian nationals under Vande Bharat Mission (May-September 2020). An air bubble agreement is operational between both the countries since 1 October 2020.

Aiding Procurement Efforts during COVID Second Wave in India

Oman's government dispatched 36 ventilators, 10 SPO2 monitors, 1000 Tocilizumab 400 mg I.V. infusion vials and other medical supplies to India to support India's fight against COVID19. The complete consignment along with Indian community's contribution was sent to Delhi on 12 May 2021 on-board Royal Air Force of Oman aircraft.

The Indian community in Oman contributed 30 Oxygen concentrators and 100 Oxygen cylinders (10 ltrs).

Oman-based Muscat Pharmacy LLC donated 100 Oxygen Cylinders (10 ltrs) and therapy sets which were shipped to India on-board INS Aditya on 20 May 2021 for transit to Mumbai.

The first consignment of 20 MT Liquid Medical Oxygen was also dispatched from Oman on 18 May 2021. It was gifted by MISCO (M/s. Moon Iron and Steel Company), an Indian Joint Venture company, and was coordinated by Indian Oil Corporation Limited.

Indian Navy sourced 1500 vials of Amphotericin B from Oman in June 2021 for use in Indian Naval Hospitals.

Embassy of India, Baghdad

Assistance Offered to Stranded Indians

Emergency consular services were rendered even during the lock-down. Regular contacts were maintained with all Indian nationals working at different sites in Iraq and all their grievances were taken up with the employers and resolved satisfactorily. All the instructions related to COVID pandemic were disseminated to the Indian diaspora in Iraq by uploading them on Embassy's website, social media handles of the Mission and interactions with Indian community organisations.

Vande Bharat Mission

The approved capacity was increased from 200 passengers per week to 400 passengers per week on 9 November 2020 under *Vande Bharat* Mission. A total of 8,253 Indians, registered with the Embassy were repatriated by chartered flights under *Vande Bharat* Mission during COVID pandemic.

Ease of Restrictions of Travel

India and Iraq entered into an air bubble agreement in September 2020 to facilitate air travel of citizens of both the countries as scheduled civil commercial airlines operations continued to be suspended by Directorate General of Civil Aviation in the wake of COVID pandemic in 2020-21. A total of 13,837 visas of different categories were issued by the Mission for medical treatment, tourism, education and business as compared to 48,000 visas issues in 2019-20.

Embassy of India, Tehran

Iran was the second country after China to be affected by the pandemic in 2020. The impact of the virus was compounded by confusion owing to lack of adequate information on the nature of COVID, lax decision making and failure to issue suitable and timely public health advisories viz. the use of masks and sanitisers, social distancing measures, etc. The overall situation was made more complex and challenging due to US sanctions on banking system of Iran barring international transactions etc. resulting in procurement delays and severe shortages of COVID testing kits, medical equipment and medicines leading to an enormous stress on the country's health care system.

Within hours of reports emerging of the first COVID infections in the nearby city of Qom, Mission took immediate precautionary measures. All Mission personnel as well as the Indian community leaders were quickly and suitably briefed on the nature of COVID and steps to be taken to mitigate its spread (frequent hand washing, compulsory wearing of masks, placement of sanitizers in all open spaces, etc). Mission personnel were instructed to strictly practise social distancing measures, all elevator services were suspended and public interactions severely curtailed. A local medical services company was contracted to carry out santizing measures across all offices and public spaces including the Consular Section.

Officer-led teams were constituted and tasked to monitor and look into various aspects. Mission also established direct liaison with the local WHO office so as to gather timely information on the spread of the virus. This enabled the Mission to carefully mark out those cities and towns which were being infected with COVID and hence suitably advise Indian nationals in those places. A dedicated control room was set-up for coordination and 24-hour helpline numbers were opened. Mission began the practise of issuing periodic health advisories on the COVID situation in Iran.

Mission's surveys showed that over 6,000 Indian nationals were living across Iran, including in far off places with poor connectivity. Several thousand Indian pilgrims were stranded in Qom and Mashhad. Over a thousand fishermen were working across Iran's southern coastal province of Hormozgan. There were several hundred Indian students in various universities and colleges around the country and, there were workers and seafarers. Officials from the Embassy and Consulate in Bandar Abbas travelled to remote places, met with the stranded Indians and put in place measures to render every possible assistance.

With regards to modalities for repatriation, Mission grouped Indian nationals based on a set of criteria viz. age, location, etc. and accordingly sequenced their return. The pilgrims and students were the initial focus. In accordance with Government of India's Health directives for mandatory RTPCR negative test result, a six-member team of Indian Council of Medical Research (ICMR) was deputed to Tehran. A sampling 'facility' was set up in the Chancery. Teams of Mission personnel assisted in the collection of swab samples which were packed in iceboxes and sent onward via charter flights to Pune for testing. Upon receipt of the results, all Indians who were COVID negative were informed and assisted with their return to India. Mission also stepped in and provided essential amenities, food and basic medicines to Indian nationals especially in Hormozgan province as the province was under lockdown. Mission also arranged accommodations and board for pilgrims, including those who had tested positive.

Under the 'Operation Samudra Setu', over 900 Indian fishermen were repatriated via two Indian Navy ships, 'INS Shardul' and 'INS Jalashwa'. Mission made necessary coordination with concerned authorities, viz. Iran Navy, Islamic Revolutionary Guard Corps Navy, Governor's Office, etc. Mission members paid several visits to port terminal areas and held meetings with port authorities. This helped develop repatriation plans including chalking out the modalities by place of domicile in India, interfacing downstream with state officials at the district level, etc.

Overall, despite being faced with a unique situation and unprecedented challenges, the efforts of Mission in Tehran helped showcase the importance and benefits of effective planning and the role played in accomplishing complex operational tasks and ability to scale.

AFRICA

High Commission of India, Dar Es Salaam

The Indian Mission in Dar Es Salaam compiled the applications/ requests received from distressed, stranded Indian nationals in Tanzania and Zanzibar, on account of various reasons related to Covid infection. The Mission examined these requests and depending on the urgency or medical condition and as per available capacity of the special aircrafts prepared list of Indians to be repatriated by special flights. As there were no Vande Bharat Mission flights to India, Mission had to get approval for the Special Evacuation Flight from Dar es salaam to different cities in India including Mumbai, Delhi, Kochi, Hyderabad, and Ahmedabad. Mission coordinated with Ministry, Civil Aviation, Air Tanzania, Health department, airport authorities in both India and Tanzania, COVID cell, concerned state government for successful evacuation. Due to non-availability of flights and closure of international borders by neighbouring countries, many Indians entered Tanzania through land (Burundi, Rwanda, Zambia), sea borders (Comoros), to catch these special flights to India, Mission also facilitated the travel of these Indian passengers from neighbouring countries. All in all, 23 special chartered flights to Mumbai, Kochi, Hyderabad, Ahmedabad, Chennai, Delhi were operated from May 2020 to September 2020 which carried 2232 passengers back to India. Besides, Mission also conducted an open house to sensitize and alert the Indian expatriates/diaspora towards countering the spread of Covid infection. Indians from across Tanzania were catered and facilitated through advice on website, email and phone thereby normalising the panic situation.

Embassy of India, Tunis

The Mission oversaw the evacuation of 25 Indians by a Tunisian military aircraft on 21 May 2020. It was perhaps the only evacuation that was done free of cost and using a foreign military aircraft to carry Indian civilians. The Tunisian aircraft thereafter picked up 40 Tunisian nationals from New Delhi. EAM subsequently wrote a letter of thanks to the Tunisian Foreign Minister thanking him for the help and cooperation of the Tunisian government. The numbers in Tunisia (around 40) were not sufficient to have a separate aircraft to go there for an evacuation. Combining Tunisia with other neighbouring countries such as Algeria/ Morocco was considered but was not found feasible. Therefore, a local solution had to be found in Tunis and Mission took up the matter with the local government to keep Mission informed when they decide to evacuate Tunisian nationals from anywhere in South/South East Asia. The Tunisian government decided to evacuate Tunisian nationals in Thailand/ Vietnam and India. Mission then approached the Tunisian government to take the stranded Indian nationals on the forward journey, to which the government acceded. It was also perhaps the first time for them that they allowed foreign civilians on a military aircraft.

High Commission of India, Yaoundé

Vande Bharat Mission and Evacuation of Stranded Foreign Nationals

The Mission in Yaoundé coordinated with local travel agent for evacuation of stranded Indian nationals in Cameroon. Out of 180 Indian nationals registered with the Mission on repat.videshapps.gov.in portal, 101 Indian nationals, who opted to go to India, were repatriated through 3 different chartered flights being operated by Ethiopian Airways.

The Mission was also involved in the evacuation of stranded Cameroonian nationals in India. One hundred eight Cameroonian nationals were evacuated from India to Cameroon by Ethiopian Airlines in September 2020. The Mission coordinated with agencies in India for facilitating the flight clearance.

Embassy of India, Djibouti

Sixteen Indian Naval Ships made port calls at Djibouti for Operational Turn-Around/anti-piracy patrol in the Gulf of Aden and the Red Sea. In addition, three Indian naval aircrafts also visited Djibouti on Operational Turn around. The Embassy of India facilitated their visits including arrangement for re-fueling, logistical support and essential repairs.

Despite challenges posed by the COVID pandemic in a country with poor medical infrastructure, the newly opened (2019) Indian Embassy in Djibouti not only completed its establishment related work but also helped Indian nationals in distress and worked to strengthen bilateral relations with Djibouti. Under the aegis of Vande Bharat Mission, the Embassy facilitated repatriation of 94 Indian nationals, including a 70-member film crew, stranded in Djibouti by a special chartered Air India Flight. The film crew was shooting a Malayalam film titled 'Djibouti' when international flights got suspended due to the pandemic. On the inbound Air India flight from Mumbai to Djibouti, 17 Djiboutian, 2 Yemeni and 2 Kenyan nationals were repatriated from Mumbai to Djibouti free of cost.

During the time of the pandemic, India provided 50 Metric Tonnes of food aid to Djibouti. The shipment was delivered by INS AIRAVAT on 11 November 2020. A consignment of medicines, weighing 5954 kg, was gifted to the Government of Djibouti on 12 April 2021 (procurement cost in India: USD 1.18 lakh). In March 2021, an MoU was signed between the Embassy and Djibouti's Ministry of Women and Family for providing a grant of USD 50,826 for vocational training of underprivileged girls and women. The project is under implementation.

As part of the diplomatic engagement with Djibouti, EAM held a video call with the Foreign Minister of Djibouti on 16 April 2020 to discuss bilateral relations and issues of mutual interest. The Embassy also facilitated port calls of 16 Indian Naval Ships and 3 naval aircrafts to Djibouti in connection with Operational Turn-Around/anti-piracy patrol. A two-member delegation from NTPC visited Djibouti on 21 January 2021 to explore cooperation in the field of renewable energy. The Embassy also organised many events involving the Indian diaspora during the pandemic time.

High Commission of India, Mbabane

On 26 June 2020, as humanitarian assistance to complement the national efforts of the Kingdom of Eswatini to combat COVID19, India donated 6,000 kg of essential medicines costing above INR 1 crore which was personally received by Prime Minister Ambrose Mandluvo Dlamini in the company of the Minister of Health and other Ministers of the Kingdom.

On 11 March 2021, High Commissioner handed over 20,000 doses of Covishield vaccines as Government of India's grant to Senator Lizzy Nkosi, Health Minister of the Kingdom of Eswatini at the Central Medical Stores, Matsapha.

Mission assisted in repatriation of a total of 22 Indian nationals from the Kingdom of Eswatini under Vande Bharat Mission, via Johannesburg during COVID-19 pandemic in 2020.

Embassy of India, Khartoum, Sudan

During the first wave of COVID in Sudan, a round the clock helpline including over Whatsapp was made functional for attending distress calls from Indian nationals stranded in Sudan. Prompt replies were given to all incoming emails/queries of Indians on a real time basis. Mission issued guidelines/advisories via social media to Indians on COVID protocol, closure/opening of airports/flights/chartered flights, etc. The Mission disseminated all information received from the Ministry and other official Indian sources through social media, website and the local newspaper, in English and the local language Arabic after translation.

As no Vande Bharat Mission flight was destined for Sudan for the repatriation of stranded Indian nationals, the Mission organised special chartered flights on 3 and 18 June 2020 and later used Badr airlines flights which were going to India to evacuate Sudanese nationals on 2, 3 and 18 July 2020. Mission facilitated evacuation of 507 stranded passengers, including 501 Indians, 2 OCI card holders, 5 Bhutanese nationals and 1 Sudanese national and back. Mission also facilitated approval from Indian authorities for several additional Badr Airlines flights sent from Sudan to India and back for the evacuation of Sudanese nationals stranded in different cities of India. Fourteen stranded Indian nationals were provided boarding and lodging from Indian Community Welfare Fund till they managed to make alternate arrangements or returned to India during the pandemic. The Mission facilitated smooth departure of Indian workers at the immigration in cases like exemption for the period with expired or non-renewed residence permit, non-availability of yellow fever cards or cases of non-registration with the police on arrival as they could not attend to these formalities due to pandemic led closure.

On 2 November 2020, 100 MT of food aid, consisting of wheat flour and sugar was handed over to the Government of Sudan in a ceremony held at Port Sudan on board the visiting Indian Naval Ship Airavat on an HADR Mission under SAGAR for the flood and pandemic affected population of Sudan. The first batch of 8,28,000 doses of AstraZeneca COVID Made in India vaccines under WHO's COVAX Facility and in collaboration with UNICEF, arrived at Khartoum on 3 March. On a request by the Federal Ministry of Health of Sudan for the supply of essential medicines related to the pandemic, an air consignment of 5,903 kg of life saving and essential medicines was gifted by Government of India to Sudan on 19 April 2021.

On the initiative of the Mission, the local media carried press releases and the news about Government of India granting permission to Indian companies to export Paracetamol, Hydroxychloroquine and other pharmaceuticals effective in COVID management to foreign countries including Sudan. The Mission informed relevant Sudanese authorities and other stakeholders about activities and progress made in India on vaccine, Co-Win platform, sharing details for all authorisation to the indigenous Covaxin and other COVID management related measures.

Under the e-ITEC, 13 Sudanese have attended e-ITEC programme on safe management of the COVID Pandemic.

As of October 2021, Mission was procuring a consignment of vaccine for in-house use to vaccinate Mission's official specially South Sudanese national who don't have access to Sudan government provided vaccine.

High Commission of India, Nairobi

EAM had three telephonic conversations with his counterpart, Cabinet Secretary of Foreign Affairs Raychelle Omamo to discuss issues of mutual interest including cooperation in healthcare especially during the time of COVID pandemic. India allowed one-time commercial export of Hydroxychloroquine tablets, at a time when it was banned for export from India. A consignment of medicines related to COVID was handed to Kenya in August 2020. Chief Administrative Secretaries (MoS level) of Foreign Affairs and Health were present at the handing over ceremony. Both Foreign and Health Ministries gave it wide publicity on their social media platforms.

An Air-bubble arrangement between Kenya and India was signed on 29 September 2020. Under the arrangement, the designated airlines, Air India and Kenyan Airways have since been operating flights. Five Air India flights and four chartered flights under Vande Bharat Mission repatriated a total of 1487 stranded Indians. These flights also brought back stranded Kenyans from India.

The Mission continued to provide consular services even during the lockdown period. The Mission proactively reached out to the community through online platforms and discussed possibilities of help from the Mission. Benefits of Yoga and Ayurveda in combating the pandemic were highlighted through social media. Government of India's efforts in combating the pandemic were shared with the media. The Mission reached out to the Government of Kenya to get an understanding on the institutional capacity for Phase-III testing and possibilities of institutional collaboration in delivery of vaccine and Phase-III testing. The Mission also shared information on the developments on vaccine trials undergoing in India. Kenyan Government was approached for possible supply of COVAXIN from India.

Kenya received 1.02 million doses of Covishield from India through the COVAX Facility and 100,000 doses of Covishield as a grant from Government of India in March 2021. The gifting ceremony was widely covered in the media. India's successes in development of indigenous vaccines, the Co-WIN platform, and the world's largest vaccination programme were suitably highlighted to the Kenyan Government and media.

Embassy of India, Brazzaville

Assistance Offered to Stranded Indians in Republic of Congo

The Mission in Brazzaville worked with the Indian Association of Brazzaville and Pointe Noire on monitoring the COVID situation and making arrangements for stranded Indians. Separate accommodations were arranged for isolation, and to attend Indian COVID patients two doctors and two nurses were kept on standby with all the requisite medicines. Arrangements were also made to keep a stock of essential groceries, toiletries, medicines, etc. for Indian nationals for emergency use during lockdown. Some Indian restaurants were authorised to provide food to the Indian nationals during isolation/mandatory quarantine.

In addition to above, the Mission received multiple requests from Indian nationals who got stranded in the Republic of Congo due to non-availability of flights. The Mission complied with all the requests as per the guidelines issued by the Ministry. In order to evacuate the stranded Indian nationals, the Mission along with the Indian Association of Brazzaville arranged for a charter flight under the framework Vande Bharat Mission which repatriated 99 Indian nationals stranded in the Republic of Congo to Mumbai in India without any complications on 10 July 2020.

Embassy of India, Harare

Assistance to stranded Indian citizens in Zimbabwe

While there were no Vande Bharat Mission flights between India and Zimbabwe, the Mission coordinated the journey home by a special chartered flight of 44 stranded Indians in Zimbabwe on 9 June and 25 July 2020 as also the return of 5 ITEC trainees from India on 19 June 2020. The Mission again coordinated the return to Zimbabwe on 13 August 2020 of 13 OCI card holders, 6 Zimbabwean students and 5 people with working visas who were stranded in India. The Mission coordinated with COVID Cell, the Ministry, Directorate General of Civil Aviation and Madhya Pradesh Government for the clearance for Private Charter flight on 13 August 2020 for Mr Narottam Somani, a prominent Indian businessman in Zimbabwe.

Vaccine assistance to Zimbabwe

In March 2021, Zimbabwe became the first country in Africa to give authorisation for the emergency use of COVAXIN.

Zimbabwe, in January 2021, supported India at WTO in sponsoring the proposed waiver of TRIPS Agreement for the Prevention, Containment and Treatment of COVID along with South Africa and other countries.

During the year, essential medicines worth USD 1.05 million were donated to the Government of Zimbabwe, besides USD 350,000 COVID related medicines. A consignment of 35,000 doses of COVAXIN were also donated to Zimbabwe on 29 March 2021.

On the request of the Government of Zimbabwe, India cleared the export of Hydroxychloroquine to Zimbabwe in the month of June 2020.

On 27 May 2021, a consignment of ten Ambulances, manufactured by M/s Mahindra of India, were handed over to Zimbabwe, as a donation from India. The Ambulances were promised during the visit of Vice President to Zimbabwe in November 2018.

The Embassy, in association with the Deputy Minister of Industry and Commerce, Mr Raj Modi, organised a free health camp on 27 August 2021 in Bulawayo. Over 350 people availed of the services at the Health Camp.

High Commission of India, Abuja

The Mission organised nearly 35 flights (including 13 Air India Vande Bharat Mission flights and 20 charter flights) to help repatriate 8,000 Indian nationals and several thousand Nigerians. Almost all flights (other than the two in Benin and Chad) departed from Lagos, Nigeria's largest city and commercial capital, having the largest concentration of Indian community and businesses in West Africa.

Officials in Lagos, with Mission's support, worked tirelessly to ensure smooth on-ground coordination and successful departure of these Vande Bharat Mission/Charter flights despite several challenges, including deficient physical and medical infrastructure, lack of Air India official presence, declaration of one flight as Aircraft of Ground (AOG), local security challenges and End SARS protests. Community associations and Indian businesses were regularly informed of the steps being taken by the Mission to ensure early and safe repatriation. Their support towards Mission's welfare activities, including set up of a COVID isolation centre, provision of accommodation/food/medicines to stranded individuals, ambulance services, etc. was noteworthy.

Nigeria received nearly 3.92 million doses of the made in India COVID vaccines, shipped via the COVAX facility, in March 2021. These were the first vaccines to have been approved by NAFDAC, Nigeria. Government of India also donated 7-tonne consignment of essential medicines and 100,000 vaccine doses (manufactured by the Serum Institute of India) to the Government of Nigeria.

Embassy of India, Malabo

India gifted 6-tonne consignment of essential medicines to Equatorial Guinea in solidarity to its fight against COVID. During the COVID pandemic, with support of Equatorial Guinea's Ministry of Civil Aviation, two special charter flights were organised and repatriated about 100 Indian citizens.

Mission helped Equatorial Guinea's Government to procure COVID's medicine 'Remdesivir' from India. Equatorial Guinea is one of the first countries in Africa which used Remdesivir for treatment of COVID patient.

Embassy of India, Antananarivo, Madagascar

The Mission facilitated three special chartered flights for evacuating stranded Indians from Madagascar and Comoros:

a. The evacuation of 85 stranded Indians from Madagascar on 17 June 2020 through a special chartered flight operated by Ethiopian Airlines.
b. The Indians who were stranded in Comoros (total 19) were evacuated by a special chartered flight on 9 August 2020.
c. The Mission coordinated the evacuation of 61 Indians who were stranded in Madagascar in a flight on 19 August 2020. The same flight evacuated the stranded Malagasy nationals in India. This was the first ever direct flight that flew between India and Madagascar, starting from Antananarivo, capital of Madagascar and landing in Mumbai, India.

INS Kesari visited the port of Antsiranana from 26-28 May 2020 to deliver the consignment of medicines meant for treatment of COVID. From 22-25 March 2021 INS Jalashwa visited the port of Ehoala to deliver the donation of 1000 MT of rice and 100,000 tablets of Hydroxychloroquine from Government of India to the people of southern Madagascar.

In response to a request for medical assistance from the Comorian side during telecon between the Foreign Minister of Comoros and EAM in April 2020, a 14-member Medical Assistance Team reached Comoros onboard INS Kesari. The team carried out medical duties from 31 May to 18 June 2020 as a gesture of India's support to Comoros in fight against spread of Dengue and COVID. The medical team visited three islands—Anjouan, Moheli and Grand Comore during this visit and held camps along with Comorian health authorities. Besides this, a consignment of medicines which included Hydroxychloroquine was also donated by India to Comoros.

The evacuation reports were published on all the social media handles of the Embassy and also in Indian media.

High Commission of India, Victoria-Mahe

HADR to Seychelles

Government of India donated two consignments of essential medicine supplies to Seychelles in its fight against COVID pandemic on 15 April 2020 and 6 June 2020 respectively. The shipment caters to most of the living saving ailments in Seychelles including Blood Pressure, Cholesterol, Diabetes, Cancer, Cardiovascular diseases apart from 50,000 tablets of Hydroxychloroquine. This was a special arrangement made in view of the exceptional relations with Seychelles to enable the supply of these medicines despite the restrictions in place due to the lockdown. This was yet another manifestation of India's unwavering commitment to Seychelles

The then President of Seychelles, Mr. Danny Faure profoundly thanked Prime Minister on both the handover ceremony of the critical medicine supplies, which were all done on a grant basis and at a critical juncture during Seychelles' fight against the first wave of COVID. The first consignment of urgent medicine supplies of 3.4 tonnes from India was airlifted and delivered to Seychelles on a war footing through a chartered Air India aircraft on 15 April 2020 and was received by Secretary of State for Foreign Affairs for Seychelles, Amb. Barry Faure on behalf of the Government of Seychelles. A second consignment despatched onboard INS Kesari as part of 'Mission SAGAR' was jointly received by Secretary of State for Health, Amb. Marie-Pierre Lloyd and Secretary of State for Foreign Affairs, Amb. Barry Faure. The timely donations reflects India's commitment to work together with its maritime neighbours and partners in the Indian Ocean Region. The total cost of these donations amount to INR 1.5 crore.

Administrative Issues and Regulatory Regime

During the handover of the first consignment supplied by BPPI, the Mission didn't receive the 'Certificate of Analysis' on time. This caused some delay in clearing the consignment. The Mission did not face similar issue with second consignment supplied by HLL Hites, as the certificate was provided with the invoice. There were no other administrative/ clearance issues faced during the process. Seychelles freely accepts medicines of Indian Pharmacopoeia' or 'IP' Standard and India is the main country of imports for pharmaceuticals to Seychelles.

THE AMERICAS

Embassy of India, Washington

Mission's engagement with the US Administration, private sector and community organisations in the context of COVID-19 pandemic

India and the United States of America have a long-standing cooperation in the healthcare sector, which has been a source of strength for both countries in combating the COVID pandemic. The solidarity and support extended by the U.S. Government, the Congress, States, the private sector and the American people in India's efforts to contain the second wave of COVID, is a reflection of the strong India-US partnership, people-to-people ties, and the strength and potential for bilateral healthcare cooperation. The Indian Mission and the five Consulates in the US played an integral role in coordinating and facilitating the COVID relief efforts from the US Government, private sector, and U.S. citizens, including the Indian American community.

US solidarity and assistance

As the second wave of pandemic hit India in April 2021, the Ambassador reached out to senior officials in the Administration, including the White House, NSC and State Department to apprise them of the COVID situation in India, India's national efforts and immediate priorities. President Biden and the Prime Minister had a telephone call on 26 April 2021, during which President Biden conveyed that just as India had helped the US in its difficult situation last year, the US will "stand shoulder to shoulder with India" and support India's efforts by quickly deploying resources. President Biden committed to provide emergency relief to India, including oxygen-related supplies, vaccine raw materials, therapeutics and identifying sources of raw materials to be made available for manufacture of Covishield vaccines in India. President's Biden's message was echoed by the entire US Administration including Vice President Kamala Harris, Secretary of State Antony Blinken, Defense Secretary Lloyd Austin, NSA Jake Sullivan, Deputy Secretary of State

Wendy Sherman, USAID Director Samantha Power and several other senior officials.

Starting 28 April, a total of seven flights carrying emergency supplies from the US Government landed in India by 17 May 2021. The overall US Government's commitment stood at USD 100 million. COVID assistance received from US Government included oxygen cylinders and ventilators, Remdesivir, masks, rapid diagnostic kits, and an oxygen generation plant. List of items received is attached in the Annexure 9b.

In addition, USAID allocated funds to purchase locally an additional 1,000 mobile oxygen concentrators.

US re-directed its own order of AstraZeneca manufacturing supplies to India to allow India to make over 20 million doses of COVID vaccines.

As the demand for COVID-related medical equipment, raw materials and critical ingredients for vaccines significantly increased during in the aftermath of the second wave, several Indian pharmaceutical companies manufacturing vaccines and drugs began to face supply chain issues vis-à-vis US suppliers. Mission continuously engaged with the US Government and Indian pharmaceutical industry to determine the priority of their orders pending with the US companies. The Ambassador held meetings with the CEOs of all major US suppliers to expedite shipment of orders and ensure that the demand was met and that there were no gaps left in the supply chain. The Ambassador also engaged with senior officials in the White House, NSC and State Department. The Mission was able to impress upon the US authorities to remove Defense Production Act priority ratings on AstraZeneca and Novavax vaccines, which allowed Indian companies to source the critical raw materials in a timely manner. The Mission had continued to follow up with the US companies to ensure that Indian pharmaceutical companies can continue to scale-up production and deliver life-saving drugs and vaccines.

The Mission and Consulates remained in continuous touch with interlocutors. The Ambassador held conversations with several Cabinet members as well as other senior officials including Director of National Institute of Allergy and Infectious Diseases Dr Anthony Fauci, Centre for Disease Control Director Rochelle Walensky, Surgeon General Dr Vivek Murthy, White House Coronavirus Response Coordinator Jeff

Zients, State Department COVID Response Coordinator Gayle Smith apprising them of the COVID situation and steps being taken by the Government to address the COVID challenges. All of them expressed their support and solidarity with India.

Bipartisan support at the US Congress

At the Capitol Hill, the Ambassador interacted with several members from the Democratic and Republican parties. There were strong bipartisan expressions of solidarity and support at the US Congress. More than 100 members from both sides of the aisle issued tweets/ statements, focusing on:

(a) Supporting US administration's efforts to assist India;
(b) Several arguing in favour of the WTO TRIPS waiver proposal;
(c) Calling for more to be done including provision of surplus AstraZeneca vaccines to India.

On 12 May 57, members of the House Caucus on India and Indian Americans wrote to President Biden urging the Administration to enhance assistance for India. In the Senate, the Indian Caucus wrote twice to President Biden urging the Administration to help India overcome the challenges posed by the second wave of infections.

To seek US support for the proposal at the WTO for a TRIPS waiver on COVID vaccines and therapeutics, the Ambassador interacted with several senior members in the Senate and House of Representatives. The Ambassador joined the South African and Kenyan Ambassadors in Washington DC, for outreach to several influential senior members who urged the Administration to support this proposal at the WTO.

In the House, 108 members wrote to President Biden urging him to support the proposal at the WTO. In the Senate 10 senior Democratic Senators led by Senators Bernie Sanders and Elizabeth Warren penned a similar letter to President Biden. This matter was discussed in the telephone conversation on 26 April between Prime Minister and President Biden. On 5 May, US Administration announced its support for the proposal of India and South Africa for a temporary waiver of IP rights on COVID vaccines.

Strong support of the US Private Sector

The Mission actively engaged with the US private sector to facilitate supply of COVID assistance including critical medicines, inputs for vaccine manufacturing, oxygen cylinders, ventilators, and concentrators to India to cope with the surge in COVID infections.

The main source of support and relief from the US private sector emanated from the Global Task Force, constituted by the US Chamber of Commerce in coordination with the influential Business Roundtable, US India Business Council and US India Strategic Partnership Forum. The Global Task Force membership includes 40 of the largest US companies across sectors. The quick mobilisation of some of the largest US companies reflected the strong business ties between India and the US. The Ambassador consistently engaged with the Global Task Force informing them about the critical areas of India's requirements. EAM's interaction with the Global Task Force members provided a timely overview of India's COVID situation and requirements and enabled better coordination. The cumulative support extended by the Global Task Force and the US private sector is estimated at around USD 400 million, making it the largest source of financial assistance to mitigate India's COVID situation. The Mission helped facilitate supplies/assistance in consultation with appropriate agencies in Government of India as well as State Governments.

In May 2021, the USISPF and the Global Task Force members mobilised 25,000 oxygen concentrators, 1 million rapid antigen testing kits, and 4 large oxygen trucks. As of May 2021, they were trying to scale up supply of oxygen concentrators up to 100,000 units. In addition, the Mission worked with the US Chamber of Commerce to facilitate supply of 1,000 Medtronic ventilators as well as 45,000 oxygen concentrators in partnership with US India Business Council. The Mission worked with member companies of the Global Task Force to coordinate their assistance such as USD 70 million from Pfizer, USD 25 million from Accenture, USD 30 million from U.S. Chamber of Commerce, USD 10 million from Boeing, USD 18 million from Google, USD 10 million from Facebook, and USD 10 million from Mastercard.

The Mission also worked extensively with the US pharmaceutical sector to coordinate supply of life-saving COVID drugs and raw materials.

Gilead Sciences, which holds the patent for the Remdesivir drug, donated 450,000 doses. They are commercially supplying more than 800,000 vials of AmBisome for treatment of invasive fungal infections associated with COVID. The Mission facilitated a contribution of 700,000 doses of Baricitinib from Eli Lilly. Roche's Genetech contributed 50,000 doses of Tocilizumab (80 mg). Separately, Genetech commercially supplied 100,000 doses of Tocilizumab.

Support from Indian community organisations/individuals

There was overwhelming expression of support and offers of assistance from the Indian Diaspora/community. While many community organisations and members supplied required relief materials directly to India based organisations and individuals, several community organisations pooled in resources to source and supply relief material including diaspora organisations, professional associations like American Association of Physicians of Indian Origin (AAPI), Federation of Indian Physicians Association (FIPA), Pan-IIT and several individual IIT Alumni Associations, Asian American Hotel Owners Association (AAHOA), SEWA International, The Indus Entrepreneur (TiE); regional organisations and cultural organisations among others.

The Indian-origin medical fraternity in the US represented by AAPI, FAPI volunteered to provide tele-medicine assistance and psychological counselling to patients in India. They worked with groups like UPS Foundation, FedEx and international airlines like Qatar Airways to facilitate transportation of relief materials. Several individuals and organisations contributed to Prime Minister CARES Fund.

The Mission/Consulates remained in regular contact with community organisations and provided timely information regarding required priority items, procedures for sending relief materials. They also coordinated their efforts on real time basis and facilitated at the Indian end in consultation with the Ministry, Ministry of Health and Family Welfare, NITI Aayog and other Government of India agencies. Nodal points of contact were designated in the Embassy and Consulates for coordination and facilitation, and details shared with community organisations/leaders.

The huge effort mounted by the community, in coordination with Mission/Consulates, led to supply of more than 18,000 oxygen

Concentrators, 2400 oxygen Cylinders/Flow Meters, several oxygen generation plants, over 200 Portable Ventilators, about 2,700 hospital beds, etc.

Harnessing India-US vaccine partnership

A parallel area of Mission's focus was accelerating the vaccine partnership with the US. Towards this, the Ambassador is regularly engaged with key interlocutors including Surgeon General Dr Vivek Murthy, National Institute of Allergy and Infectious Diseases Director Dr Fauci, CDC Director Dr Walensky and US vaccine manufacturers. The vast network of institutional engagements brought scientific communities of the two countries together to jointly respond to COVID research and its management.

Indian vaccine companies have collaborated with US based agencies to develop and produce vaccine against COVID. At least seven vaccine candidates are being developed through bilateral engagement including one vaccine being developed using mRNA platform. The India-US partnership in battling COVID remains a part of a larger framework of engagement on healthcare and will play a crucial role in confronting global COVID pandemic.

High Commission of India, Ottawa

Vande Bharat Mission

In Canada, Mission and Posts were proactive in managing the pandemic, first by facilitating the evacuation of stranded Indians through the Vande Bharat Mission flights. Between 23 May 2020 and 23 April 2021, the Mission helped the travel of 70,500 people on Vande Bharat Mission flights. The Mission and the Posts also played a significant role in mobilising the Indian community in Canada towards generating support and assistance for Indian students and other Indian nationals who had been stranded and needed support during the initial phase of the pandemic.

Outbound HADR and Vaccine Maitri

The Mission played a significant role in promoting Vaccine Maitri which saw India provide half a million doses of Covishield vaccine to Canada in March 2021, a gesture that was deeply appreciated by the Canadian leadership. Canada was the only G-7 country to receive such vaccines from India. This helped change political attitudes as well. The Mission was also instrumental in promoting India's position as the pharmacy of the world by facilitating supply of Paracetamol and Hydroxychloroquine to Canada in June 2020, which generated tremendous goodwill among the Canadians.

Procurement

Mission and Posts in Canada were able to quickly mobilise support from Canadian Federal Government, Provincial and non-governmental organisations, particularly the Indian origin associations and generating substantial resources including emergency medical equipment, pharmaceutical supplies and funds towards support for India's efforts in managing the second wave of COVID pandemic.

The High Commissioner addressed letters to the Prime Minister of Canada and Premiers of Canadian Provinces informing them of the priority requirements in India. Following this, the Canadian government made a grant of C$ 10 million (USD 8 million) (27 April 2021) to Canadian Red Cross Society which was designated as the main Canadian platform to support the Indian Red Cross Society which had been designated as the nodal point in international COVID related assistance by Government of India.

The Federal Government sent an immediate shipment of 25,000 Remdesivir doses as well as 350 specialised oxygen concentrators/ ventilators, air-lifted by special Canadian Air Force plane on 08 May and 13 May 2021. The Mission also identified a manufacturer of large hospital and ward level oxygen generating plants in Canada and worked with the equipment manufacturer to modify these plants for use in Indian conditions and with the Canadian Red Cross for supply of 16 such plants to India.

Posts in Toronto and Vancouver also mobilised support from Canadian provincial governments. CG Vancouver liaised with the Province of Saskatchewan which sent 100 ventilators. Similarly, the Province of British Columbia announced a grant to the Red Cross, as did the territory of Yukon.

Consulate in Toronto worked closely with the Province of Ontario, the largest province of Canada, to provide 5000 ventilators, 500 oxygen concentrators, 80 cylinders and 7 mini-oxygen generators to India. This shipment was delivered in 11 tranches by special and commercial flights to New Delhi between 12-24 May 2021. The province of Quebec also announced a grant towards supporting pandemic relief in India.

The High Commissioner and Consulate Generals reached out to the Indian community which actively organised a number of initiatives for raising resources and supplying required material to India. Mission officials worked with such voluntary organisations in Canada to coordinate the shipment of supplies to India in accordance with the instructions given by the Ministry by liaising with various Indian and Canadian organisations. High Commissioner personally addressed several major conferences to brief the Canadian public and Indian community about the situation in India and to ensure that the supplies and resources being raised was tuned to the requirements of the Government of India.

The Mission and Posts also reached out to over 100 Canadian companies and suppliers for commercial procurement of essential materials as directed by the Ministry. More than 60 quotations for supply of various products, medications and equipment were sent by the Mission to the authorities concerned India for due verification. The High Commissioner made a special outreach to corporate Canada, especially large business with presence in India to support relief efforts in India and major corporates like Fairfax Holdings and McCain Foods announced contributions on an urgent basis. Several other corporates were similarly encouraged to contribute by the Mission and the Posts.

The Mission also worked with Canadian pharmaceutical companies in setting up joint ventures, including for joint production of vaccines in India (Biological E Ltd, Hyderabad, India and Providence Therapeutics of Calgary, Canada) and in Canada (Bharat Biotech of India and Vaccigen Ltd, Canada).

Outreach

Mission and Posts used innovative communication and outreach strategies including effective use of social media to not only mobilise sympathy and support in Canada for dealing with the COVID pandemic in India but also for providing a correct and factual picture about the efforts being made by India to effectively combat the pandemic.

The High Commissioner gave interviews to the media including the prime time 'Power and Politics' show (6 May), spoke to prominent news channels and radio stations. Consulate Generals in Toronto and Vancouver similarly had strong outreach through media and social media. The High Commissioner and Consulate Generals addressed many conferences organised by Indian community organisations and associations to spread awareness. As part of the wider outreach, the Mission and Posts coordinated with local Canadian authorities which led to positive messages of solidarity with some of Canada's iconic landmarks such as Niagara Falls, City Hall Halifax, Hamilton Sign and Brampton City Hall being illuminated with Indian colours in a show of solidarity.

The Mission answered queries, identifying and reaching out to Canadian entities and organisations with the required capacities and supplies and advising Canadian contributors and donors with regard to best possible channel for assisting with the efforts in India. In continuous consultation with the Ministry, regular coordination was maintained with key Canadian organisations including the federal government, provincial governments, airport authorities, airline authorities, cargo handling services and the Canadian Red Cross.

The strong mobilisation of the federal and provincial governments in Canada and the unprecedented wave of goodwill and support for India among the Canadian public was due in part to the positive impact of India's efforts earlier in supporting Canada combat its own COVID pandemic. In June 2020 India had provided pharmaceutical supplies to Canada, especially Paracetamol and Hydroxychloroquine. Following the request made by the Canadian Prime Minister to the Prime Minister during a telephone conversation on 10 February 2021, India had also agreed to allow shipment of AstraZeneca vaccines manufactured by Serum Institute of India with the first tranche of vaccines arriving in Canada on 3 March 2021 under the Vaccine Maitri Initiative. This gesture generated tremendous positive feelings for India in the Canadian public and the Canadian leadership. This goodwill was instrumental in mobilising the immense wave of public sympathy for India in the subsequent months and was an important reason for the rapid action by Canadian government and organisations in providing assistance to India when approached by the Mission and the Posts.

A list of some of the headline supplies/assistance is placed at Annexure 9A.

Embassy of India, Santiago

Chile was placed under a state of Emergency in March 2020 when the first COVID case was detected in the country. To accommodate distressed Indians during the COVID outbreak, Embassy of India, Santiago, established a temporary shelter in the old Chancery building at Triana. During the period from May 2020 to January 2021, 13 distressed Indians were accommodated in the shelter. While the Mission incurred expenditure from Indian Community Welfare Fund on electricity, water charges of the shelter and for providing electric heaters, cooking stove, gas etc., Indian community helped them by providing beds, kitchen items, groceries, etc.

The Mission coordinated with various agencies in Chile and India to facilitate repatriation of 75 Indians who were affected by the COVID pandemic. However, the expenditure on repatriation was met by the passengers themselves.

High Commission of India, Georgetown (concurrently accredited to Antigua and Barbuda, and St. Kitts and Nevis)

Guyana

Under Vaccine Maitri initiative,India donated 80,000 doses of Covishield to Guyana on 7 March 2021. The procurement and despatch of these doses were arranged by the LAC Division and the Mission facilitated its receipt, delivery and handing over in Georgetown.

India also donated USD 1 million to Guyana in 2020 under India-UN Development Partnership Fund to upgrade its critical healthcare infrastructure to combat COVID19 which helped them to procure over 34 ventilators, thousands of protection equipment and emergency care medicines, etc. Besides, India provided 30,000 Hydroxychloroquine tablets to Guyana in 2020.The procurement and despatch of these were arranged by DPA-II Division and Mission facilitated its receipt, handing over and delivery in Georgetown.

Antigua and Barbuda

Under Vaccine Maitri, India donated 40,000 doses of Covishield to Antigua and Barbuda on 1 March 2021. The procurement and despatch of these were arranged by the LAC Division in the Ministry and the Mission facilitated its receipt, delivery and handing over in St. John's. India also donated USD 1 million aid to Antigua and Barbuda in 2020 for upgrading health infrastructure to combat COVID19. This assistance of USD 1 million from India under India-UN Development Partnership Fund was used for improving health infrastructure, for procurement of life-saving medical supplies and equipment. Besides, India provided 10,000 Hydroxychloroquine tablets to Antigua and Barbuda, the procurement and despatch of which were arranged by the DPA-II Division and the Mission facilitated its receipt, handing over and delivery in St. John's.

St. Kitts and Nevis

India donated 20,000 doses of Covishield to St. Kitts and Nevis on 1 March 2021. The procurement and despatch of these were arranged by the LAC Division and Mission facilitated its receipt, delivery and handing over in Basseterre. India also provided an amount of USD 300,000 under the Government of St. Kitts and Nevis's proposal to utilise the "Quick Impact Community Development Projects" Fund of USD1 million for 'Support on COVID Response'. This funding under India-UN Development Partnership Fund was used for procurement of life-saving medical supplies and equipment like Ventilators, masks, infrared thermometers, defibrillators test kits, medicines and Personal Protective Equipment. As of October 2021, St. Kitts and Nevis Government's proposal for part funding to the tune of the balance amount USD 700,000 from the India-UN Development Partnership Fund for construction of St. Peters Health Centre at a total cost of USD 1,815,555.28, is under process with PMI New York. India also provided life-saving medicines and medical supplies worth USD 100,000 and 10,000 Hydroxychloroquine tablets to St. Kitts and Nevis. The medicines and medical supplies thus provided include Azithromycin, Amikacin injections, Cefotaxime Sodium injections,

Ceftazadime Injections, Lopinavir/Ritonavir Tabs., Oseltamivir Caps., Amoxicillin + Clavulanic Acid Susp., Levocetrizine, Mannitol, Metronidazole, Metronidazole inj., Ceftriaxone injection, Paracetamol, Intra Venous Paracetamol, Ibuprofen, Vitamin C Tabs., Thermometer, Surgical gowns, Over shoes, Surgical gloves, Cape hood, Sampling Tubes and Swabs. The procurement and despatch of these items were arranged by the DPA-II Division and the Mission facilitated its receipt, handing over and delivery in Basseterre.

Embassy of India, Panama (concurrently accredited to Costa Rica and Nicaragua)

At the start of the pandemic last year, a group of India Trade Promotion Organisation sponsored delegation comprising of five women and a man got stuck in Panama airport while in transit. The Consular Officer visited them and rendered help in re-booking the flights and facilitated them while in transit in coordination with the airport authorities and airlines.

There are no direct flights between India and Panama/Costa Rica/Nicaragua. The travel related protocols and restrictions were in place. The Vande Bharat flights were not operating from these countries. The professionals, businessmen, students, tourists and seafarers from various states of India viz. Andhra Pradesh, Delhi, Punjab, Karnataka and Uttar Pradesh got stuck in these countries during the pandemic. Mission created Whatsapp groups for them to keep them updated about the travel related measures in force in India and transiting countries. The Mission coordinated with airlines and Embassy of India in Paris to find best routes for them depending on the visa for the transiting country in order to ensure their safe travel to India. A total of 70 Indians were repatriated from three countries during the first wave which entailed a hard work of almost two months by the Embassy officials. Paris was found the most suitable and available connection at that point of time. In coordination with the Embassy in Paris, Indian Association in Costa Rica and Airlines, Mission successfully repatriated all the deserted Indians.

In the second wave, two Indian nationals while in transit got stuck in Panama due to cancellation of flights and also due to technical problems with their travel documents. The Mission coordinated with the airport authorities to ensure that their hardship is minimised while in transit and also helped in getting the PCR tests done at the airport for exiting the country. Financial assistance for food was sourced from the Indian Community Welfare Fund.

Embassy of India, Lima

The Governments of Peru and Bolivia acted swiftly in the month of March 2020 to contain the spread of COVID with drastic measures like suspension of international and domestic air travel with just a day's notice, sealing of borders, lockdown, strict enforcement of health protocol etc. The Embassy immediately established a 24×7 Helpline to assist stranded Indian nationals as well as members of the Indian community. Contact was established with the Host Governments and relevant organisations to secure necessary information, clearances and cooperation.

Two dedicated online platforms were created with senior officers of the Embassy personally monitoring and responding to the requests from Indian nationals in need of help. A group of businesspersons and officials of India Trade Promotion Organisation who could not travel out of Lima were facilitated boarding and lodging with the support of India Trade Promotion Organisation. Medical and other assistance was extended to the Indian nationals who contracted COVID as well as to those suffering from other ailments.

Help was extended to people stranded in remote parts of the country far away from the Capital through local Governments and NGOs to reach the Capital and later to exit the country for India. Financial assistance was extended to those in real need with the help of Indian Community Welfare Fund. In the absence of regular commercial flights, the Mission explored all possible options, made special efforts to tie up with a Diplomatic Mission of another country and organised return of Indian nationals in groups, in coordination with the Ministry, Ministry of Home Affairs, Directorate General of Civil Aviation and States. In the process, elderly persons, pregnant women and Indian nationals with compelling reasons were given priority.

EUROPE

Embassy of India, Paris

France is one the few countries which manufactures quality oxygen generator plants. During the peak second wave of COVID pandemic in

India, the demand in India for liquid medical oxygen, zeolite molecular sieves Oxygen Concentrators, Oxygen Cylinders, Oxygen Tanks, Ventilators, Oxymeters, flow meters, Remdesivir, Heparin, ECMO Machine and various ingredients that go into manufacturing Remdesivir and other lifesaving medicines suddenly increased. Missions were asked by the Ministry to survey local market for sourcing these much-needed items.

The Mission explored companies in France capable of supplying these anti-COVID equipment and material. Mission reached out to a number of companies, including Air Liquide, Gaz Systemes, Novair, Mil's, Linde, Scaleo Medical, Boemedical, Cryolor, SOS Azote, Wika, Eurotainer, Azote Services, Cryo Diffusion, Posaconazole, etc. to identify availability of products, quotations and delivery schedules for various equipment/ items.

The list containing range of products, including oxygen generators, molecular sieves, ingredients for life saving medicines, along with cost was updated regularly and shared with various Government of India entities, state governments, NGOs, businesses, chambers and associations, including from Singapore and the USA, in response to various offers of assistance for India. This information got eventually translated into delivery from France to India, of more than 70 oxygen generating plants, 200 tonnes of high-grade molecular sieves and thousands of oxygen concentrator ordered by various French and Indian businesses, associations and governments.

The Mission closely coordinated with the French company Arkema to finalise supply orders of close to 600 metric tons of crucial high-grade zeolite absorbers—a key component in oxygen generating plants. The Mission negotiated for maximum supply to India, through both increased capacity and redirection of supplies meant for other parts of the world.

The Mission also closely followed up on Bharat Biotech's order with French company Biowest for supply of 2.5 million litres of 'Dulbecco's Modified Eagle Medium' (DMEM)—a crucial component in vaccine production. In response Biowest was able to ramp up its production to be able to fulfil all requirement from India at the rate of 400,000 litres per month.

The Mission closely followed up on an order of 4 tonnes of Betadex-a crucial raw material for the production of Remedesivir, ordered by

Zydus Cadila from the French company Zach Systems. Zach systems was able to augment its production capacities to fulfil this order in a timely fashion.

The Mission intervened to facilitate an early conclusion of long unsettled arbitration between the French company Air Liquide and Rashtriya Ispat Nigam Ltd over a steel plant in Visakhapatnam which could also serve as a producing unit of medical grade oxygen. The negotiations have picked up after Mission's rigorous follow up.

The Mission facilitated direct contact between oxygen plant generating companies and the Indian Armed Forces. The Air Force was able to order and airlift five oxygen generating plants and close to 200 concentrators in its C17 flight from Bordeaux.

The Mission facilitated coordination and transportation of 20 oxygen generating plants for use by the Delhi government ordered from the French company Novair.

Given the close strategic ties between India and France and large presence of French companies in India, the French Government mobilised about 60 French companies which contributed in different capacities to deliver 8 Oxygen Generation Plant, 18 OSIRIS Transport Respirators, 5 Liquid Oxygen Container, 200 Electric Syringe Pumps and many Respirators for Intensive Care.

Embassy of India, Sofia

The Mission maintained constant liaison with the Ministries of Foreign Affairs of Bulgaria and North Macedonia to check the latest regulations concerning travel and entry of Indian nationals. The details were disseminated through the Embassy website and social media platforms in real time. Three 24×7 helpline numbers were instituted for promptly responding to Indians in distress/emergency. WhatsApp Support Groups were created for Indian community and Indian students. Individualised clarifications and assistance were provided through telephone calls and emails to Indian nationals in finding the best travel route back home prior to imposition of lockdown measures by various countries in March 2020. More than 20 stranded Indians (1 from North Macedonia and rest from Bulgaria) were provided assistance in travelling back to India through Vande Bharat Mission flights via Frankfurt.

The Ambassador undertook multiple conferences for students and Indian diaspora in Bulgaria and North Macedonia to address their concerns and needs. The Mission was in touch with university authorities in Bulgaria to ensure they were responsive to the Indian students' requirements and well-being. The Mission also corresponded with several concerned parents to reassure them about well-being of their children. Due to the Mission's interventions the Bulgarian Government extended the validity of residence cards issued to Indian citizens for a period of 6 months which were due to expire between 13 March and 31 October 2020.

Relief and ration packets were distributed during pandemic to Indian workers working at various factories in Sofia and Stara Zagora in Bulgaria.

The Mission also assisted the host government in organising evacuation flights from India to Bulgaria for Bulgarian and EU citizens. This included obtaining necessary clearances from the Ministry and Directorate General of Civil Aviation. One flight took off on March 27, and another on 9 April 2020.

Embassy of India, Prague

The Mission issued advisories and press releases from time to time through its website and other social media platforms, to keep updated the Indians as well as others in the Czech Republic.

The helpline numbers including the regular emergency contact of the Mission were widely publicised through website, social media and local Indian Associations.

Concerned Czech authorities were approached inquiring about Indian nationals affected by COVID.

Those Indian nationals, who could not move to India due to non-availability of flights and whose Czech/Schengen visas expired, were helped by the Mission to have their stay validated till the date of their departure.

More than 200 students studying in various institutions of Czech Republic were supplied with food and grocery items by the Mission from Indian Community Welfare Fund in April 2020. Masks and sanitizers were also distributed among the Indian student community.

Since the Mission was covered under 'Hub and Spoke Model' operating at Frankfurt airport by Embassy of India, Berlin, requests of stranded Indians were shared with the Mission in Berlin for further collaboration with Air India. The Mission made a continuous push to prioritise cases of pregnant women, small kids, people who had suffered deaths in the family, etc. Many of them were able to make use of special flights under Phase-II of the Vande Bharat Mission.

Later when Paris and London were opened for stranded Indians in Czech Republic under Vande Bharat Mission scheme, the Mission assisted several Indians to move from those hubs also. Over 100 stranded Indians were, thus, helped to reach their home.

Embassy of India, Belgrade

Serbia imported 150,000 AstraZeneca vaccine from India in February 2021. Serbia also imported gloves from India in early stages of the pandemic in 2020.

The Mission assisted 30 Indian nationals to travel to India through Vande Bharat Mission. The expenses were borne by the Indian nationals. The Mission assisted in providing boarding and lodging from Indian Community Welfare Fund to 6 Indian nationals during COVID lockdown in Serbia.

Embassy of India, Athens

The Mission assisted the Greek authorities in the procurement of emergency medicines—for instance the import of five tons of hydroxychloroquine in its fight against COVID in the last week of March, and 300 kg of Chloroquine sulphate in April, 2020. When the COVID cases spiked in India, the Greek Government was quick in donating 90 oxygen Cylinders with total capacity of 440 liters with various sizes of cylinders and some medical protection devices (Mask, Gloves, etc.) to India, through EU. India accepted 10 cylinders of 10 kg capacity.

The Mission arranged repatriation of 40 stranded Indian nationals including seafarers through Vande Bharat Mission flights via Frankfurt/Paris in June and July. Mission also provided accommodation and dry ration to stranded nationals including 10 Indian students. Air tickets were also provided to one student and 1 stranded Indian.

The Mission also worked with Armed Forces. The Greek Foreign Ministry extended its full support and cooperation in granting overflight clearances to the Indian Army aircrafts in a timely manner, even at odd hours/weekends, for carrying COVID related relief supplies from various countries.

Embassy of India, Madrid

Setting up of seven dedicated COVID-19 helplines to respond to queries 24×7 was undertaken. The Mission promptly responded to queries via Twitter, Facebook, Instagram and WhatsApp. Conference calls with student representatives and Community Leaders were conducted and latest COVID-19 developments in India were shared regularly. Essay Competition for the Indian Community on the topic 'Will the World Remain Flat After the Curve Flattens?' and webinars were organised for the Indian Community with eminent personalities from Medicine, Bollywood, Business and Cultural sectors as the Guest Speakers. These sessions engaged the Indian community positively, encouraged them to be creative and helped to calm their nerves.

Separate online registrations were enabled for Indian students, Indian Professionals and Indian Nationals in Spain. The Mission sent advisories and updates to the community through mass emailing and social media. Special WhatsApp group for Community Representatives effectively coordinated to assist any Indian in their vicinity. The Food Solidarity Network by Indian Origin Senator Robert Masih Nahar and Indian restaurant Indali was given a financial assistance of EUR 5000 to aid in the supply of food and medicines for the Indian students and stranded Indians in Barcelona. Financial assistance provided to solidarity initiatives in Valencia to provide food and medicines to the Indian community, and 80 food packets were distributed to tourists, students and community in Madrid through diaspora volunteers. The Embassy together with Indian Association of Barcelona donated masks to the Community Representatives in Madrid and Valencia to be distributed among tourists, students and community. Ambassador penned letters to the Indian Community calling for cooperation and calmness and Indian community members shared posts and videos in support of this communication. The Embassy organised one Vande Bharat Mission flight on 31 May 2020 carrying 247 passengers and one chartered flight by a shipping company with 227 crew members on 5 June 2020.

During the second COVID-19 wave in India, the Mission facilitated Spanish Government assistance [141 ventilators, 10 oxygen concentrators], a special relief flight by the Regional Government of Catalonia, a shipment of 28 oxygen concentrators by an NGO 'World in Harmony', and 3 oxygen concentrators were contributed by Mission officials.

WORKING WITH THE ARMED FORCES

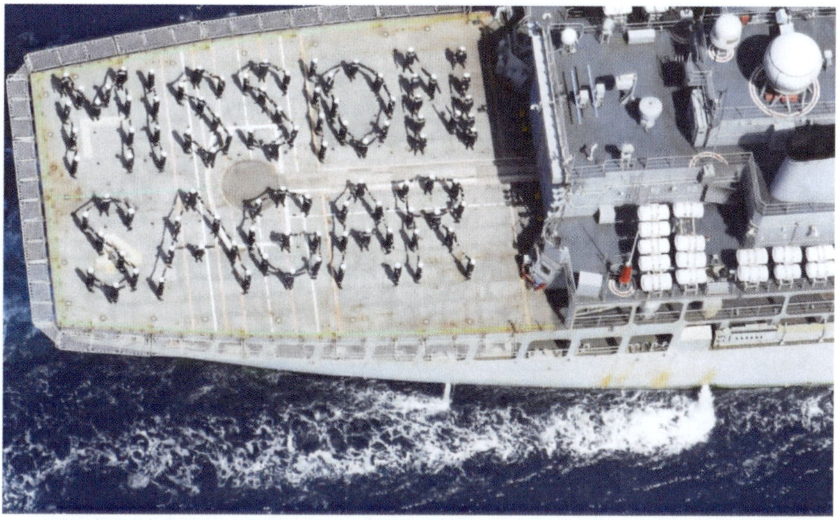

Mission Sagar: INS Kesari returned to Kochi upon completion of Mission Sagar, India's outreach amidst COVID-19 pandemic, in line with Prime Minister's vision of Security & Growth for All in the Region.

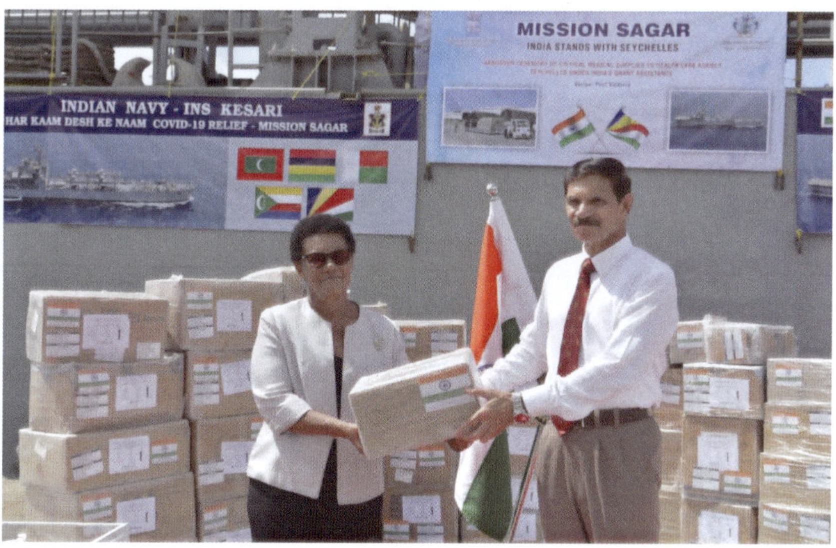

Mission Sagar: Handing over of medicine supplies consignment that reached Seychelles onboard INS Kesari, as a part of Mission Sagar

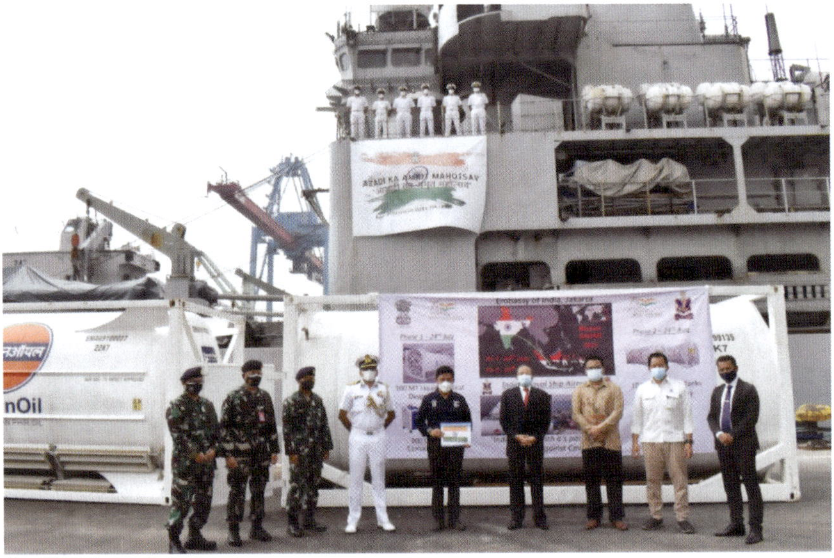

Mission Sagar: Indian Navy's Landing Ship Tank (Large) INS Airavat arrived at Tanjung Priok Port in Jakarta, Indonesia on 24 August 2021 to deliver 10 Liquid Medical Oxygen, based on the requirement projected by the Government of Indonesia.

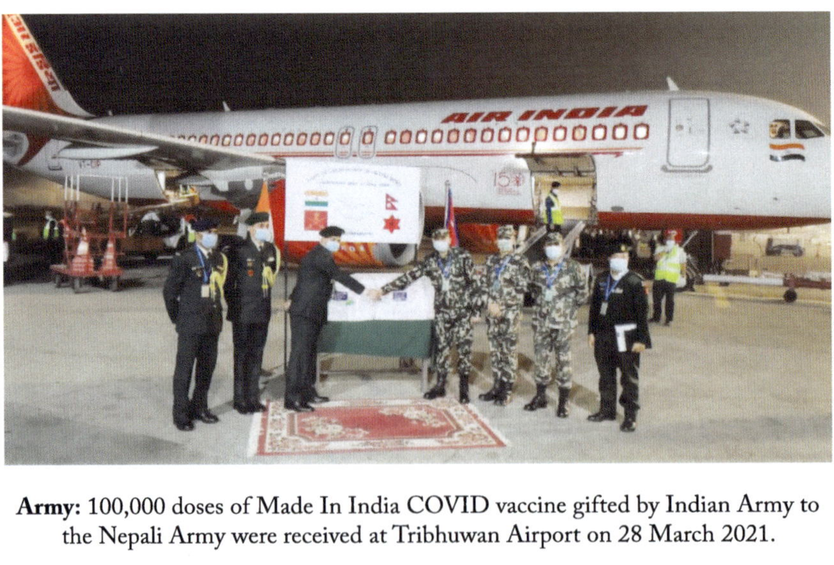

Army: 100,000 doses of Made In India COVID vaccine gifted by Indian Army to the Nepali Army were received at Tribhuwan Airport on 28 March 2021.

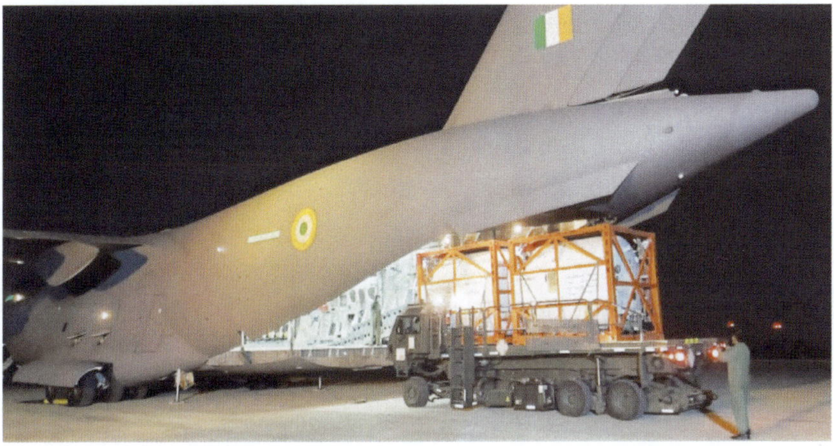

Air Force: IAF C-17 airlifted 6 Cryogenic oxygen containers from Dubai and landed at the Panagarh Air Base.

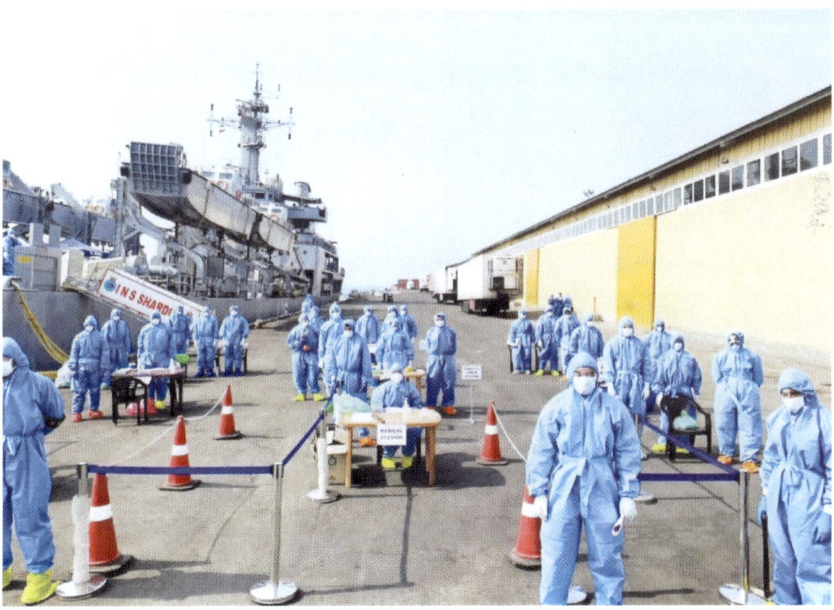

Operation Samudra Setu: INS Shardul at Bandar Abbas, Iran for Operation Samudra Setu, with crew carrying out pre-embarkation preparations, checks and briefings

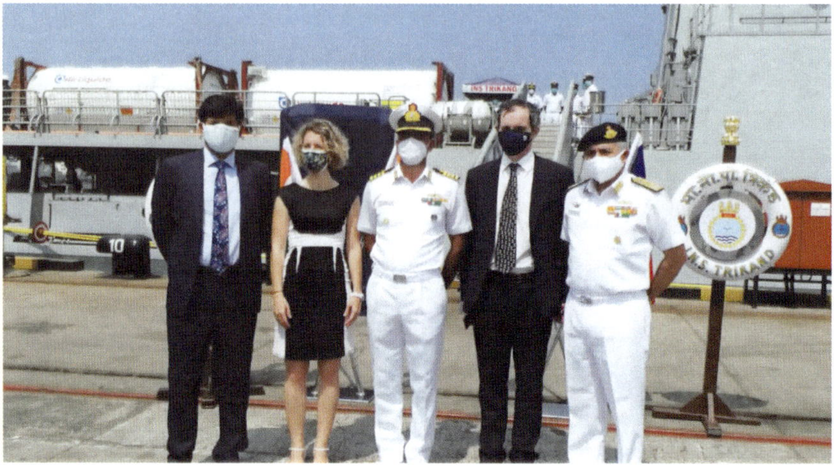

Operation Samudra Setu II: A joint endeavour across the seas, wherein INS Trikand carried 2 cryogenic tankers with 20 MT liquid medical oxygen each filled in Qatar by France's Air Liquide Group to Naval dockyard, Mumbai

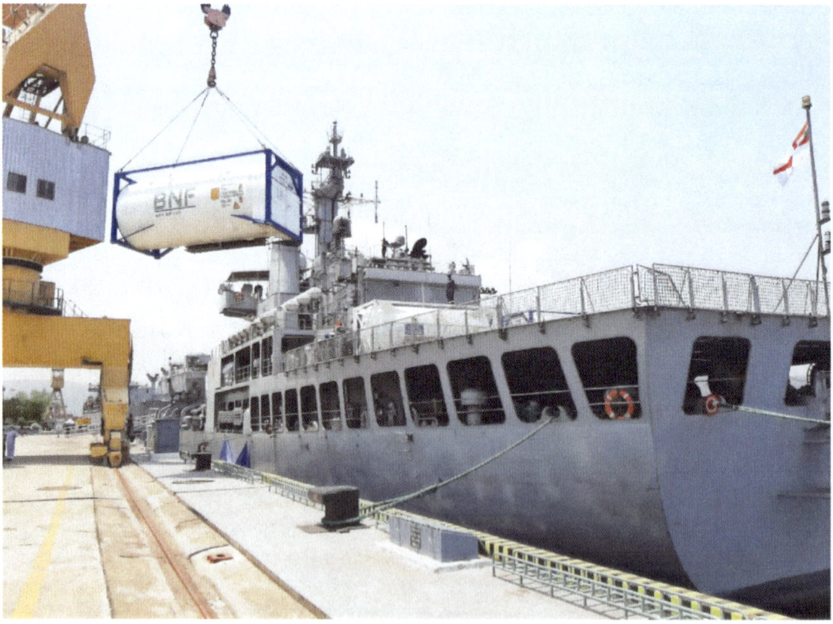

Operation Samudra Setu II: INS Airavat in Visakhapatnam brings 8 cryogenic oxygen tanks, over 3500 oxygen cylinders and other medical equipment from Singapore

10

WORKING WITH THE ARMED FORCES

MISSION SAGAR

Launched in May 2020, Mission Sagar was India's initiative to deliver HADR and COVID related assistance to the countries in the Indian Ocean region, over three phases. Mission SAGAR is a major milestone in India's engagement with the countries in the Indian Ocean Region, in line with the Prime Minister's vision of 'SAGAR- Security and Growth for All in the Region'.

This HADR operation involved the deployment of Indian naval assets to deliver assistance to India's maritime neighbors in dealing with the COVID crisis. Indian Naval Ship (INS) Kesari successively completed visits to Maldives, Mauritius, Madagascar, Comoros and Seychelles. India's humanitarian assistance included supplies of essential food items, medicines, Ayurvedic medicines and deployment of Medical Assistance Teams to Mauritius and Comoros.

Following the success of Mission Sagar-I, Mission Sagar II was launched in November 2020. As part of Mission Sagar-II, INS Airavat delivered food aid to Sudan, South Sudan, Djibouti and Eritrea.

Following this, India carried out Mission Sagar III wherein India offered HADR assistance to Friendly Foreign Countries in Southeast Asia during the pandemic. INS Kiltan arrived at Nha Rong Port, Ho Chi Minh City on 24 December 2020 as part of Mission Sagar-III. It delivered 15 tonnes of HADR Stores for the flood-affected people of Central Vietnam, which was handed over to Vietnam's Central Steering Committee for National Disaster Prevention and Control. INS Kiltan arrived at Sihanoukville Port, Cambodia on 29 December 2020 and delivered 15 tonnes of HADR Stores for the flood-affected people of Cambodia, which was handed over to Cambodia's National Disaster Management Committee.

OPERATION SAMUDRA SETU

Operation Samudra Setu, which was launched on 5 May 2020 as part of the national effort to repatriate Indian citizens from overseas during the COVID pandemic brought 3,992 Indian citizens back to their homeland by sea. Indian Naval Ships Jalashwa (Landing Platform Dock), and Airavat, Shardul and Magar (Landing Ship Tanks) participated in this operation which lasted over 55 days and involved traversing more than 23,000 km by sea.

The greatest challenge for the Indian Navy was to avoid any incident of outbreak of infection onboard the ships during the evacuation operation. Rigorous measures were planned and medical/safety protocols unique to the operating environment of ships were implemented. These were strictly followed onboard the ships undertaking Operation Samudra Setu.

Operation Samudra Setu was undertaken utilising Indian Naval ships best suited for the operation, catering for COVID related social distancing norms vis-à-vis medical arrangements and carrying capacity. Ships used for the operation were specially provisioned and the Sick Bay or the clinic onboard was especially equipped with COVID related equipment and facilities. Women Officers and military nursing staff were on duty to help the women passengers. Basic amenities and medical facilities were provided to all evacuees during sea passage on these ships.

Indian Naval ships Jalashwa, Airavat, Shardul and Magar steamed more than 23,000 km during Op Samudra Setu and undertook the evacuation operation in a smooth and coordinated manner. Details of the evacuation are as follows:

Ship	Date Embarked	Port of Embarkation	Number of Citizens	Date Disembarked	Port of Disembarkation
Jalashwa	8 May	Malè	698	10 May	Kochi
Magar	10 May	Malè	202	12 May	Kochi
Jalashwa	15 May	Malè	588	17 May	Kochi
Jalashwa	1 June	Colombo	686	2 June	Tuticorin
Jalashwa	5 June	Malè	700	7 June	Tuticorin
Shardul	8 June	Bandar Abbas	233	11 June	Porbandar
Airavat	20 June	Malè	198	23 June	Tuticorin
Jalashwa	25 June	Bandar Abbas	687	1 July	Tuticorin

Along with other Government agencies, the Indian Navy has also been at the forefront of national efforts to assist citizens. Indian Naval IL-38 and Dornier aircraft were used for ferrying of doctors and COVID related material across the country. Indian Naval personnel also developed innovative equipment such as Personnel Protection Equipment NavRakshak, hand-held temperature sensors, assisted respiratory system, 3-D printed face shield, portable multi-feed oxygen manifold, ventilators, air-evacuation stretcher pod, baggage disinfectants, etc. Most of these innovations were carried onboard the ships undertaking Operation Samudra Setu and niche equipment was also provided to host countries from where evacuation was undertaken.

The Indian Navy utilised its amphibious sea-lift ships for Operation Samudra Setu, which has reinforced the flexibility and reach of these multi-faceted platforms. Whilst Jalashwa, Magar, Airavat and Shardul were undertaking Operation Samudra Setu, another Landing Ship (Tank) Kesari undertook 'Mission SAGAR', carrying 580 tonnes of food aid and medical stores including ayurvedic medicines to Maldives, Mauritius, Madagascar, Comoros Islands and Seychelles, covering over 14,000 km in 49 days. One medical team each was also deployed at Mauritius and Comoros Island as part of the mission.

The 3,992 Indian citizens evacuated during Operation Samudra Setu were disembarked at various ports as indicated in the table above and entrusted to the care of respective state authorities. This operation was undertaken by the Indian Navy in close coordination with the Ministry, Ministry of Home Affairs, health and various other agencies of the Government of India and State Governments.

OPERATION SAMUDRA SETU-II

In late April 2021, when the extraordinary surge of the second wave of COVID put tremendous pressure on the country's health infrastructure and capacity, the Indian Navy launched *Operation Samudra Setu-II* to augment the national mission for meeting medical oxygen requirements. Ten Indian Navy warships from all three Naval Commands in Mumbai, Visakhapatnam and Kochi were deployed for shipment of LMO filled containers, concentrators, PPE, COVID test kits, Ventilators and other medical equipment from friendly foreign countries across the expanse of the Indian Ocean Region, from Persian Gulf to Southeast Asia. As the name of the operation 'Samudra Setu' suggests, this maritime Bridge by the Indian Navy ships ensured critical medical supplies to the country.

Indian Naval Ships *Kolkata, Kochi, Talwar, Tabar, Trikand, Tarkash and Aditya* from the Western Naval Command, *Shardul* from the Southern Naval Command, and *Jalashwa and Airavat* from Eastern Naval Command were deployed for the Mission ferrying critical stores from Bahrain, Brunei, Kuwait, Qatar, Saudi Arabia, Singapore, Brunei, Oman, UAE and Vietnam, the details of which are as follows:

S. No.	Unit	Embarkation Port		Disembarkation Port		Distance Covered (nm)	Manpower Involved
		Port	Date of Departure	Port	Date of Arrival		
1	Talwar	Manama (Bahrain)	30 Apr	New Mangalore	05 May	3217	256
2	Kolkata	Doha	02 May	Mumbai	10 May	3422	425
3	Kolkata	Kuwait	04 May	New Mangalore	10 May		
4	Airavat	Singapore	02 May	Vizag	10 May	3146	340
5	Kochi	Kuwait	05 May	New Mangalore	11 May	3422	304
6	Tabar	Kuwait	05 May	New Mangalore	11 May	3422	231
7	Trikand	Doha	05 May	Mumbai	10 May	2566	215
10	Tarkash	Doha	07 May	Mumbai	12 May	2566	230
11	Jalashwa	Brunei	10 May	Vizag	23 May	4478	268
12	Aditya	Muscat	10 May	Mumbai	23 May	1706	151
13	Shardul	Kuwait	12 May	Kochi	24 May	4210	141
14	Trikand	Doha	17 May	Mumbai	23 May	2566	215
8	Tarkash	Manama (Bahrain)	20 May	Mumbai	24 May	3178	230
16	Airavat	Ho Chi Minh	24 May	Vizag	03 Jun	4360	170
17	Tarkash	Kuwait	31 May	Mumbai	08 Jun	3230	230
18	Shardul	Kuwait	12 Jun	Mumbai	23 Jun	3230	141
19	Airavat	Vietnam	20 Jun	Vizag	02 Jul	4640	160
						53359	

Deployed for nearly two months, Indian Naval warships made overall 17 trips, traversed more than 53,000 nm (nearly 100,000 km) to bring more than 1100 metric tonnes of LMO, more than 14,000 oxygen cylinders with 314 kiloliters of oxygen, 23 Empty Oxygen containers (20 MT) and other critical medical aid like Oxygen concentrators (173), RAD Test Kits (10,000), PPEs (450) and Ventilators (140), thereby significantly contributing to the improved oxygen availability in the country. Operation Samudra Setu II involved extensive coordination between all agencies involved viz. the Ministry, Missions abroad, Ministry of Defence, Indian Navy, Indian Air Force and Indian expatriate Community. Ship wise details of medical stores brought to India are as follows:

S. No.	Ship (Port of Embarkation)	Details of Medical Supplies
1	*Talwar* (Manama)	• **40 MT LMO**
2	*Airavat* (Singapore)	• 08 Empty containers • Rapid Antigen Kit – 10000 • PPE Kit – 450 • 07 OxygenConcentrator • Filled oxygen Cylinder– 500 • Empty oxygen cylinder – 3150
3	*Kolkata* (Kuwait and Doha)	**Kuwait** • **40 MT LMO** • 500 filled oxygen Cylinders • 04 Oxygen Concentrators **Doha** • 200 filled oxygen cylinders • 43 Oxygen Concentrators
4	*Trikand* (Doha)	• **40 MT LMO**
5	*Kochi* (Kuwait)	• **60 MT LMO** • 800 filled oxygen cylinders • 03 Concentrators
6	*Tabar* (Kuwait)	• **40 MT LMO** • 600 filled oxygen cylinders
7	*Tarkash* (Doha)	• **40 MT LMO** • 232 filled oxygen cylinders

8	*Jalashwa* (Brunei and Singapore)	• **300 MT LMO** • 03 Empty Containers • 800 Filled oxygen cylinder • 2850 Empty oxygen cylinder
10	*Trikand* (Doha)	• **40 MT LMO** • 100 Filled oxygen cylinder
11	*Aditya* (Muscat)	• 100 empty oxygen cylinders
12	*Tarkash* (Doha and Manama)	• **40 MT LMO** • 760 Empty oxygen cylinder • 10 Concentrators
13	*Shardul* (Kuwait and Fujairah)	• **270 MT LMO** • 1200 filled oxygen cylinders
14	*Airavat* (Singapore and Vietnam)	• **140 MT LMO** • 450 filled oxygen cylinders • 2272 + 1176 empty oxygen cylinders • 10 + 100 Ventilators • 75 oxygen Concentrators
16	*Tarkash* (Doha)	• 785 filled oxygen cylinders • 300 empty oxygen cylinder • 50 concentrators
17	*Shardul* (Kuwait and Qatar)	• **40MT LMO** • 7640 filled oxygen cylinders. (Kuwait) • 15 Concentrators
18	*Airavat* (Vietnam and Singapore)	• **60 MT LMO** • 08 Empty Containers • 250 oxygen cylinder • 09 Concentrators • 30 Ventilators

Incidentally, most of the warships which participated in this operation were already Mission deployed in the Indian Ocean Region and were given this additional task of ferrying LMO from friendly foreign countries in the region. A case in point, INS Talwar, the first warship to ferry LMO from Bahrain to New Mangalore, was Mission Deployed in the Gulf and quickly diverted to meet the emerging requirement. The agility, reach and versatility of a warship afford it the inherent advantage, wherein it can be utilised for multiple tasks concurrently. Operation Samudra Setu has demonstrated the merits of 'Mission Based Deployments (MBD)' which the Indian Navy had commenced in 2017. MBDs enabled the ships, in this instance, to immediately adapt to the new requirements swiftly and transform their roles from military to HADR—a testament to the Navy's resolve to deliver—*Har Kaam Desh Ke Naam.*

The Indian Navy, being a professional service with experience in all manners of operations, is always mission ready. However, a unique mission like '*Samudra Setu*' in an unprecedented situation had its own set of challenges which required a re-alignment of operating procedures. Operation Samudra Setu II, during the second wave of the COVID pandemic, required additional safety precautions in terms of social distancing and medical cover. Physical distancing is extremely challenging onboard warships and submarines. Each mission was, therefore, undertaken under the spectre of COVID, with naval crews sparing no precaution in keeping themselves and others on board safe.

The 'bridging of the sea' by the Navy, under 'Samudra Setu II', exemplifies how the Indian Navy can overcome the tyranny of distances, to connect India with its regional friends, in a meaningful and abiding manner.

Arindam Bagchi
@MEAIndia

🇮🇳🇩🇪
Collaborating with our trusted partner & friend 🇩🇪 to address this global pandemic. Grateful to Germany for gift of 120 ventilators.

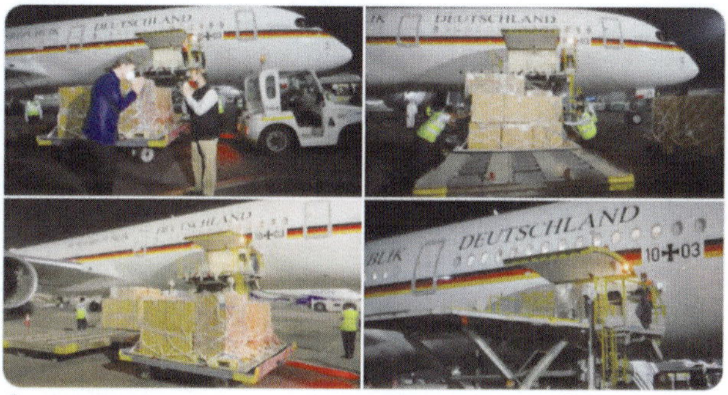

India in Germany and German Embassy India

10:44 PM · May 1, 2021 · Twitter for iPhone

1,008 Retweets **48** Quote Tweets **8,941** Likes

Arindam Bagchi
@MEAIndia

🇮🇳🇩🇪🇫🇮🇬🇷🇪🇺
Spirit of solidarity & cooperation - a hallmark of India-EU relations. Aircraft arrives carrying 176 ventilators from Germany, 324 O2 cylinders from Finland & 10 O2 cylinders from Greece. Value the continuing support from our EU 🇪🇺 partners.

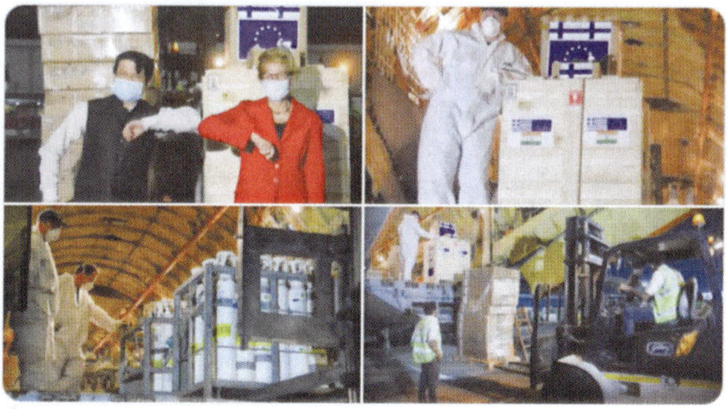

India in Germany and 5 others

5:31 AM · May 13, 2021 · Twitter for iPhone

329 Retweets **22** Quote Tweets **2,730** Likes

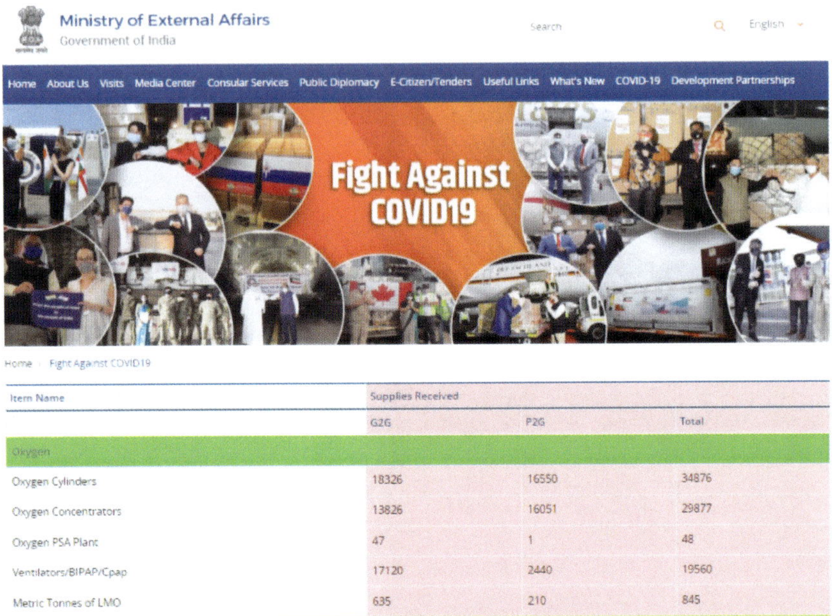
Ministry of External Affairs
Government of India

Search

English

Home | About Us | Visits | Media Center | Consular Services | Public Diplomacy | E-Citizen/Tenders | Useful Links | What's New | COVID-19 | Development Partnerships

Fight Against COVID19

Home › Fight Against COVID19

Item Name	Supplies Received		
	G2G	P2G	Total
Oxygen			
Oxygen Cylinders	18326	16550	34876
Oxygen Concentrators	13826	16051	29877
Oxygen PSA Plant	47	1	48
Ventilators/BIPAP/Cpap	17120	2440	19560
Metric Tonnes of LMO	635	210	845

A dedicated tab on MEA's website to document the aid received from foreign countries was created

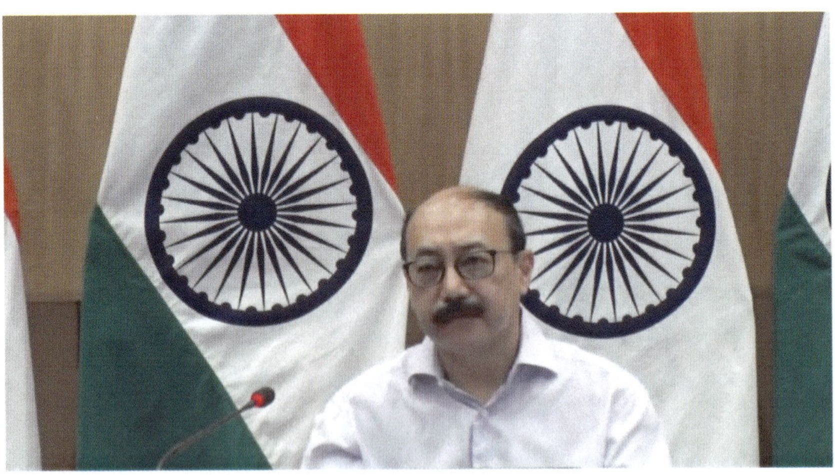

Special Briefing by Foreign Secretary on International Cooperation on COVID Pandemic (29 April 2021)

11

PUBLICITY AND OUTREACH

INTRODUCTION

An important element of Ministry's COVID related activities was publicity and outreach, largely handled by the XP Division of the Ministry.

The need to keep both domestic and global audiences informed of activities and developments was realised early on in the pandemic. Given India's population size, there was global interest in how India was handling the pandemic. In some cases, lack of authentic and timely information was leading to negative speculation and misinformation. Such an outreach also helped share the Ministry's crucial role in this national effort.

The principal challenges were getting timely and accurate information and visuals, coordination with multiple stakeholders at different locations, as well as functioning effectively on the ground in a COVID environment. Apart from the Missions and the COVID Cell, real time coordination was needed with other Ministries, foreign Missions in India, private companies/industries, hospitals, armed forces, etc. Such coordination was done at various levels.

Paradoxically, the Ministry was also deluged by information and visuals that did not provide a clear or comprehensive picture of the actual situation. Hence, efforts were required to stitch simpler narratives from the information. Such a narrative building exercise also helped counter incorrect information.

Social media (Facebook, Twitter, Instagram and YouTube channels of the Ministry) was the principal medium for dissemination information. Media briefings (mostly virtual due to COVID restrictions) were also used to reach out to traditional media. In addition, background briefings continued to be a key element of outreach. Apart from the weekly media briefings by JS (XP), special briefings were conducted periodically by OSD (COVID) and Foreign Secretary.

XP teams worked round the clock to ensure information capture and dissemination. A lot of the activities need presence on the ground, particularly for the in-house visual media teams, which was a particular challenge during COVID. Distinct and non-interacting groups were made within XP Division to avoid the risk of complete shutdown of operations when someone tested positive or came in contact with a COVID positive patient.

Regular media outreach efforts were supplemented by human interest or focused stories, such as the role of individual Embassies and Heads of Missions, the impact on common man, last mile delivery confirmation, etc. Direct guidance from EAM and Foreign Secretary on these narratives helped ensure coherence with overall Government of India messaging.

Thanks to a well thought out media strategy, and a willingness to adapt and modify it as required, visuals of repatriation of Indians, export of India-made vaccines and securing oxygen related supplies from abroad, recorded some of the defining moments of the battle against the pandemic.

Some specific activities and perspectives are outlined below:

WUHAN EVACUATION

This was the initial phase of the pandemic and lack of verified information about COVID made it very difficult to ensure visual coverage and putting out the right narrative. Despite that, real time coverage of these initial operations was ensured.

Close coordination with the Embassy helped in getting visuals quickly.

VANDE BHARAT MISSION

Ministry's COVID Control Room was duly publicised through traditional and social media.

From the inaugural flight, Ministry obtained hundreds of visuals related to COVID-protocol at airports, flights taking-off, experiences of Indians being repatriated, and bytes of key officials from the Missions and Posts. These visuals found enormous resonance in India.

There were various positive human interest stories that emerged from individual repatriations—example repatriation of pregnant ladies, sick workers, sailors stuck in ships in harbours, etc. XP Division sought details of such cases from COVID Cell and disseminated that information informally.

Weekly media briefings by JS XP commenced with read-outs on Vande Bharat Missions. Significant milestones like 1 million repatriations in August 2020, 3 million repatriations in November 2020 and 5 million repatriations in January 2021 received a wider coverage as they were highlighted in briefings.

Messages by leadership (Prime Minister and EAM) and other high level officials about the commitment that Indians would be brought back were highlighted across platforms to generate confidence.

VACCINE MAITRI

Prior coordination with Missions helped capture arrival visuals. Visuals of departure from India proved to be more challenging as the flights were taking off from Mumbai for Covishield and from Hyderabad for Covaxin. XP Division relied upon ANI to fill this gap, but close coordination with GVK, GMR and BCAS was required, particularly for tarmac deployment of camerapersons.

Operation Samudra Setu also carried Indian vaccines to various countries. Close cooperation with the Indian Navy ensured availability of visuals on an immediate basis.

Arrival of Indian vaccines abroad generated massive positive coverage in recipient countries with local leadership, celebrities and common people appreciating the support. XP Division requested Missions to procure such video bytes, which were compiled and publicised. For example, the message from Prime Minister of the Commonwealth of Dominica and a tweet from Cricketer Kevin Peterson, became viral sensations on social media.

Private media was put in touch with Indian vaccine manufacturers. This helped create greater interest in the Vaccine Maitri story, and also in sharing details of Indian vaccine manufacturing to a wider audience.

AID DURING SECOND WAVE OF PANDEMIC

Initial media coverage during this period was uniformly negative, with a focus on the overstretched health system in the country and the large number of deaths.

A conscious decision was taken to share as much information as possible on the efforts being made by the Ministry to obtain oxygen related equipment and supplies from abroad. This helped reassure the public that the world was with India in her time of need, and that help was on its way.

XP Division worked 24X7 in covering supplies from abroad, from the point of departure till final deployment in India.

Missions helped obtain visuals at departure points, apart from visuals of diaspora organisations extending support. In-house coverage teams of photographers and videographers were deployed at Delhi airport round the clock to capture arrival visuals of flights from all 53 countries that supplied relief material.

Given the severe COVID restrictions, such visuals became not just the earliest arrival images, but also an authentic source of information on equipment and material that was actually received.

Access for coverage teams of other countries, private media and press teams of other Ministries was also facilitated.

Most of the foreign aid arrived at stations outside Delhi. To capture those visuals, XP Division coordinated with Air Force Stations (Panagarh, Hindon, Chennai), Airport Operators (GVK, GMR), Indian Customs, Naval Bases (Mumbai, New Mangalore), Air Liquide Group and news agencies (DD, ANI).

Intensive coordination was required to secure end to end coverage from arrival till deployment.

The in-house coverage team also captured visuals of deployment of Oxygen plants, concentrators, testing kits, etc. from the ICU wards of hospitals. This was at a time when even private media was averse to providing such coverage due to fear of infection. Details of deployment of the foreign aid were obtained in coordination with the Ministry of Health and Family Welfare and various State Governments. Visuals were compiled in the form of video bytes and shared extensively.

COUNTERING FALSE INFORMATION

Each major operation viz. Vande Bharat Mission, Vaccine Maitri or Aid from Abroad was met with misinformation. Immediate efforts were required to counter such false information.

At the initial stage of Vande Bharat Mission, there were reports of infected Indian nationals being repatriated. Immediately, media outreach was conducted to convey that all the protocols were being followed at departure points in consultation with the local authorities.

There were some media reports in neighbouring countries about Indian vaccines having a severe adverse impact. Media briefings from the

Ministry of Health and Family Welfare were shared with Missions and Posts to counter such narratives.

The Delta variant of COVID virus was erroneously called 'Indian variant' in various media reports. A media campaign was launched to convey that WHO had not classified any variant based on any country.

When media reports emerged about foreign aid supplies lying unutilised at airports, visuals were obtained from numerous hospitals across the country (including by requesting doctors to shoot with their mobile phones). Since most private media was avoiding hospitals due to fear of infection, this timely dissemination of visuals played a key part in countering the false narrative about unused oxygen related supplies.

A dedicated tab was created on the Ministry's website (accessible from the home page) to document the aid received from foreign countries. This provided granular details of supplies received and was used extensively by the media.

INTERAGENCY PROCESS AND INTERACTION WITH OTHER AGENCIES

Close coordination was undertaken with the Ministry of Information and Broadcasting, Ministry of Health and Family Welfare, News Agencies and Foreign Missions in India.

For Operation Samudra Setu, contact was maintained with the Indian Navy. Visuals were also obtained Indian ports and destination directly. Similarly, the Indian Air Force was extremely helpful in providing access and facilitating coverage on their premises.

Close coordination with the COVID Cell resulted in the coverage of all the flights/ships despite constant change in departure/arrival for passengers' flights, vaccines flights or aid from abroad. The COVID Cell as the central hub for logistic information helped in adjusting to even the last minute changes in departure/arrival.

XP Division worked closely with the Director General of Civil Aviation, Bureau of Civil Aviation Security and Central Industrial Security Forces to facilitate access of departure/arrival coverage not just for the Ministry but also for private media and media team of other countries.

News Agencies like DD and ANI have presence all around the country and their resources were helpful in securing coverage from airports, naval bases and hospitals outside Delhi.

SOPS THAT EMERGED FROM PANDEMIC EXPERIENCE

- **Matrix Structure within the Division**: In-house coverage team was stretched during coverage of aid from abroad as the flights were arriving round the clock so the Press Relations team had to draw officers and staff from other wings. The officials from other wings of the Division also gained experience on coverage of visuals.
- **Establishment of a single point of contact:** A single nodal person from COVID Cell was in touch with a single nodal person in XP Division constantly. This helped in avoiding any misinformation about departure/arrival.
- **Easing of accessibility:** Coverage team initially took access permission from the airport authorities for each flight during coverage of Vaccine Maitri and aid from abroad. As the intensity increased, a blanket approval for 15 days was sought from Delhi and Mumbai Airport Authorities.
- **Establishment of database:** A database has been created of nodal contacts from Airport Authorities, Naval Bases, Air Bases, Customs, important hospitals and security agencies. This database would be very helpful in any such future exercises.

BEST PRACTICES

Influencers played a huge role in highlighting various aspects of operations and generating goodwill from the pandemic response. Large numbers of influencers conveyed their appreciation for Vande Bharat Mission for helping Indians coming back. Similarly, a large number of global leaders conveyed their appreciation for the support extended during the pandemic. An important lesson was to compile such appreciation in the form of video bytes and sharing them with the media. It helped in quicker and more intense projection which brought more focus from media in general and from people on social media.

EAM and Foreign Secretary shared various aspects of India's response to COVID through their interactions at various forums. These virtual events were carried live on the Ministry's social media platforms. They helped in allaying misconceptions and sharing authentic information directly to the public.

MEDIA OUTREACH (PRESS BRIEFING, BULLETIN, WEBPAGE)

Along with the core task of facilitating the movement of foreign aid, the Ministry's COVID Task Force conducted comprehensive media outreach to disseminate information about the aid being received from the global community.

A ***'Special Briefing by Foreign Secretary on International Cooperation on COVID Pandemic'*** was conducted on 29 April 2021, describing the efforts being made by the Government of India in collaboration with partner countries to address resource constraints in the fight against the second wave of COVID. Foreign Secretary also informed that the EAM held regular video meetings with Heads of Missions all over the world, and Heads of territorial divisions in the Ministry, with the objective of directing them on what they needed to do for meeting priority health system requirements.

On 7 May 2021, officials from various ministries/agencies including OSD COVID Cell participated in the regular Press Briefing and shared information about medical supplies received from various countries and their allocation process. The Press Briefing touched on various aspects including coordination efforts with Missions, structure and members of the coordination cell, standard operating procedures for receiving donation from abroad, allocation criteria, role of various stakeholders especially the Ministry.

OSD COVID Cell highlighted the active engagement by Indian Missions in mobilising support for India's fight against pandemic. He thanked all countries for their generous support and expressed that this was a reflection of India's good will globally. He described the Ministry's Standard Operating Procedures including initial vetting, receivable, allocation/distribution and sharing of information on COVID related medical supplies with resident Missions. He clarified that all consignments received have already been sent for distribution in a seamless manner. They were being individually monitored and tracked so that they reached the final destination. He reaffirmed that Government of India is open and transparent in sharing all the information.

OSD's remarks answered some misplaced anxieties and fears regarding the allocation and distribution of the medical supplies in India by the government. It brought out that government agencies were working together and ensuring that all received medical supplies were distributed to specific places without delay or pilferage.

A dedicated webpage on the Ministry's website to document the aid received from foreign countries can be accessed from its home page (mea.gov.in) by clicking on the tab "COVID" and then choosing the drop down option "Fight against COVID" or by directly going to the URL: https://mea.gov.in/fight-against-covid-19.htm. The webpage contains tabular details on Supplies received from foreign countries (under G2G and P2G modes), list of Partner Countries, Press Releases and links of Press Briefings, photographs of consignments being received, consignments being flagged off by Missions, and of equipment in use. The webpage also contains the list of important points of contact from the Ministry, IRCS, HLL, etc.

Press Briefings by Ministry of Health and Family Welfare: Regular physical press briefings were being organised by Ministry of Health and Family Welfare to provide information on the efforts made by the Government to fight the COVID pandemic. Updates were provided by it on the medical aid received from foreign countries. Ministry of Health and Family Welfare was assisted by senior officials from the Ministry and NITI Aayog during the press briefings. The press briefings are available online on the Youtube channel of Press Information Bureau (PIB). Daily Press Bulletins by Ministry of Health and Family Welfare are also being issued. These can be accessed at URL: https://pib.gov.in/newsite/bulletinn.aspx

Since a few foreign resident Missions were insisting on the end use of donations received, territorial heads of divisions including JS AMS, JS EW, and JS EA had been continuously in touch with the respective foreign Missions and informing them about the destinations where the medical aid had gone and was being utilised. JS EW organised a special meeting with EU Ambassadors and other diplomatic representatives on how the aid has been received and distributed. All the foreign Missions expressed satisfaction on the way the foreign aid was handled by the Inter-ministerial group.

12

ADMINISTRATION

INTRODUCTION

The Ministry was the principal instrument for dealing with the international dimension of dealing with the pandemic. It had to rapidly adapt and respond to new realities. In March 2020, as COVID began spreading across the world and countries imposed lockdowns, the Ministry created the COVID Cell, headed by an Additional Secretary to respond to concerns of Indians stranded abroad and foreigners in need of assistance in India. The primary functions of the COVID Cell included analysing global trends of the spread of the COVID virus and how other countries were tackling it; media briefings; parliamentary briefings; attending to Public Interest Litigations (PILs); coordinating supply of medicines and medical equipment to foreign countries; facilitating repatriation of Indians abroad; evacuating foreigners in India; and to assist in the clearance of air ambulances for treatment of patients with serious medical conditions in India.

In order to respond swiftly timely to the large number of queries coming in from all over the world a decision was taken to set up a 24×7 the Ministry COVID Control Room on 16 March 2020 with operations from two locations, Situation Room in South Block, and from Jawaharlal Nehru Bhawan. The COVID Cell was manned by 19 Officers at any given point of time (1 Additional Secretary, 3 Directors, 5 Deputy Secretaries and 10 Under Secretaries). Apart from this5 teams of 3 members each (1 Officer, 2 Staff) manned the Control Room 24×7 on a rotation basis. 30 Officer Trainees of the 2019 batch were also deployed in shifts in the Control Room in the early stages. In total, about more than a hundred officers and staff members, including officers on training of the 2019 batch, worked in the Control Room.

On 24 March, a nationwide complete lockdown was imposed in the hope that a strict lockdown will prevent the spread of the virus. The lockdown was initially meant to be imposed for 3 weeks but remained in force with extensions till end May. The COVID Cell monitored the spread of the virus in various parts of the world on a daily basis based on the inputs received from Missions. These global trends summarised in report form with graphs, tables and analysis were shared with Prime Minister's Office, Cabinet Secretariat, Home Ministry, Health Ministry and other line Ministries. Often presentations were made to the 'Committee on Strategic Issues relating to Lockdown' to better understand global developments and what lessons they hold for us for tackling the COVID challenges.

Questions relating to testing, quarantine, travel, medicines, family reunions among others were responded to. Foreigners stranded in India were given assistance.

The Ministry received offers of assistance from around 40 countries committed to providing India with critical items including oxygen cylinders, concentrators, and medicines such as remdesivir, favipiravir, etc.

The Ministry's operations were guided by an objective to be transparent and accountable. Information was constantly shared, through RTI applications, and by placing information in the public domain. This was of particular importance in respect of the donations that were received and the allocation and distribution of medical equipment and supplies States.

The Inter-ministerial Group and Ministry COVID Task Force started functioning on 26 April 2021 and met regularly for smooth and effective coordination.

EXPENDITURE INCURRED ON SPECIAL FLIGHTS AND SHIPS

Assistance was provided in the form of airlifts and transportation by Indian Navy Ships. This was done with the approval of Empowered Group-2 or directly arranged through DM Division, Ministry of Home Affairs.

In the meeting of Empowered Group-II on 13 May 2021, the Ministry made a presentation on proposal with details of costs and charges being incurred by Indian Missions on transport of items from overseas to India. Actual expenditures incurred on: (i) fuel, (ii) ground and cargo handling charges, (iii) in-flight catering for crew, (iv) items required for personnel as per local protocols (e.g. PPE, Masks, sanitizers, etc.). It was decided that these expenditures incurred by the Indian Missions on the transport of items from overseas through special Indian Air Force/Air India flights would be debited to Ministry of Health and Family Welfare. Information on expenditures on additional expenditure by Indian Missions/Posts as per a uniform template was collated and shared with Ministry of Health and Family Welfare every week for regularisation and sanctions.

PORTALS

Repat

The Ministry created a dedicated data portal, named Repatriation Portal, or REPAT, on the instructions of Foreign Secretary, that could capture data of returning Indians. This would capture the data of returning Indians category-wise and make it available to all stakeholders, especially the relevant Ministries/Departments, State Governments and Missions which were involved in the welfare of the returning persons. With the help of an experienced team of consultants, EG and IT Division designed, in-house, the 'REPAT Portal'. Joint Secretary (eG&IT) coordinated these activities.

This portal "mapped" Indians abroad who wished to return and provided that data to various agencies, ranging from Airlines, Immigration to State Health Ministries, District Administrations and even airport authorities. The Portal captured data about various categories of stranded Indians who were classified according to domicile. Missions asked local stranded Indians through emails to provide data about themselves in pre-formatted Excel sheets that were linked to REPAT Portal. A real-time picture thus developed that allowed COVID Cell, at the click of a mouse, to plan flights directly to relevant specific locations in India in different States from multiple points of origin abroad.

States were able to see data in real time and were able to plan for the arrivals of flights. The portal and the real-time data it provided was useful for state governments, immigration and health officials to plan logistics such as screening, testing, quarantine and transportation for arriving passengers. This was essential to ensure proper compliance with quarantine protocols issued by Ministry of Health and Family Welfare. To facilitate smooth registration of people stranded abroad on the Repatriation Portal, the flight schedule prepared by Air India was carefully converted into an easily understandable format devoid of technical jargons. The schedule was regularly updated and continues to be published even to date, on the Ministry website.

Logistics Management System Portal

(a dedicated portal for monitoring the medical aid)

A dedicated portal was also developed to manage the logistics of incoming medical assistance during the second wave. It collated data and tracked arrival and distribution of critical medical equipment such as Oxygen concentrators, Ventilators, Oxygen cylinders, lifesaving drugs like Remdesivir, etc. received from the various countries and their distribution within the country by the.

The highlights of the portal included the following:

(i) It was user friendly;

(ii) The dashboard gave the figures of total consignments, arrived as well as expected; it gave details of the number of items received;

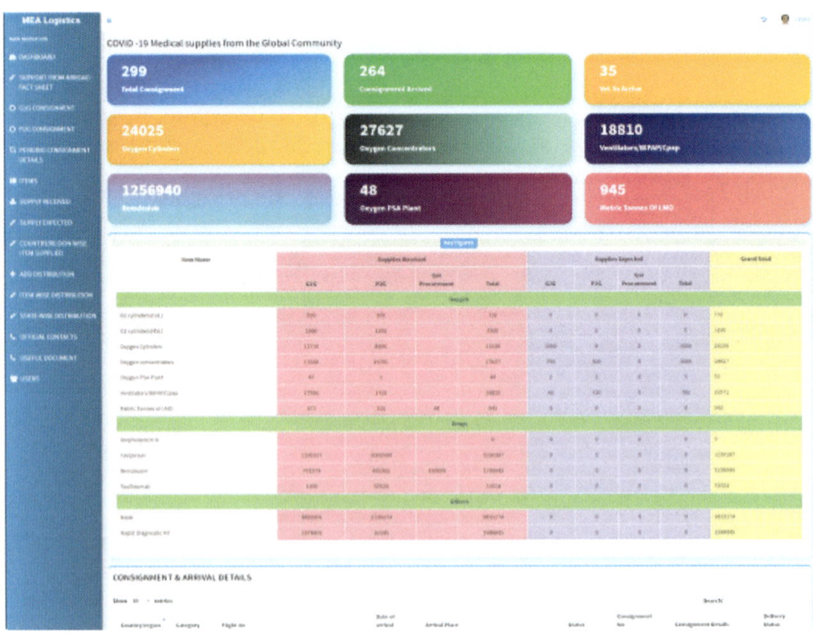

(iii) The portal gave country-wise and item-wise data;

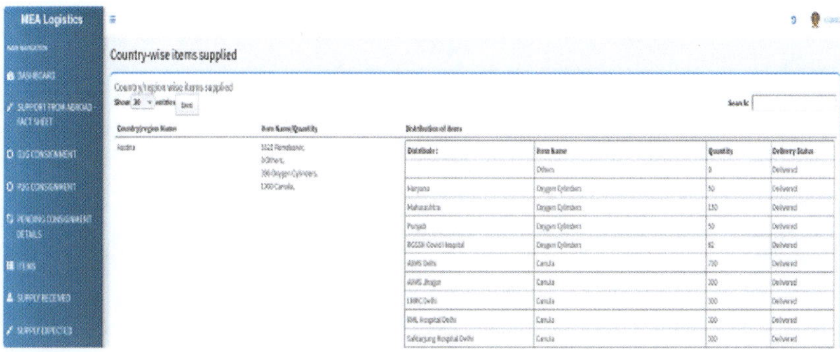

(iv) Most importantly the items delivered to any particular State could be tracked;

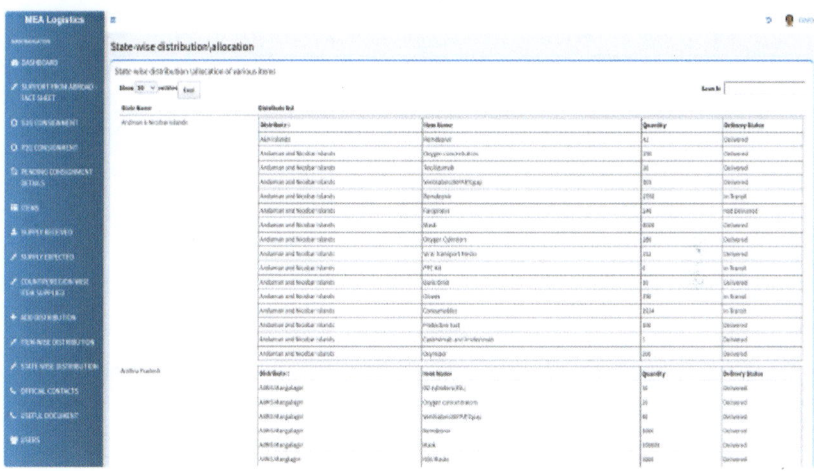

(v) Government-to-Government and Private-to-Government data could be accessed separately on the portal;

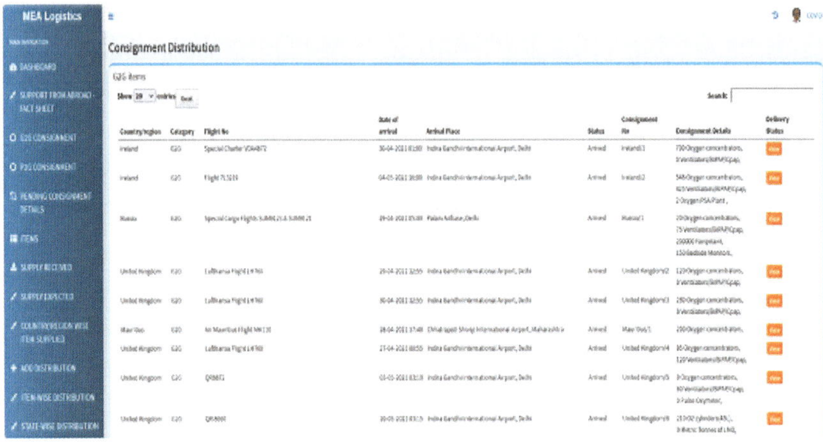

(vi) All important documents including Standard Operating Procedure were uploaded real time on the portal, which helped guiding the Missions.

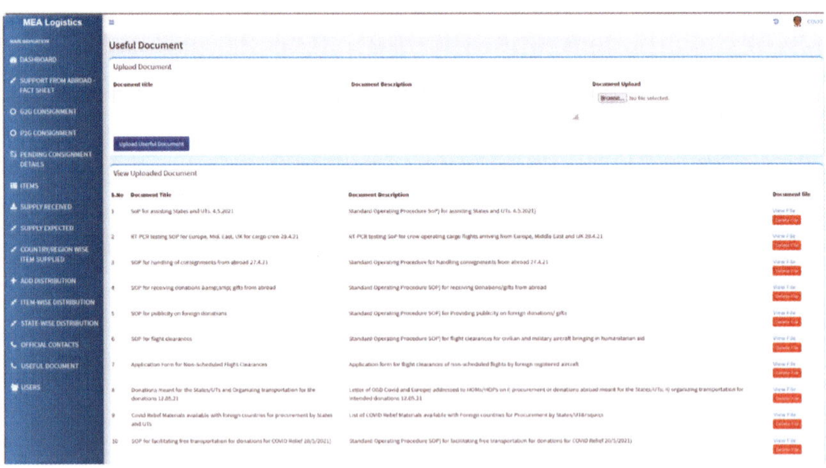

To populate the portal with information was not an easy task. A team of around 10 officers worked almost on a continuous basis to secure the data, verify it and upload it. Maintaining information on receipt of consignment, allocation and distribution of medical aid; further tracking it down through the State Governments till the ultimate end-user and feeding that data on portal was a continuous operation.

The data being maintained by the Ministry was concurrently shared with Ministry of Health and Family Welfare, NITI Aayog, Ministry of Home Affairs, Prime Minister's Office and all other relevant Ministries and Departments. All territorial heads of divisions and Missions from where aid was received could access the portal.

The portal helped in real-time monitoring of the arrival of consignments, allocation and distribution of medical aid received from abroad. Since the data posted on this portal was accessed by all the stakeholders, it ensured uniformity in data maintained by all the departments, which was used for answering RTI queries, parliamentary questions, submitting reports to relevant parliamentary committees, and to judicial authorities.

RESOLVING RTI QUERIES AND PUBLIC GRIEVANCES

Great importance was given to sharing information and to answering Right To Information (RTI) queries. The objective was to be transparent and accountable with regard to the donations received and the allocation and distribution of medical equipment and supplies to states. It was also an effort to assure the public that each and every item that was received as a donation was accounted for and utilised promptly. The COVID Task Force's work also made public as much up to date information as it could in the public domain including on the Ministry's social media handles and website. The RTI requests were swiftly answered. In the same spirit, the COVID task force also undertook special efforts for resolving public grievances. These were resolved through coordination with the concerned divisions in the Ministry and Indian Missions around the world.

13

CASE STUDY ON OUTSOURCING: HLL LIFECARE LTD.

(Input directly from HLL Lifecare Ltd)

HLL Lifecare Ltd, a Government of India enterprise was responsible for managing incoming consignments. HLL collected the required documents from different agencies like Indian Red Cross Society/ Ministry of Health and Family Welfare/the Ministry of External Affairs for the IGST exemption as well as for timely customs clearance. For the same, HLL engaged Custom House Agents at different places. Once the items were cleared at customs, the same were transferred to the respective warehouses.

All international shipment arrived either at cargo warehouse or depot at Gurugram (which is managed by HLL). Once the consignment arrived, cargo teams did physical verification as per invoice and made entries in the computer system. All medicines which required cold storage facility were sent directly to cold room warehouses. Rest of the items were sent to the non-cold chain warehouses. For the loading and unloading of the items, machinery like Forklift, Hydra, etc. were arranged by HLL.

Ministry of Health and Family Welfare prepares an allocation plan, which was shared with the HLL team for further execution. Based on allocation order by Ministry of Health and Family Welfare, HLL made arrangements for dispatch of all items within 24 hours. HLL's central team prepared a daily dispatch sheet after consolidation of allocation order and shared with cargo warehouse team to execute it. HLL's central team decided the mode of transportation (Air/Road/Courier) based on factors like requirement of items, distance, weather condition, etc. Proper coordination with Transporter, NDMA/NDRF, CONCOR, State Nodal Agencies, etc. were made by HLL for the successful dispatch of the items.

HLL empanelled vendors to handle the transportation throughout India. Once warehouse teams received the dispatch sheet, they started the process of sending out the items to designated locations of end users. At the same time DC (Delivery Challan) was prepared which includes details of items, vehicle number, driver number, etc. for actual tracing. DC was shared with State agencies for follow up of consignment.

Prior to the dispatch of the items, warehouse personnel ensured proper labeling on boxes for proper traceability. The items were palletised and shrink wrapped as per the requirement at the warehouse level. E-Way bills, Delivery challans, Declaration statements, etc. were prepared and handed over to the transporter. Proper acknowledgment of the items received was obtained from the transporter. The total operation was controlled through SWIMS software. After successful delivery of the items at the customer end, the transporter collects Proof of Deliveries (PoDs) and shares it with HLL. The same was uploaded in the SWIMS Software.

HANDLING OF P2G AND P2P DONATIONS

Missions on the receipt of information on offers from private individuals/ Indian associations/Companies/NGOs informed NITI Aayog, Ministry of Health and Family Welfare, and the Ministry. NITI Aayog is the nodal body for coordinating P2G donation offers. Missions would vet such offers, including verification of antecedents of donors before forwarding proposals.

On offers of donations to the Government of India, including to PSUs, Indian Red Cross Society (IRCS) was the consignee. Such offers were given blanket exemptions from Customs, IGST and other mandatory clearances. The offers of donations would adhere to the minimum threshold for effective use and expeditious clearance on arrival. The specifications were ascertained by NITI Aayog as per the guidelines issued by Ministry of Health and Family Welfare. For internal distribution to end users, NITI Aayog coordinated with Indian Red Cross Society and HLL.

Donations meant for private use were also coordinated by NITI Aayog. Such consignments were cleared by an agency designated by NITI Aayog and its distribution came under the direction of NITI Aayog.

Documentation required for dispatch of donation includes Airway Bill, Commercial Invoice, List of items, carton-wise, Donation/Gift Certificate.

RECEIVING OF CARGO BY RESPECTIVE DIVISIONS (PROTOCOL)

It was ensured that a Joint Secretary level officer from the Ministry Headquarters, preferably the one heading the concerned Territorial Division, would receive the first consignment coming in from different countries. The first consignment would have representatives from the donor country local resident Missions, often at the level of Ambassadors, and concerned officers present at the time of arrival of these consignments. Having senior officers receive these donations right at the tarmac, through the day and through the night, lent a human face to the Government's expression of gratitude to the donor countries for this timely support.

While consignments arriving in Delhi were received by officers from Headquarters, for consignments arriving via ships to Mumbai/Mangalore etc., it was ensured that colleagues posted in the respective Regional Passport Offices or Branch Secretariats would be present to receive the ship loads of help and assistance.

ASSISTANCE PROVIDED BY HLL FOR COVID PANDEMIC MANAGEMENT

By the middle of April 2021, the second wave of the COVID pandemic struck India. In order to fight the unprecedented surge in COVID cases, the Government of India received significant donations and aid in the form of medical supplies and equipment from different countries and organisations world over. HLL was again assigned with the task of handling the logistics and distribution of the donations thus received from various overseas countries. (In 2020, during the emergence of the first wave of COVID pandemic in India, the Ministry of Health and Family Welfare nominated HLL as the Nodal Agency for the Procurement and supply of Emergency Medical items to fight against the pandemic. HLL took up this mammoth task in a project mode and executed the same by building an institutional mechanism to handle the imports and distribution of emergency supplies across India.)

All the donation materials from abroad were received by the Indian Red Cross Society or Niti Aayog on behalf of the Government of India and then handed over to HLL for further distribution. HLL was responsible for the warehousing, storage, logistics and distribution of donation items across all states and Union Territories as per the allocation plan issued by Ministry of Health and Family Welfare. Apart from handling the donations, HLL, on behalf Ministry of Health and Family Welfare also offered its support to the Ministry for the procurement of medicines like Remdesivir and Liposomol Amphotericin B from different overseas suppliers/manufacturers. As on date HLL received donation items (listed in Annexure 13a) through 402 shipments and 2228 dispatches have been made to 161 destinations in India, which includes hospitals, government institutes, government medical college, depots coming under the state government, etc.

Team Formation

The following teams were made swift into action on an emergency basis for the timely and smooth execution of distribution of medical supplies.

- **Import coordination team:** An exclusive team to coordinate the imports of emergency medical supplies with the Ministry, Ministry of Health and Family Welfare and IRCS
- **Warehouse management team:** Integrated Warehouses with Logistics facilities at 7 strategic locations in India to facilitate hassle-free and timely dispatch of Donation materials.
- **IT support team:** IT enabled Warehouse Management System (called SWIMS) as a comprehensive solution for efficient logistics management, which includes warehouse management, warehouse automation, transportation and contract management, shipping logistics for the safe transportation and delivery of materials to various beneficiary locations in the country.
- **State Nodal officers:** Deployed a dedicated team of Nodal Officers in every State and a taskforce was formed for sourcing, logistics, dispatch and data maintenance
- **Central Team:** Overall administration, monitoring and control

Operations

The following were the important operations being executed by HLL:

1. Receipt of Donation Materials

The details of grant-in-aid consignments being sent to India were communicated to HLL by the Ministry, to ensure timely clearance at Airport and acceptance of the material. The import coordination team handled the customs clearance by way of submission of required documents in coordination with the Ministry, Indian Red Cross Society and Ministry of Health and Family Welfare. HLL had engaged Clearing Housing Agents (CHA) at Delhi, Mumbai and Visakhapatnam for clearance of material. Once the items were cleared by customs, based on the nature of material, the same gets transferred to the pre-planned warehouses—Cargo warehouse or at a Cold storage warehouse.

2. IT Enabled Warehouse Management

All donation materials were brought either at Cargo Warehouse Logistics (CWL) at IGI Terminal in New Delhi, or depot of AWL, Gurugram. Once the consignment arrives, the warehouse team does the physical verification as per the documents and takes inward receipt of the consignment in the SWIMS software. All medicines, which need cold storage facilities, go directly to the cold room warehouses. All related data is uploaded in the cloud by the warehouse management team. The SWIMS software, which is implemented across all warehouses, ensures proper accounting of the receipt of items, its dispatch to various destinations and acknowledgement of receipt of donation items at destination. The entire logistics operations were monitored and controlled through SWIMS Software. A dashboard named **"CHAKSHU"** was developed to provide real-time MIS.

3. Distribution

As mentioned earlier the allocation plan prepared and issued by Ministry of Health and Family Welfare is shared with the HLL team for further execution. Based on allocation, HLL plans for the dispatch of donations items within 24 hours. The central team prepares a daily dispatch plan on the basis of the allocation order received and shares it with the warehouse team for execution. On the basis of important factors like urgency of requirement of items, current situation of pandemic in state, distance to be covered, local weather conditions etc. and also as per the directions or guidelines received from NITI Aayog/Ministry of Health and Family Welfare/Empowered group, the Central team decides the mode of transportation to be used (Air/Rail/Road/Courier). Proper coordination with the transporter, NDMA/NDRF, CONCOR, State Nodal Agencies etc. were also ensured.

Indian Air force on behalf of NDRF/NDMA did a commendable job by transporting the relief material which ensured meeting the turnaround of delivery time of 3 days across any part of the country. Flight operations were made from Palam, Bengaluru, Chennai, Vizag, Kolkata and Mumbai airports to various destinations across the country. While transporting cold chain items to ensure maintenance of optimum temperature, data loggers were installed in the reefer vehicles along with proper packing.

Once the warehouse team received the dispatch plan, the dispatch process commences. A Delivery Challan (DC) with item details, Vehicle number, Driver number, etc. was prepared for traceability. The same DC was shared with the state for consignment tracking. Prior to the dispatch of items, Warehouse personnel arrange the items as per the allocation sheet and ensure proper labeling on the box for traceability. The items were palletised and shrink wrapped as per the requirement. E-Way bills, Delivery Challans, Declaration statements, etc. were prepared and handed over to the transporter. The warehouse team also ensured proper acknowledgment of the receipt of items by the transporter. The total operation was controlled through SWIMS software. After successful delivery of the items at the customer end, the transporter collected Proof of Deliveries (PoDs) and shared it with HLL. The same was uploaded in the SWIMS Software and automatically reflected in the Dashboard.

4. Monitoring and Reporting

On a daily basis, a report on the actual dispatches undertaken and any concern/issue pertaining to dispatch or allocation or stock was submitted to Ministry of Health and Family Welfare by the HLL central team. Nodal officers were appointed at different States/UTs to coordinate with the State/UT/Institutional Level personnel for ensuring successful receipt of consignment and for obtaining proper acknowledgement towards its receipt. Also, other details like availability of manpower, space, Cold Chain

Equipment, material handling Equipment, etc., at the destination, were collected and required measures put in place with proper coordination with the State Level people well in advance, so that the items can be easily unloaded on its receipt.

A centralised call centre operating 24x7 was set up in Delhi which helped with the consolidation of information and timely submission of MIS to Ministry of Health and Family Welfare updating the receipt, acknowledgement, dispatch and delivery details of all consignments. The call centre numbers were provided to all state nodal officers for receiving real-time information as well as clarifications on various other details like type of items dispatched; destination address, etc. In addition to this, one WhatsApp group was also created as a helpdesk, where any state or institutions put their queries on the items received or any other concern and resolution for the same was expected from the concerned team within a stipulated time frame.

This is a brief outline on the interventions made by HLL for the successful distribution of COVID relief material received on behalf of Ministry of Health and Family Welfare during the second wave of the pandemic in the country. HLL could successfully handle the distribution of emergency medical supplies to nearly 161 destinations in India which includes hospitals, government institutes, government medical colleges, depots coming under state government, etc. HLL's prior experience during the first wave has really helped in the smooth execution of the project. The major donation items received through 402 shipments (as on date) are available in Annexure 13a and 13b.

UTILISATION OF COVID RELATED EQUIPMENT BY STATES AND UTS

Battling COVID pandemic has been an unprecedented challenge, and in this fight against the pandemic, the significance of ensuring timely availability of the medical aid and equipment to the various states and UTs in the country cannot be emphasised enough. In this effort, the role played by the Ministry in acting as the nodal agency for channelising the help that poured from foreign partner countries, Indian associations, private individuals and companies abroad, and coordination with the Indian Missions and Consulates abroad has been pivotal. It was this aid in the form of the medical equipment that through a proper channel involving various agencies and organisations reached the states and UTs, where these were then made available to the patients in need. Various state agencies, departments and the state nodal officers for COVID played a vital role as an essential linchpin in giving shape to the fight against the pandemic. Following are the experiences shared by some states and Union Territories in their fight against COVID.

Chandigarh

Highlighting that the medical aid and equipment from foreign countries was of high quality and met the needs/requirements, Chandigarh expressed gratitude towards the countries that offered the much needed help at the time of necessity, and HLL life care for providing the essential support to fight the pandemic in the UT. Following is what the state conveyed.

"The donation received through HLL life care (CPSE) for Management and Containment of COVID in Chandigarh were of great help in tiding over the Second surge in the UT. These donations were used to augment the resources in Government hospitals and the COVID Care Centers in Chandigarh, more so at the level 2 facilities, where the Oxygen Concentrators played a significant role. These donations were also issued to Government Medical College and Hospital, sector 32, Chandigarh and Government Multi-specialty Hospital sector 16, Chandigarh and its allied units".

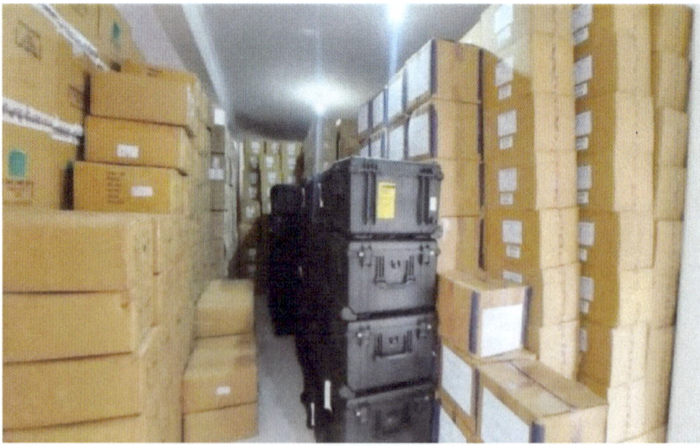

Medical Supplies received by Chandigarh

Himachal Pradesh

Pointing out issues like—non-fitting of Oxygen Cylinder valves, colour coding of cylinders and different sizes of a few cylinders, Himachal Pradesh nevertheless underscored the importance of receiving the life-saving essential medical aid in time. It shared the following experience.

"The D-Type Oxygen Cylinders have been very useful during the peak of the second wave in our state, as these cylinders were not available anywhere and we were facing difficulty in procuring/arranging these precious life-saving Oxygen Cylinders. We have received portable ventilators and ICU ventilators as foreign aid. The Oxygen Concentrators received as foreign aid is ready to use and have been distributed throughout the state and they have proved to be very beneficial and lifesaving for the suffering patients".

Odisha

Stating that the supplies received in the form of foreign aid helped in augmenting the existing stock of medical equipment, Odisha highlighted that these supplies helped the state in fighting the second wave of the pandemic of COVID effectively. Following is the experience shared by Odisha.

"The state started receiving critical and essential items required for effective management of COVID from the Government of India on a no-cost basis from 6 May 2021. Items like the BiPAP/CPAP ventilators and their accessories, High Flow Nasal Cannula and Oxygen Concentrators provided immediate assistance to the Dedicated COVID Hospitals—both in the purely government run hospitals as well those being operated in PPP (Public Private Partnership) mode. Critical drugs, especially Tocilizumab, were instrumental in further enhancement of the state's own reserves. Most of these items have been issued and utilised by the various health facilities. Some portions of these items have been maintained at the central reserve in the central store of Odisha State Medical Corporation Limited (OSMCL) to maintain a strategic buffer for possible deployment to meet any emergent need.

Some issues were encountered in the beginning, including dispatch of certain drug items without the necessary requirement of a cold chain. However, these were rectified in the subsequent dispatches. Also, some oxygen cylinders did not have the compatible accessories which were resolved by procuring valves locally. Overall, the assistance received from the Government of India on a no-cost basis has been very helpful in meeting the challenge of the second wave of the pandemic of COVID ".

Sikkim

Expressing gratitude towards the Ministry in the role it played in ensuring the availability of vital medical equipment and consumables from various foreign governments and agencies, Sikkim shared the following experience in utilising the aid to fight the pandemic.

"There existed excellent coordination between all the people involved in sending and receiving the aid materials. Materials reached the state hospitals, district hospitals and primary health centers timely. Oxygen Cylinders were one of the most needed items and their timely receipt contributed greatly in managing the COVID patients in Sikkim hospitals".

Tripura

Expressing gratitude towards the countries that extended support to India and the state of Tripura in fighting this deadly disease, Tripura also presented appreciation for the efforts put in by the Ministry team for arranging and providing all the necessary aid in such times. Following is the experience Tripura shared.

"As on date, more than 61,782 people have been tested positive in this small state since the beginning of this pandemic and a total of 619 people have lost their lives to COVID so far. Due to the sudden rise in the number of cases and quick spreading of the pandemic, there was a strong need for provision of essential items, like—life saving equipment, Oxygen Cylinders, Oxygen Concentrators, Drugs, Protective gears and Testing kits.

It was a grave situation and the state was struggling to arrange all the essentials. It was from May 2021 that huge support regarding all-important COVID related items from the Ministry, through HLL was received by the state. This came as a big blessing for this state. Tripura received various life-saving equipment, like—Ventilators, BiPAPs machines etc. donated by nations like Canada, Vietnam and others. These were shifted to the Dedicated COVID care Hospitals (DCHCs), TMC and BRAMT Hospital, AGMC and GBP Hospital, RCC Hospital and IGM Hospital.

Most of these have been put to good use, and for some, the installation process is underway. The most important equipment received—Oxygen concentrators, 445 in number from Ireland, Switzerland, Qatar, Bahrain, Hong Kong, are being used at the DCH, DCHC and in the COVID Care Centers (CCCs) across the state. Healthcare workers also received benefits with donation of the Protective gears like—Gloves, Face Shields, masks and Hand-rub solutions.

Thanks to this huge donation the state has received, now there is no shortage of Oxygen concentrators in our State.

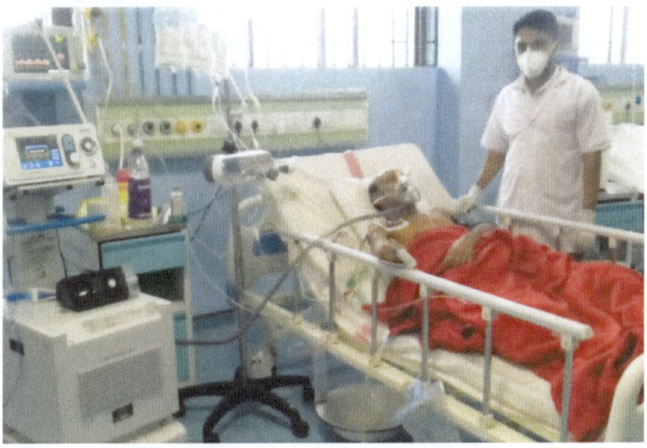

BiPAP Machine at RCC ICU, Tripura

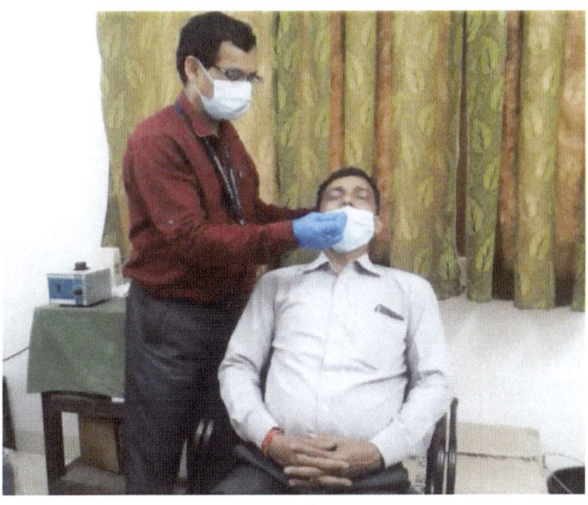

RAT being performed using RAT kit (South Korea) at Lab, AGMC and GBP Hospital. Surgical Mask (Myanmar) and Gloves (Myanmar), Tripura

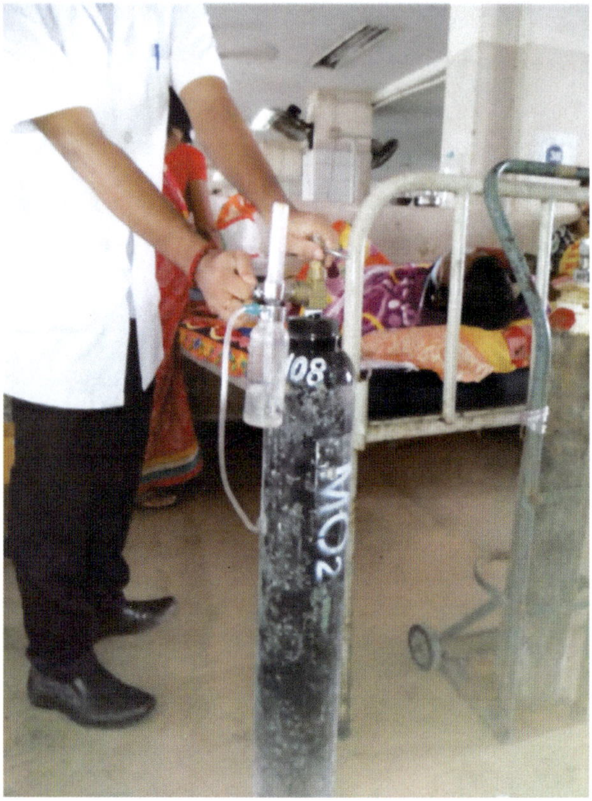

Oxygen Cylinder (Kuwait) in use at a General ward of GPB Hospital, Agartala

Inputs and photographs provided by:

- Dr. Paramjeet, Medical Superintendent, Chandigarh
- Dr. Ramesh Chand, Deputy Director, Health Services (Procurement), Directorate of Health Services, Shimla, Himachal Pradesh
- Ms. Yamini, COVID Nodal Officer, Odisha
- Rinzing Chewang Bhutia, Secretary, Coordination, Home Department, Government of Sikkim
- Dr. Russel Bhattacharjee, Branch Officer (Procurement), NHM and State ASHA Nodal Officer, Tripura

14

COVID TIMELINE

2019					
Dec		First COVID death reported in China			
2020					
Jan	17	GoI travel advisory for travellers to China to follow public health measures at all times			
Feb	31	Evacuation flight from China			
Feb	1	Evacuation flight from China			
Feb	26	Evacuation flight from China			
March	11	WHO declares pandemic			
March	12	COVID Cell created			
March	13	Visa and OCI travels privileges suspended			
March	15	Video Conference of SAARC Leaders			
March	16	24×7 Control Room operational			
March	18	Travel from EU, EFTA, Turkey, Afghanistan, Philippines, Malaysia& UK suspended			

March	19	International flights suspended			
March	24	National Lockdown			
March	26	PM participates in G20 Leaders Summit			
March	30	PM addresses Indian HoMS worldwide			
Apr		Vande Bharat Planning			Outbound evacuation
Apr		Procurement First Wave Starts			
Apr	4	DGFT bans HCQ export	Vande Bharat Mission	Procurement Phase I	
Apr	11	RRTs dispatched to Kuwait			
May	5	Mission Samudra Setu launched			
May	7	Vande Bharat launched			
May	9	SAARC COINEX launched			
May	10	Mission Sagar launched			
May	26	INS Kesari in Madagascar			
May	31	INS Kesari in Comoros			
Jun	4	PM addresses Global Vaccine Summit			
Jun	6	INS Kesari in Seychelles			

Jun	18	Export restrictions on HCQ, including APIs/ formulations lifted			
Aug	7	IX 1344 crashes in Kozhikode			
Sep	26	PM addresses UNGA			
Oct	2	India and South Africa propose TRIPS waiver at WTO			
Nov		Mission Sagar II launched			
Nov	2	INS Airavat in Port Sudan			
Nov	11	INS Airavat in Djibouti			
Nov		Briefing to foreign HoMs in Delhi on India's vaccine program			
Dec		EG2 begins to identify LMO sources in Asia and Oceania			
Dec		Mission Sagar III launched			
Dec	9	Foreign HoMs visit vaccine facilities in Hyderabad			
Dec	24	INS Kiltan in Cambodia			

2021				
Jan		CDSCO approves restricted use of two COVID vaccines		
Jan	20	NEGVAC formed		
Jan	20	Vaccine Maitri begins	Vaccine Maitri	
Mar	12	Prime Minister participates in Quad Leaders Meeting		
Mar	12	Quad Vaccine Experts Group formed		
Mar	22	INS Jalashwa in Madagascar		
Apr		DCGI approves restricted use of Sputnik V		
Apr		Inter-ministerial group formed with senior officials from MEA, MOHFW, MHA, Customs, MCA, Niti Aayog, HLL, IRCS		
Apr	16	HLL issues shot term tender for procurement of 50000 MT of liquid oxygen		
Apr	26	Inter-ministerial group and COVID Task work starts functioning		
Apr	27	First SOPs for accepting gifts/ donations issued		
Apr	28	EAM briefs HoMS on requirements of Indian healthcare system		
Apr	30	Seven emergency airlifts from US deliver medical supplies		
Apr	30	Mission Samudra Setu 2 launched		

May		MOHFW requests MEA to identify sources of Remdesivir, Tocilizumab & Favipiravirtreatment of COVID & Liposomal Amphotericin B, Posaconazole & Isavuconazole for treatment of Mucormycosis.		Procurement Phase 2
May	1	1.5 lakh Sputnik V doses arrive		
May	3	140 MT LMO and 7 ISO containers from UAE arrive at Mundra Port		
May	3	EAM visits the UK		
May	5	40 MT LMO and 2 ISO from Bahrain arrive at Mangalore		
May	10-11	60 MT LMO and 3 ISO tankers from UAE arrive at Mundra Port		
May	10-14	215 MT LMO arrive from Kuwait		
May	24-25	210 MT LMO arrive at Mangalore on INS Shardul from Kuwait		
May	24-28	Visiting the US, EAM informs about requirements of Indian vaccine manufacturers		
Jun		India chairs Quad Vaccine Experts Group		
Jun	12	PM participates in the first Outreach Session of G7 Summit		
Jun	16	72nd and last WHO weekly India Situation report published		
Jul	5	PM addresses CoWIN Global Conclave		

ANNEXURES

Annexure 1a: "Compelling cases"/Preferences for VBM flight boarders from amongst all distress cases

Ministry of External Affairs
COVID 19 Cell
***

ANNEX I

Criteria for Compelling Cases

1) Those facing deportation by foreign governments
2) Migrant workers/Labourers who have been laid off
3) Non-Permanent Residents/Short-Term Visa holders faced with expiry of visas
4) Those faced with medical emergency/seeking treatment for terminal illness
5) Pregnant Women/Elderly
6) Those required to return to India due to death of a family member
7) Tourists/ visitors stranded abroad
8) Students - if their educational institutes/hostels are closed

***

Annex III

Undertaking

To,

Embassy of India,
....

Subject: Consent Form for evacuation from ....(City, Country)

1. I, ... (name, city, country) holding valid Indian passport .... (passport number), confirm my willingness to return to India.

2. I confirm my readiness to follow all instructions given by the officials of Government of India/Embassy of India/Aircraft crew/medical personnel on arrival.

3. I am also willing to undergo a 14 days mandatory quarantine on my arrival in India at my own expense as per the protocols framed by the Government of India.

(Signature with date)
Name: ....
Passport Number:......................................
Mobile :.................................
Email :.....................................

Annexure 1b: Undertaking provided by VBM passengers citing compelling reasons due to which they boarded flights on a priority basis

UNDERTAKING

(To be filled in by passengers seeking a booking in Air India Flight No...............from..................... to .... on ....(date))

1. I am a citizen of the Republic of India/ I am an Overseas Citizen of India.
2. I am in possession of a valid Indian passport No. ..../OCI Card No...............
3. I wish to return to India by Air India under 'Vande Bharat Mission'.
4. I have registered with the Indian Embassy/High Commission/Consulate at .... for returning to India.
5. I shall follow all protocols framed by Government of India under 'Vande Bharat Mission'.
6. I am willing to undergo mandatory quarantine upon my arrival in India as per the SOP of 24 May 2020.
7. I am willing to pay for all expenses with respect to my airfare and quarantine in India.
8. I certify that I meet the criteria of compelling reasons to return as outlined by Government of India.
   (Please tick the relevant category and submit supporting documents)
   (i) Migrant worker/ labourer laid off work (ii) Non-permanent resident/short-term visa holder (iii) Medical emergency (iv) Pregnant woman/Elderly (v) Tourist stranded abroad (vi) Student stranded abroad (vii) Deportee (viii) Death of family member in India
9. I have registered my request for repatriation to India and provided all requisite personal details to the concerned Embassy/ High Commission/ Consulate General of India for uploading on the online portal of 'Vande Bharat Mission'.
10. I certify that I am domiciled in the State of ....in India.
11. I voluntarily give my consent to travel by the repatriation flight under 'Vande Bharat Mission' while fully being aware that I may be inadvertently exposed to any infection, including Covid-19.
12. If any of the above conditions are found to have been not met by me, I agree not to be allowed to board the flight.

I certify that the information provided by me above is true and complete to the best of my knowledge.

(Signature)
Date.............................
Name ....
Mobile No. (in India) ....
Mobile No. (abroad) ....
E-mail id ....

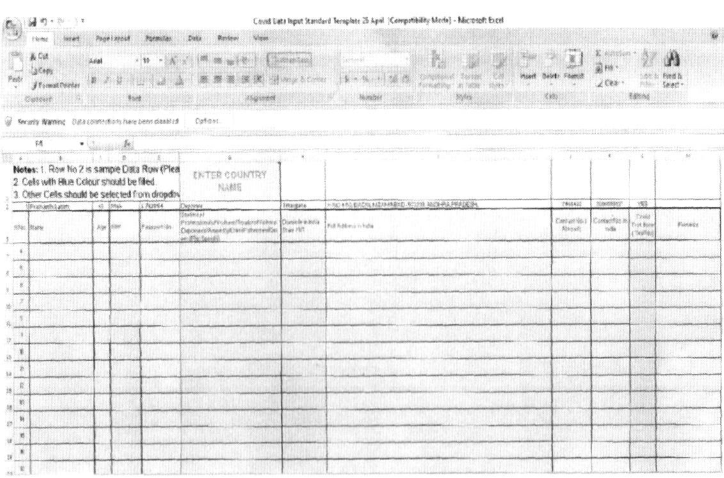

Annexure 1c: MHA Standard Operating Procedures (SoPs) to operate VBM flights, amnesty flights, deportee flights, naval ships

No.40-3/2020-DM-I (A)
Government of India
Ministry of Home Affairs

North Block, New Delhi-110001
Dated 5th May, 2020

ORDER

In continuation of Ministry of Home Affairs' Orders No.40-3/2020-DM-I(A) dated 1st May 2020 and in exercise of the powers, conferred under Section 10(2)(I) of the Disaster Management Act, the undersigned, in his capacity as Chairperson, National Executive Committee, hereby issues Standard Operating Protocols (SOPs), for ***movement of Indian Nationals stranded outside the country and of specified persons to travel abroad, as Annexed*** herewith, to Ministries/Departments of Government of India, State/Union Territory Governments and State /Union Territory Authorities with the directions for its strict implementation.

5/5/2020
Home Secretary

To: **(As per list attached)**

1. The Secretaries of Ministries /Departments of Government of India.
2. The Chief Secretaries/Administrators of States/Union Territories.

Copy to:

i) All Members of the National Executive Committee.

ii) Member Secretary, National Disaster Management Authority.

Annexure to Ministry of Home Affairs' (MHA) Order No.40-3/2020-DM-I (A) dated 5th May, 2020

A. Standard Operating Protocol (SOP) for movement of Indian Nationals stranded outside the country

In order to contain the spread of COVID-19 pandemic, international travel of passengers has been prohibited under MHA's Orders related to lockdown measures. As per information available, many Indian Nationals who had travelled to different countries before the lockdown, on various purposes such as employment, studies/ internships, tourism, business, etc., are stranded abroad. Due to their prolonged stay abroad, they are facing distress and are desirous of returning to India urgently. Apart from the above cases, there are other Indian Nationals who need to visit India in medical emergencies or death of a family member.

2. In order to facilitate the movement of such Indian Nationals, the following SoP is hereby laid down:

i. Such persons will register themselves with the Indian Missions in the country where they are stranded, along with necessary details as prescribed by MEA.

ii. They will travel to India by non scheduled commercial flights to be arranged by Ministry of Civil Aviation (MOCA); and, naval ships to be arranged by Department of Military Affairs (DMA). Only those crew and staff, who are tested COVID-19 negative, will be allowed to operate these flights/ ships.

iii. Priority will be given to compelling cases in distress, including migrant workers/ labourers who have been laid off, short term visa holders faced with expiry of visas, persons with medical emergency/ pregnant women/ elderly, those required to return to India due to death of family member, and students.

iv. The cost of travel, as specified by MoCA/ DMA will be borne by such travellers.

v. Based on the registrations received, MEA will prepare flight/ ship wise database of all such travellers, including details such as name, age, gender, mobile phone number, place of residence, place of final destination; and information on RT-PCR test taken and its result. This data base will be shared by MEA with the respective State/ UT in advance.

vi. MEA will designate State/ UT wise nodal officers, who will co-ordinate with the nodal officers designated for this purpose by the respective States/ UTs.

vii. MEA will display with at least two days notice, the schedule (day, place and time of arrival) of the incoming flight/ ship, on their online digital platform.

viii. Before boarding, all travellers shall give an undertaking that they would undergo mandatory institutional quarantine for a minimum period of 14 days on arrival in India, at their own cost.

ix. All travellers will also be required to give an undertaking that they are making the journey at their own risk.

x. At the time of boarding the flight/ ship, MEA will facilitate thermal screening as per health protocol. Only asymptomatic travellers would be allowed to board the flight/ ship.

xi. Passengers arriving through the land borders will also have to undergo the same protocol as above, and only those who are asymptomatic will be enabled to cross the border into India.

xii. Self-declaration form (with health and personal details) in duplicate will be filled in advance by all passengers coming from any point of entry, i.e., land, sea or airports, and a copy of the same will be given to Health and Immigration officials present at the airport/ seaport/ landport.

xiii. While on board the flight/ ship, the health protocol of MoCA/ DMA will be strictly followed. This would include wearing of masks, environmental hygiene, respiratory hygiene, hand hygiene etc. to be observed by airline/ ship staff, crew and all passengers.

xiv. On arrival, thermal screening, as per health protocol, would be carried out in respect of all the passengers by the Health officials present at the airport/ seaport/ landport.

xv. All passengers shall be asked to download *ArogyaSetu* app on their mobile devices.

xvi. The passengers found to be symptomatic during screening shall be immediately taken to medical facility as per health protocol.

xvii. The remaining passengers shall be taken to suitable institutional quarantine facilities, to be arranged by the respective State/ UT Governments. These facilities may be as far as possible, in the district headquarters, of the district to which the arriving passengers belongs.

xviii. These passengers shall be kept under institutional quarantine for a minimum period of 14 days.

xix. If they test negative after 14 days, they will be allowed to go home and will undertake self-monitoring of their health for 14 more days as per protocol. The remaining persons will be shifted to the medical facility by the State/ UT Government.

***

B. Standard Operating Protocol (SOP) for movement of persons stranded in India who are desirous to travel abroad

In order to contain the spread of COVID-19 pandemic, international travel of passengers has been prohibited under MHA's Orders related to lockdown measures. As per information available, many persons are stranded in India who desirous to travel abroad urgently for various purposes.

2. In order to facilitate the movement of such persons, the following SoP is hereby laid down:

- **i.** Such persons will apply to Ministry of Civil Aviation (MoCA) or to any agency designated by MoCA for this purpose, along with necessary details, including the places of departure and arrival, as prescribed by MoCA.
- **ii.** Only those persons shall be allowed to travel to the destination countries, who are citizens of that country; who hold visa of at least one year duration of that country; and green card or OCI card holder. In cases of medical emergency or death in the family, Indian Nationals holding six month visa can also be allowed.
- **iii.** Before the tickets of such persons are confirmed, MoCA will ensure that the destination country allows entry of such persons in that country. The conditions, if any, imposed by the destination country, will have to be fulfilled by the person intending to travel.
- **iv.** The travel from India shall be by on the non scheduled commercial flights that are being arranged by MoCA for bringing back stranded Indian Nationals from abroad.
- **v.** The cost of travel, as specified by MoCA, will be borne by such travellers.
- **vi.** At the time of boarding the flight, MoCA will ensure that all travellers undergo thermal screening as per health protocol. Only asymptomatic travellers would be allowed to board the flight.
- **vii.** While on board the flight, health protocol as issued by MoCA will be strictly followed. This would include wearing of masks, environmental hygiene, respiratory hygiene, hand hygiene etc. to be observed by airline staff, crew and all passengers.

***

No.40-3/2020-DM-I(A)
Government of India
Ministry of Home Affairs

North Block, New Delhi-110001
Dated 22 August, 2020

ORDER

In continuation of Ministry of Home Affairs' Order No.40-3/2020-DM-I(A) dated 29th July, 2020 and in exercise of the powers, conferred under Section 10(2)(I) of the Disaster Management Act, 2005, the undersigned, in his capacity as Chairperson, National Executive Committee, hereby issue Standard Operating Protocol (SOP), for ***international travel on non-scheduled commercial flights under Vande Bharat Scheme and Air Transport Bubble arrangement,*** in supersession of MHA order of even number dated 24th May, 2020 to Ministries/Departments of Government of India, State/Union Territory Governments and State/Union Territory Authorities with the directions for its strict implementation.

22/08/2020
Home Secretary

To: (**As per list attached**)

1. The Secretaries of Ministries/Departments of Government of India
2. The Chief Secretaries/Administrators of States/Union Territories.

Copy to:

i) All Members of the National Executive Committee.

ii) Member Secretary, National Disaster Management Authority.

Annexure to Ministry of Home Affairs' (MHA) Order No.40-3/2020-DM-I (A) dated 22nd August, 2020

Standard Operating Protocol (SOP) for travel on Vande Bharat and Air Transport Bubble flights

In order to contain the spread of COVID-19 pandemic, Central Government had taken a series of steps to curtail the inward/ outward movement of international passengers (both foreigners and Indians) in a calibrated manner. Further international air travel of passengers (except as permitted by MHA) has been prohibited under MHA's Orders related to lockdown/ Unlock guidelines. For bringing back Indian Nationals stranded abroad, Government of India has launched '***Vande Bharat***' mission. In addition, Ministry of Civil Aviation (MOCA) has entered into the '***Air Transport Bubbles***' arrangements with few countries to allow limited commercial passenger services on reciprocal basis, when regular international flights are suspended as a result of the COVID-19 pandemic.

2. In order to facilitate the movement of persons on these limited international non-scheduled commercial flights, the following SoP is hereby laid down:

A. In-bound flights:

i. The category of persons, who will be eligible to travel on these flights, will be as permitted by MHA from time to time.

ii. Persons desirous to travel to India *on Vande Bharat* flights, will register themselves with the Indian Missions in the country where they are stranded/ residing, along with necessary details as prescribed by MEA. Such a registration may not be required on flights operating under Air Transport Bubbles arrangements.

iii. They will travel to India by non-scheduled commercial flights as allowed by Ministry of Civil Aviation (MOCA); and ships as allowed by Department of Military Affairs (DMA)/ Ministry of Shipping (MOS). Only those crew and staff, who are tested COVID-19 negative, will be allowed to operate these flights/ ships.

iv. SOP for the operations of these flights/ ships will be as issued by MOCA/ DMA or MOS from time to time.

v. Priority will be given to compelling cases of in distress, including migrant workers/ labourers who have been laid off, short term visa holders faced with expiry of visas, persons with medical emergency/ pregnant women/ elderly persons or those required to return to India due to death of family member, and students.

vi. The cost of travel, as specified by the carrier, will be borne by such travellers.

vii. Based on the registrations received for Vande Bharat flights, MEA will prepare flight/ ship wise database of all such travellers, including details such as name, age, gender, mobile phone number, place of residence, place of final destination; and information on RT-PCR test taken and its result. This data base will be shared by MEA with the respective State/ UT in advance.

viii. In case of flights operating under air transport bubbles, passenger manifest containing the same details as given above for Vande Bharat flights or in a revised format as may be finalised by MEA with the country concerned, will be submitted by the airlines to the Indian Mission in the country concerned before operation of each flight with a copy to the State/ UT Government of the destination airport in India.

ix. MEA/ MOCA will designate State/ UT wise nodal officers, who will coordinate with the nodal officers designated for this purpose by the respective State/ UT, both for the Vande Bharat flights as well as for the flights operated under air transport bubbles.

x. MEA and MOCA will display with at least two days' notice, the schedule (day, place and time of arrival) of the incoming flight/ ship, on their online digital platform.

xi. All travellers will also be required to give an undertaking that they are making the journey at their own risk.

xii. While on board the flight, required precautions such as wearing of masks, environmental hygiene, respiratory hygiene, hand hygiene etc. are to be observed by airline staff, crew and all passengers.

xiii. Passengers arriving through the land borders will also have to undergo the same protocol as above.

xiv. The Guidelines on health protocols and quarantine for international arrivals, as issued by Ministry of Health & Family Welfare (MoHFW), from time to time, will be observed.

B. Out-bound flights:

i. The category of persons, who will be eligible to travel on these flights, will be as permitted by MHA from time to time.

ii. MOCA will display on its website the category of persons eligible to travel out of India.

iii. Such persons will apply to MoCA or to an agency/ agencies designated by MoCA for this purpose, along with necessary details, including the places of departure and arrival.

iv. The travel from India shall be on the non-scheduled commercial flights, as are allowed by MoCA.

v. Indian seafarers/ crew seeking to accept contracts to serve on vessels abroad, can travel on the non-scheduled commercial flights as allowed by MOCA or the flights arranged by their employers subject to clearance given by the Ministry of Shipping.

vi. Before the tickets of such persons are confirmed, the airline concerned will ensure that the destination country allows entry of such persons with valid visa in that country. The conditions, if any, imposed by the destination country, will have to be fulfilled by the person intending to travel.

vii. The cost of travel, as specified by the carrier, will be borne by such travellers as prescribed.

viii. At the time of boarding the flight, MoCA will ensure that all travellers undergo thermal screening as per health protocol. Only asymptomatic travellers would be allowed to board the flight.

ix. While on board the flight, required precautions such as wearing of masks, environmental hygiene, respiratory hygiene, hand hygiene etc. are to be observed by airline staff, crew and all passengers.

Annexure 1d: Example of details of assistance provided by Missions to stranded Indians abroad

S. No.	Country	Details of measures taken by the mission to help Covid affected Indians abroad
1.	Austria	Mission provided grocery items/dry food items to the stranded students during lock down period. Mission also helped stranded Indians in identifying suitable accommodation for stay. Few of them were accommodated on concessional rates, whereas some were accommodated by Indian community organization. Mission also took steps to repatriated stranded Indians by providing financial assistance for their return journey.
2.	Bahrain	Data of COVID affected individuals are shared by the local authorities. However mission has set up 24×7 COVID-19 emergency helpline for all kind of assistance the grievants. Indian nationals were provided with masks and sanitizers, food kits etc. The Indian national were kept updated of the designated hospitals and labs. Facilitated the cremation-burial of the mortal remains of Indian nationals who past away due to COVID-19. Regular follow-up were made with companies which notified cases of Covid affected Indian nationals
3.	Belarus	Belarus has very small Indian community and no lockdown was imposed in the country during 2020. However the Mission was in constant touch with the Indian student community to extend all possible support in case any need arose. The Ambassador chaired several video conferences with the students and faculty of the Universities to assess the situation on the ground and extend support where required. Emergency number to contact the Embassy staff was also shared with them and the representatives of Medical Universities.
4.	Bangladesh	1. Timely dissemination of Government guidelines on health preventive measures. Medical testing facilities and travel in consultation with host Govt. 2. Assistance to stranded Indians by providing food items, transport, air tickets, etc. 3. Repatriation of stranded Indian Nationals under Vande Bharat flights and through ICPs in coordination with Ministry and Bureau of Immigration, MHA, GoI and Host Government. 4. Intervened positively with immigration authorities of host Government to sort out visa extension issues during pandemic. 5. Liaison with host Govt. for successful introduction of Air Bubble Scheme between both the countries.

5.	Canada	To help Indians affected by COVID pandemic, Mission took several measures viz., Opening of automated Chatbot for answering queries related to COVID-19; HCI Diaspora WhatsApp group created with leaders of Community Organizations across Canada to better coordinate support and assistance to distressed Indians and Indian Students; Established Dedicated mobile phone helpline 24×7 for answering queries related to COVID-19; Mission also worked with local Indian community organizations as well as student associations to mobilize volunteer's to assist with social work; Several restaurants/grocery shops/pharmacies have been encouraged by the Mission to provide support by providing food delivery to needy students.
6.	Chile	The Mission established a Shelter at Embassy's old premises to accommodate stranded Indian nationals where 18 affected Indians were provided with BL facilities.
7.	China	Authorities accordance with regulations in this regard. However, Embassy was in touch with them and provided assistance as asked for by Indians regarding the issue. As there was a shortage of masks in China during the initial period of COVID, Post obtained masks from Indian and had them distributed to the local Indian community. Post also made arrangements for food for some of the Indian students who had run out food supplies during the initial days of the COVID outbreak in China. Indian nationals in distress including Indian students were assisted in terms of getting their local visas extended. Post intervened with universities in China to help students get their completion certificates including attestations of medical certificates in a timely manner. During the lockdown in China, the Post facilitated the movements of Indian nationals who to travel inter-city or intracity to catch flights. As and when required timely counseling of students and other stranded Indians were done telephonically. The Indians who were under medical observation and quarantine were also helped through and in consultation with the concerned Provincial Foreign Affairs Offices.

8.	Germany	1. A 24-hour Covid helpline was created by the Embassy of India, Berlin to help distressed Indians affected by Covid-19. The helpline was manned round the clock by Embassy Staff and necessary guidance was provided to all the distressed Indians in respect of seeking medical aid, making travel arrangements for travelling back to India and other personal issues. 2. EoI Berlin worked in close coordination with Indian Community and Student Associations to help Indians affected by COVID-19 in Germany. A COVID-19 Relief Fund was created to help distressed Indians and majority of the contribution in the Relief Fund was made by EoI Berlin. Indian Community and Students associations were closely involved in directing relief to distressed Indians through the Covid Relief Fund. The fund was used for providing food coupons, health insurance and aid for medical treatment to the affected Indians. 3. EoI Berlin was also in touch with local medical teams of doctors and paramedics to guide the Indian patients for the requisite medical aid. 4. Information on Covid test centres, doctors and medical process in Germany were provided to the affected patients approaching the Embassy.
9.	Indonesia	As reported by the ministry of Health, three Indians contracted COVID-19. In one of the cases, Mission was in constant touch with the individual and facilitated his treatment at a prominent hospital, when beds were difficult to come by. However, the other individuals and/or their families did not contact the Embassy. In general, Mission worked around the clock to assist fellow Indians in all respects curing lock down in India. 08 Indians were provided boarding and lodging assistance under ICWF to the tune of INR 35,878.47. Mission issued recommendation letters to the immigration authorities requesting for extension of visas to stranded Indians until lock down was lifted in India, based on which their visas were extended. Some Indians who were stranded in Indonesia, during the period, were also provided basic sustenance like groceries and items of daily use. Similarly, many Indians were also assisted by the Gurudwaras and Indian Communities in Indonesia for food and related assistance in collaboration with the Mission.

10.	Iran	1. Setting up of ICMR COVID-19 testing laboratory. 2. Hiring of dedicated quarantine facilities. 3. Provision of food and accommodation. 4. Arrangement of visit by doctors twice a day. 5. Arrangement of Emergency Medical Care (EMC). 6. Provision of items of medical hygiene viz., masks, gloves, sanitizers, etc. 7. Close monitoring of affected nationals by Mission members'. 8. Dissemination of MoHFW and MoAYUSH health advisors. 9. Provision of transportation. 10. Overseeing safe return to India.
11.	Ireland	1. 24×7 helpline established for addressing concerns/ queries via calls/emails/social media, advising to follow necessary health measures as prescribed by HSE Ireland and informing about flights to India under VBM/air bubble agreement with UK, Germany, Netherlands and France. 2. Advisories and necessary information updated on Mission's website. Facebook/twitter handle on regular basis. Ambassador also addressed the community through regular video messages with updates appealing for collective community efforts. 3. Indian Community Support Groups (CSGs) have been formed with members from various provinces where there are large Indian communities including students. Community members represent different profession including medical, business and university professors. CSGs are accessible via calls/emails for addressing needs and providing required help. CSGs are spending lot of time counseling students going through anxiety and other issues. Ireland has around 5000 students.
12.	Israel	Upon receipt of intimation of Indian national(s) being Covid-19 affected, Mission remained constant touch with (i) the patient(s) (ii) their family members in India (iii) relative, colleagues, community people in Israel (iv) local health authorities, and (v) regularly monitored their status until their full recovery and resumption of job by them s also extended help in repatriation to India as per need.

13.	Italy	Mission was regularly in touch with Indians affected by COVID in Italy as well as their family members. Regular updates were received from local authorities, particularly hospitals, regarding the state of health of affected people and to keep their families informed. Assistance was also provided in terms of food distribution, support to local communities and repatriation flights. A medical team from India also joined the mission to take swab tests and help students and stranded Indians to come back to India safely.
14.	Kenya	The High Commission was in constant touch with the Indians in Kenya during the lock down including with the community associations. Various advisories for maintaining COVID protocol were issued and circulated. Stranded Indians and distress were helped with food and accommodation with the help of community associations/ Gurudwaras. Additionally, laid off employees were assisted by approaching their employer for giving them their dues. Anybody who called the Mission's emergency number with COVID related issues/queries were duly entertained/assisted by the Mission staff handling the emergency number.
15.	Kuwait	Food kits were supplied with the help of the Indian Community Supported Group floated by Indian Embassy medical assistance was provided with the help of IDF, shelter and legal advice was provided to the stranded Indians and air tickets from ICWF were provided on means-tested basis.
16.	Lebanon	The Embassy has been extending all possible assistance to the Indian community members and is also providing help in the form of financial assistance to various Gurudwaras and local community organization. The Mission also facilitated provision of dry ration through local community volunteers. The Embassy regularly takes up with the company officials for the recovery of salary dues, insurance claims, etc. in care of the two COVID-19 death the Mission facilitated local burial as transportation of mortal remains to India was not allowed.

17.	United States	All possible help to distressed Indian students/nationals for various needs, including provision of temporary accommodation to Indian students whose colleges closed down and moved to online format of instructions and were asked to vacate hostels/dormitories. 1. While the community organization and individuals came forward to accommodate and help the Indian students in need. Asian American Hotel Owners Association (AAHOA) and other Indian Hotel owners came forward and provided free accommodation and food to the needy students. 2. A series of advisories for Indian students in the US were issued, which were regularly updated to apprise and guide the students in the context of obtaining circumstances. 3. Peer-to-Peer helpline was also started to provide counselling and guidance to the Indian students. 4. Mission organized a Live Chat session with distressed Indian students on Instagram, wherein students were assured of all possible help from the Embassy/ Consulates and emphasized on the need to stay safe and healthy by following all prescribed medical precautions. 5. Outreach was made to Indian community doctors in the US to provide medical help to those in need, including visiting parents, who had to defer/ reschedule their travel because of travel restrictions and evolving medical conditions. Apropos outreach. American Association of Physicians of Indian Origin (AAPI) dedicated resources including online/on phone consultation to those in need. 6. 24×7 helpline was established by the Embassy and the US Government to clarify and consider requests for visa status/extension because of inability to travel or getting stranded. 7. Formed terms in Embassy and Consulates to specifically deal with such requests and advise them and help in the obtaining situation. 8. Closely coordinated with Community and other groups to assist the distressed people in the best possible manner. Extensive outreach and publicity to such efforts was given to ensure that those in need are aware of the efforts and thus able to get possible relief.

Annexure 1e: SoPs for operating Charter Flights

AV-13029/1/2020-A-MOCA
Government of India
Ministry of Civil Aviation
****

'B' Block, Rajiv Gandhi Bhawan,
New Delhi, the 26th May, 2020

To,
Directorate General of Civil Aviation,
(Kind Attn.: Shri Arun Kumar, Director General),
Opp. Safdarjung Airport,
New Delhi-110003

Sub: Standard Operating Protocol (SOP) for Private aircraft and Charter operations on international sectors in view of COVID -19 pandemic

Sir,

The Ministry of Home Affairs vide order no. 40-3/2020 – DM – I(A) dated 24th May 2020, has permitted international charter operations and operations by private aircraft to bring back stranded Indian nationals to India. The MHA has also permitted certain categories of OCI Card holders to come to India in terms of the Ministry of Home Affairs Order No. 25022/24/2020-F.V/F.I dated 22nd May, 2020.

2. In order to facilitate the movement of stranded Indian nationals and certain OCI Card holders, a Standard Operating Protocol (SOP) for Private aircraft and Charter operations on international sectors in view of COVID -19 pandemic has been prepared by this Ministry. The same is enclosed herewith for strict compliance.

3. This issues with the approval of Hon'ble Minister of State(IC) for Civil Aviation.

Yours faithfully

APant
(Anup Pant)
Under Secretary to the Government of India
Tel.011-24617547

Copy for information to:

1. Ministry of Home Affairs [Kind Attn: Shri S.K. Jindal, Joint Secretary(DM); Email: jsdm@nic.in]
2. Ministry of External Affairs [Kind Attn: Shri Dammu Ravi, Additional Secretary(DM); Email: d.ravi@mea.gov.in]
3. Ministry of Health & Family Welfare [Kind Attn: Shri Lav Agarwal, Joint Secretary; Email: alav@ias.nic.in]
4. Chairman, Airports Authority of India [Shri Arvind Singh; Email: chairman@aai.aero]

Standard Operating Protocol (SOP) for Private aircraft and Charter operations on international sectors in view of COVID -19 pandemic

1. **Objective**

a. In order to contain the spread of COVID-19 pandemic international travel of passengers has been prohibited under Ministry of Home Affairs' orders related to lockdown measures. Many Indian nationals who had travelled to different countries before the lockdown on various purposes such as employment, studies / internship, tourism, business etc. are stranded abroad. Due to their prolonged stay abroad, they are facing distress and are desirous of returning to India urgently. Apart from the above cases, there are Indian nationals who need to visit India in medical emergencies or death of a family member.

b. Vide Ministry of Home Affairs' order no. 40-3/2020 – DM – I(A) dated 24th May 2020, the Government has permitted international charter operations and operations by private aircraft to bring back such stranded Indian nationals to India. The Government has also permitted certain categories of OCI Card holders to come to India in terms of the Ministry of Home Affairs Order No. 25022/24/2020-F.V/F.I dated 22nd May, 2020.

c. In order to facilitate the movement of Indian nationals and certain OCI Card holders, the following SOP is hereby laid down.

2. **General**

a. Such persons will register themselves with the Indian Mission in the country where they are stranded, giving all necessary details as prescribed by MEA.

b. The cost of travel will be borne by such travelers or their employers/hiring firms or by any other entity.

c. Before boarding, all travelers shall give an undertaking that after landing in India, they would undergo COVID-19 related protocols/guidelines issued by the Government of India (Ministry of Home Affairs, Ministry of Civil Aviation, Ministry of Health & Family Welfare and the Ministry of External Affairs) and the State/UT Government concerned.

d. At the time of boarding the flight, only asymptomatic travelers will be allowed to board after thermal screening.

e. All passengers shall be advised to download Aarogya Setu app on their mobile devices.

f. Self-declaration form in the format prescribed by the Ministry of Health (**Annexure 1**) shall be filled in duplicate by each passenger in the flight and handed over to Health and Immigration officials present at the airport.

3. **Flight Clearance**

a. Only the persons registered with the Indian Mission in the country of origin of flight shall be carried on the flight.

b. The operator or the hirer of the charter will submit the flight details at least 4 days in advance to the Indian Mission with a complete list of passengers along with their personal details mentioned in clause 2(v) of part A of the annexure to MHA's order dated 24.05.2020 referred above and obtain an NOC/recommendation from the Mission for the list of passengers to be carried.

c. The operator will also obtain an NOC for the flight from the State/UT Government of the destination airport, either directly or through MEA or through the Indian Mission in the country from where the passengers are to be evacuated.

d. After receiving the NOC/recommendation from the concerned Indian mission for passengers to be carried, the concerned State/UT Government's clearance and slot clearance from the concerned airport, the operator will apply to DGCA for flight clearance, with an undertaking that the applicable guidelines of the Government of the country of departure, the Government of India and the State Government concerned shall be complied with and the passengers shall be fully informed about the same.

e. On receipt of the flight clearance request as per (d) above, the flight shall be cleared by DGCA as per extant rules and guidelines.

f. Ground handling agency engaged by the operators or State/UT Governments to ensure its staff is fully briefed and regularly updated as per existing orders on COVID-19 related protocols/guidelines issued by the Government of India (Ministry of Home Affairs, Ministry of Civil Aviation, Ministry of Health & Family Welfare and the Ministry of External Affairs) and the State/UT Government concerned.

g. The operator shall furnish the passengers manifest of each flight in the format prescribed below to the concerned State/UT Government:

Seat Number (In Sequence)	**Name of the Passenger**	**Contact Number**	**Destination Address**	**Pin code of the Destination Address**

4. **Crew Protocol**

a. Cabin crew serving the passengers to wear Personal Protection Equipment (PPE) which include medical protective masks, medical rubber gloves, goggles / face shield, disposable medical caps, disposable protective clothing.

b. Flight crew members to use surgical masks and goggles. Disposable protective clothing can also be worn if so required by a specific task.

c. PPE wearing/taking-off procedure:

- **Donning**: clean and disinfect hands - wear cap - wear facial mask - wear gloves- wear protective clothing - wear goggles / face shield - wear shoes cover - clean and disinfect hands.
- **Doffing**: clean and disinfect hands - take off goggles / face shield - clean and disinfect hands - take off protective clothing including shoe cover - clean and disinfect hands - take off facial mask - clean and disinfect hands - take off cap – take off gloves - clean and disinfect hands.

d. The mask should be close to the face, covering the nose and mouth completely. When the mask is on or being removed, the crew must not touch the outer layer of the mask with hands to avoid hands contamination. Once dampened by secretions or contaminated by other contaminants, facial masks must be replaced immediately with new ones, and hands should be cleaned with sanitizer both before and after the replacement.
e. Flight crew members should wear masks while in the cockpit and crew rest area. All crew members should change their masks at regular intervals in case of long and ultra- long-haul flights.
f. All disposable protective equipment, after their use, should be placed in yellow medical waste bags. After the flight, they should be sprayed or sprinkled with disinfectant before cleaning, and packed in a tightly knotted plastic bag for centralized disposal as medical wastes.
g. The crew can use alcohol-based disinfection wipes or non-alcohol rinse free hand sanitizer to clean and disinfect hands. When crew members are not sure whether their hands are clean, they should avoid touching their noses, mouths and eyes with their hands. When sneezing or coughing, one should try to lower the head or turn away from passengers and crew members nearby, and cover the mouth and nose with tissue or flexed elbow. After touching or disposing wastes, hands should be cleaned with soap or hand sanitizer under running water followed by hand cleaning and disinfection.
h. Goggles should be promptly sanitized and dried every time after use.
i. Crew members should reduce their entry/exit of the cockpit and use intercom system for communication whenever they can to avoid close contact. They should avoid two of them dining at the same time to the greatest extent possible. They should use rinse free hand sanitizer to clean and disinfect hands before meals.
j. Cabin crew should be assigned to provide service in their designated areas, avoid close contact with passengers and only provide necessary in-flight service. Cabin crew also to be designated to provide basic service for flight crew members when needed.
k. There shall be no sale of any item on board in order to minimize interaction of the crew with passengers.
l. Lavatory should be sanitized once every hour, or after being used 5 times whichever is earlier, during flight, and after disinfection, hands should be cleaned and disinfected.

5. **Passenger Boarding Protocol**

a. During boarding and at the airports, all possible measures to ensure social distancing to be ensured.
b. Each passenger at the time of boarding would be handed over a safety kit containing at least 2 three-layer surgical masks, face shield and pouches / small bottles of hand sanitizer.
c. Cabin crew / boarding staff to ensure that each passenger at the time of boarding has his hands sanitized and wears a fresh mask and face shield before entering the aircraft.
d. The passengers would be seated in the aircraft sequentially from rear to front,

with passengers on windows being seated first so as to prevent any crowding or crossing over in the aisles.

e. Passengers would be sensitized by way of repeated announcements, during boarding as well as during flight about various precautions w.r.t. prevention of spread of COVID-19. The precautions include use of hand sanitizer, continuous wearing of mask and face shield, minimum use of lavatories with all precautions of sanitization, no or restricted movement during the flight and sanitizing hands before taking meals and after use of lavatories.
f. No newspapers / magazines or other non-essential loose items to be carried on board. In-flight entertainment to be switched off to minimise touch on aircraft surfaces.
g. If a bus is being used for boarding, the operators shall ensure that the bus is not crowded. Also, the bus should be sanitized continuously.
h. The operators should ensure that there is no crowding on the step ladder. The grab rails of the step ladder should be sanitized continuously.

6. **Catering / Meals Protocol**

a. No or minimum catering (pre packed cold meals / snacks – depending on the duration of flight). No tea coffee service shall be available.
b. Water bottles and pre-packaged food (wherever required) would be placed on passenger seats before passenger boarding to minimise passenger interaction with the cabin crew. Additional water bottles would be available in galley area on self-service basis. The same is also to be informed to the passengers during boarding and in-flight announcements.

7. **Medical Emergency Protocols**

a. In case of ill passenger or a passenger showing COVID-19 symptoms like fatigue or cough, high fever etc., the passenger should be isolated from the other passengers and a dedicated crew in complete protective gear be assigned to handle the case.
b. A specific area of the aircraft should be reserved as a quarantine area for handling possible in-flight emergencies. Special protections like PPE and sanitizers to be used by crew for handling such cases. Adequate quantity of PPE to be available for a possibility of more than one such case.

8. **Disembarkation / Arrival Protocol**

a. After arrival in India, the disembarkation would be staggered and sequential to ensure social distancing.
b. As far as possible, entry of ground staff and cabin crew to the cockpit should be restricted to minimum possible.
c. After disembarkation, the passengers and crew members will be subject to the COVID-19 protocols/guidelines issued by the Government of India (Ministry of Home Affairs, Ministry of Civil Aviation, Ministry of Health & Family Welfare and the Ministry of External Affairs) and the concerned State/UT Government.

9. **Disinfection of aircraft**

a. Suitable precautionary measures such as environmental sanitation and disinfection shall be ensured within the flights.

Ministry of Health & Family Welfare
Government of India

SELF DECLARATION FORM TO BE FILLED BY ALL INTERNATIONAL PASSENGERS
(TO BE PRESENTED AT THE HEALTH & IMMIGRATION COUNTER)

All persons coming to India are required to fill up the Proforma in duplicate & submitting a copy each to Heath and Immigration Counter

Personal Information

1.	Name of the Passenger	
2.	Seat No.	
3	Flight No.	
4.	Passport No.	
5.	Nationality	
6.	Age(in years)	
7.	Date of Arrival	
8.	Port of Origin of journey	
9.	Port of final destination	

Contact Address in India for All Travellers:

1.	House Number	
2.	Street/Village	
3	Tehsil	
4.	District/City	
5.	State	
6.	PIN code.	
7.	Residence Number	
8.	Mobile Number * (mandatory field)	
9.	Email-ID	

(Part-A)

a. Details of the cities/ countries visited in last 28 days_______________

b. Do you presently have any of the following symptoms:

☐ Fever ☐ Cough ☐ Respiratory Distress

- Are you suffering from (Please indicate)-(Hypertension, Diabetes, Bronchial Asthma, Cancer, Under Immunosuppressive therapy, Post- Transplant patients or any other illness).

- I am not suppressing any relevant/ material facts and all the above stated information is correct to the best of my knowledge. Non-disclosure/ suppression of information may attract penal provisions.
- I undertake this journey at my own risk of contracting any disease including COVID 19 and Air India will not be liable for any costs incurred or damages suffered upon, either direct or indirect, as a result of or incidental to such illness and I release Air India from any liability of any kind arising there from. I shall follow Quarantine and/or any other instructions as prescribed by health authorities, at prescribed location, at my own cost on arrival at destination (14 days as prescribed currently).

Signature of the passenger

In case you develop symptoms such as fever and cough within 28 days of leaving this airport, restrict your outdoor movement and contact MoHFW'S 24 hours helpline number 011-23978046. Call operator will tell you whom to contact further, in the meanwhile keep yourself isolated in your house/room.

Annexure 1f: A Snapshot of Flights and Arrivals during the VBM Phases

S. No	Phase	Number of flights	Estimated Number of Pax*
1.	Phase 1: 7-17 May 2020	84	15296
2.	Phase 2: 18 May – 10 June 2020	260	50594
3.	Phase 2 Additional: 26 May – 12 June	186	34112
4.	Phase 2++: 10-22 June 2020	690	127319
5.	Phase 3: 23 June -3 July 2020	862	167217
6.	Phase 4: 4 July – 1 August 2020	1673	368433
7.	Phase 5: 2 August – 31 August 2020	1712	333090
8.	Phase 6: 1 – 30 September 2020	1871	330201
9.	Phase 7: 1-31 October 2020	2114	419252
10.	Phase 8: 1 November – 31 December 2020	4687	1140214
11.	Phase 8+: 1- 31 December 2020		
12.	Phase 9: 1- 31 January 2021	2002	497502
13.	Phase 9+: 1 - 28 February 2021	2215	445375
14.	Phase 10: 1 – 26 March 2021	3537	725746
	TOTAL	**20715**	**4498739**

*Calculated from data avaibale on repat Portal and Daily Reports of MEA for the concerned time periods.

Annexure 1g: Deployment of Senior Officer at the rank of Additional Secretary and Joint Secretary to each State/Country

MINISTRY OF EXTERNAL AFFAIRS
Administration Division
****

No.JS(AD)/MEA/3/2020 Dated 3 May 2020

Sub: **MEA TEAMS FOR REPARTRIATION OF INDIANS FROM ABROAD**

Ministry is planning to facilitate the return of Indians who are stranded abroad owing to COVID-19 situation at an appropriate time. This involves close coordination with various Ministries and Departments in the Government of India, foreign governments, and State Governments with the active participation of our Embassies in the different countries. I am directed to convey that the following teams from MEA are being constituted to undertake the coordination of this exercise.

STATE LEVEL COORDINATORS

S.No.	State	Coordinator Mr./Ms./Dr.	Assisting officer Mr./Ms./Dr.
1.	Andhra Pradesh	Harish Parvathaneni, AS (ED & States)	Sowmya Nair, US (FSI)
2.	Bihar	Alok Ranjan Jha, JS (Estt)	Manoj Bihari Verma, US (DPA-IV)
3.	Delhi/Haryana	Neena Malhotra, AS (Indo Pacific)	Nitin Pramod, US (DPA-II)
4.	Gujarat	Dinesh Patnaik, DG, ICCR	Rajesh Kumar Jain, US Conference
5.	J&K and Ladakh	Yogeshwar Sangwan, JS (OIA-I)	Pankaj Phukan, US (CCCS)
6.	Jharkhand	Manish, JS (OIA-II)	Mukesh Kumar, DS (EAF)
7.	Karnataka	Nagma Malik, AS (Africa)	Vinesh Kalra, DS (PV)
8.	Kerala	Vikram Doraiswami, AS (IO)	Asha Anthony, US (LAC)
9.	Maharashtra	Suresh Reddy, AS (Europe)	Vaibhav Tandale, US(MER)
10.	Orissa	Rahul Srivastava, JS (FSI)	Seema Pujani, US (WA)
11.	Punjab	Virander Paul, AS (BSN)	Saravjit Soodan, DS Maldives
12.	Rajasthan and Goa	Manoj Bharti, AS (AD)	Gince K. Mattam, DS (IP)
13.	Tamil Nadu	C. Rajasekhar, OSD	Sivaguru, DS (IOR)
14.	Telengana	Bala Bhaskar, Joint Secretary	Pawan Tripathi, UC(CD)
15.	UP and MP	Akhilesh Mishra, AS (DPA)	Sandeep Kumar, DS (PAI)
16.	West Bengal	Arun Chatterjee, JS (PSP)	Sandeep Kumar, US (Extradition)
17.	Rest of India	Robert Shetkintong, JS (Coord)	P.K. Vaish, US (CCCS)

COUNTRY LEVEL COORDINATORS

S.No.	Country/Region	Coordinator Mr./Ms./Dr.	Assisting officer Mr./Ms./Dr.
1.	South East Asia/Australia/NZ/Pacific Island Nations	Vishvas Sapkal, JS (South)	Kumar Gaurav, US (Vig)
2.	Americas	Gouranglal Das, JS (AMS)	Devika Lal, US (D&ISA)
3.	Europe	Sandeep Arya, JS (EW)	Ram Karan Verma, Dir (CE)
4.	Russia/Central Asian Republics/Baltics/Armenia/Georgia/ Ukraine	Manish Prabhat, JS (ERS)	Prashant Kumar Das, DS (SCO)
5.	UAE/Bahrain/Oman/Iraq	Nagendra Prasad, JS (Gulf)	Aparna Ganesan, US (DPA-III)
6.	Kuwait/Saudi Arabia/Qatar/Yemen	Nikhilesh Giri, JS (WANA)	Ashish Sharma, DCP (C)
7.	Nepal/Bhutan	Piyush Srivastava, JS (North)	Northern Division Officer
8.	Afghanistan/Iran	Deepak Mittal, JS (PAI)	PAI Division Officer
9.	Bangladesh/Myanmar	Smita Pant, JS (BM)	BM Division Officer

The State and Country level coordinators would be further assisted by their respective Divisions, in addition to the officers attached as above. In addition, Heads of Branch Secretariats and RPOs in the respective States would assist the State Coordinators in their outreach to the States.

This issues with the approval of Foreign Secretary.

(G. Balasubramanian)
Joint Secretary (Administration)

Distribution:

All concerned.

Annexure 1h: MEA's Structural Reponse & Mobilisation of exisiting resources by activating a flat "matrix"

Deployments related to COVID Cell

No.	Order No.	Date of Order	Order
1.	5955/FS/2021	05-May-21	It has been decided that Shri Anurag Bhushan (IFS: 1995), Joint Secretary (DPA-III) will hold additional charge as Joint Secretary in COVID Cell with immediate effect, until further orders.
2.	5904/FS/2021	01-May-21	It has been decided to deploy Shri Jayant Khobragade [IFS: 1995] as Joint Secretary in the Covid Cell with immediate effect
3.	5194/FS/2021	09-Apr-21	Consequent upon their promotions to Grade-I of Indian Foreign Service, the following officers are re-designated as follows: c) Shri Dammu Ravi as OSD (Europe and Covid-19)
4.	14615/FS/2020	12-Nov-20	It has been decided to make the following deployment with immediate effect: (ii) Shri Dammu Ravi (IFS: 1989) as Additional Secretary (Europe &COVID-19).
5.	8168/JS(AD)/2020	22-Oct-20	In partial modification of Office Order No.7878/JS(AD)/2020 dated 12 October 2020, Shri Sohan Lal [Grade-I of IFS(B)], US (COVID Cell) is redeployed as Under Secretary in OIA-II Division with immediate effect.
6.	7878/JS(AD)/2020	12-Oct-20	It has been decided to make the following deployments with immediate effect: 33. Shri Sohan Lal, US (Admin Pool) [Gr I of IFS (B)] as US (Covid Cell)
7.	5106/JS(AD)/2020	21-Jun-20	It has been decided to make the following deployments with immediate effect: b) Shri R.N. Jayant [Grade-I of IFS (B)] as Under Secretary in COVID Cell vice Ms. Amita Bansal who has already been redeployed;
8.	3842/JS(AD)/2020	19-Jun-20	Reference Office Order of even number dated 05 June 2020. The said Order may be read as follows: Shri Raj Kumar (YOA: 2011) as Under Secretary in OIA-I Division vice Shri Nishi Kant Singh (IFS:2010), DS, who will continue to assist AS (COVID) in repatriation related work.
9.	3842/JS(AD)/2020	05-Jun-20	It has been decided to make the following deployment: (a) Shri Raj Kumar [Grade I of IFS(B)] as Under Secretary in OIA-I Division vice Shri Nishi Kant Singh [IFS: 2010], DS, who will continue to assist AS (COVID) in evacuation related work
10.	3644/JS(AD)/2020	23-May-20	It has been decided to temporarily deploy the following officers to assist AS(IO) in Covid-19 repatriation related work: 1) Ms. Deepti Jharwal, DS(SCO); and 2) Shri Rishi Pal, US, Administration pool.
11.	3490/JS(AD)/2020	16-May-20	In partial modification of Office Order No. 483/JS(AD)/2020 dated 15 May 2020, it has been decided to temporarily deploy Mr. Gajraj Singh Bhati, Under Secretary in Admin Pool, to assist Additional Secretary (IO) in Covid-19 repatriation related work, vice Shri Karun Bansal, DS, BM Division.
12.	3483/JS(AD)/2020	15-May-20	It has been decided to temporarily deploy the following officers to assist AS(IO) in Covid-19 repatriation related work: 1) Shri Karun Bansal, OS, IOR Division; 2) Shri Vikram Vardhan, US, CPV Division; and 3) Shri Ved Prakash Singh, US, ERS Division.

13.	**3292/JS(AD)/2020**	**05-May-20**	It has been decided to deploy Shri Yatin Patel, Deputy Secretary in XPD Division, to assist Additional Secretary & Coordinator for COVID-19 until further orders. He may report to AS(Covid) with immediate effect.
14.	**3062/JS(AD)/2020**	**20-Apr-20**	It has been decided to make the following deployments: 2. Ms. Rachita Bhandari (IFS: 2005) as Director (AMS) vice Shri Kartik Pande; She will continue to assist COVID Cell.
15.	**3043/JS(AD)/2020**	**16-Apr-20**	It has been decided to deploy Dr. Venkatachalam Murugan (IFS: 2005), Director, to assist Additional Secretary & Coordinator for COVID-19 until further orders. He may report to AS (COVID) with immediate effect.
16.	**1015/US(FSP&Cadre)/2020**	**03-Apr-20**	Further to earlier orders in this regard, it has been decided to deploy the following officers / staff to assist Additional Secretary & Coordinator for COVID-19 from 4 April 2020 until further orders: 1. Ms Kiran Khatri, Under Secretary (E&SA Division) 2. Dr Vined Gaikwad, Under Secretary (Southern Division) 3. Shri Deepak Bansal, Under Secretary (CE Division) 4. Ms Suman Sonkar, Under Secretary (L&T Division) 5. Shri Sandeep Grover, Under Secretary (PSP Division) 6. Shri Lijo Thomas, Steno, L& T Division 7. Shri Sanjay, MTS, Pension Section
17.	**3008/JS(AD)/2020**	**30-Mar-20**	The following officers have been temporarily deployed with immediate effect to DPA-II Division to assist JS (DPA-11) in COVID-19 related activities: (a) Shri Gaurav Kumar Thakur (IFS: 2011), US (LAC); and (b) Ms. Soumya Gupta (IFS: 2013), US (ED & States) 2. These officers will work from home in coordination with JS (DPA-II) and may be required to report for duty at the Ministry depending upon circumstances to be decided by JS (DPA-II).
18.	**2903/JS(AD)/2020**	**19-Mar-20**	The following officers are deployed to assist Additional Secretary & Coordinator for COVID-19 with immediate effect and till further orders: 1. Shri Kartik Pande, Director (From AMS Division) 2. Ms. Rachita Bhandari, Director (From Indo-Pacific Division)
19.	**2748/JS(AD)/2020**	**16-Mar-20**	It has been decided to deploy Shri Mohd. Shahid Alam, Deputy Secretary in Gulf Division, to assist Additional Secretary & Coordinator for COVID-19 until further orders, vice Shri Shishir Kothari, Under Secretary.
20.	**2655/JS(AD)/2020**	**12-Mar-20**	It has been decided to deploy the following officers to assist Additional Secretary & Coordinator for COVID-19 until further orders: 1. Dr. Amit Telang, Director (from EA Division); 1 2. Shri Mahesh Kumar, Deputy Secretary (from XPD Division); 3. Shri Shishir Kothari, Under Secretary (from Administration Division); and 4. Ms. Arnita Bansal, Under Secretary (from Administration pool).
21.	**4065/FS/2020**	**07-Mar-20**	Given the developments related to the prevalence of COVID-19, it has been felt that a full-time senior officer is required to coordinate efforts in this regard. It has, therefore, been decided to deploy Shri Dammu Ravi (IFS: 1989) as Additional Secretary and Coordinator for efforts to contain COVID-19 until further orders. 2. Shri Dammu Ravi will be the focal point for all interface between Missions abroad and the Ministry, and between this Ministry and the rest of the Government on matters concerning COVID-19.

Annexure 1i: Presentation made to Prime Minister on Evacuation Strategy by Foreign Secretary

Developments leading to lockdown

Indians Passengers' Arrival		Evacuation of Indians By spl. Flights (Jan-Mar)	
January	22,98,210	China	723
February	18,23,925	Japan	119
March	10,16,310	Iran	1142
		Italy	481
Total	51,38,445	Total	2,471

Date	Measures
13 March	All existing visas suspended; free travel by OCI cardholders put on hold
15 March	All passengers movement through Land Check Posts suspended
18 March	Flights suspended - EU, EFTA, Turkey, Afghn, Ph'pines, Malaysia and UK
22 March	All International flights suspended
24 March	Complete Lockdown imposed

Compelling Reasons

- Consequences of lockdown – Indians stranded abroad
- Labour layoff, Expiry of work permit, Amnesty
- Educational institutes closed
- Separated from families / emergencies – Death, illness
- Indian shipping crew; stranded fishermen
- Threat of sanctions and penalties
- PILs in domestic courts
- Shortage of medical facilities; preference given to locals
- Internal Lockdown in countries abroad

Overview of Indians abroad

Region	Indian Passport Holders	Compelling cases (Short Term)	
Gulf	88,92,633	91,102	1.02%
Russia & Central Asia	80,000	27,967	34.96%
South East Asia & Others	11,74,500	26,909	2.29%
North America	20,41,000	21,200	1.04%
South Asia & IOR	6,60,849	12,892	1.95%
Europe	7,50,585	9,380	1.25%
Africa	1,10,000	2,762	2.51%
South America	5,768	756	13.11%
Total	1,37,43,305	1,92,968	1.40%

Region wise Returning Indians

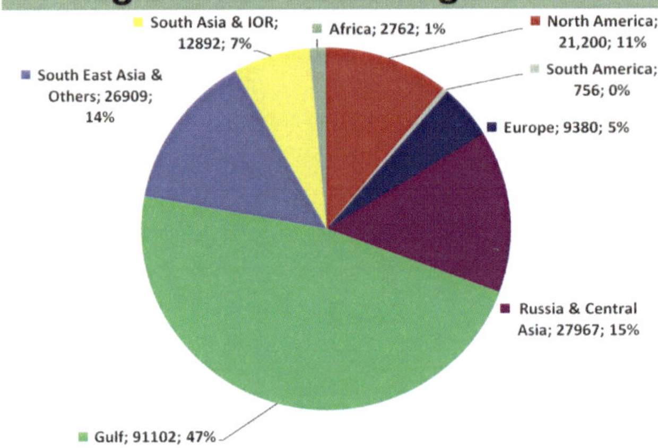

Category of Returning Indians

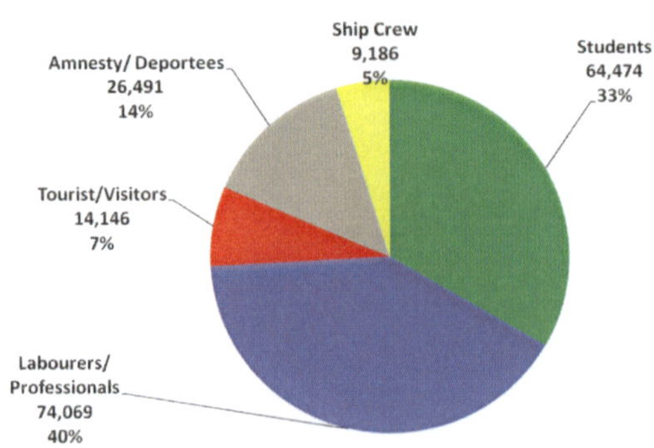

Countrywise-Category of Returning Indians

S.No.	Country	Students	Prof./Workers	Tourists/ Visitors	Amnesty / Deportees	Ship Crew/ fishermen	Total
1	Kuwait		12484	272	24984+260		38,000
2	Oman	66	2576	843	49		3,533
3	S. Arabia	300	6000	687	713		7,700
4	UAE	2709	25000	2291		157	30,157
5	Qatar		8,699	473			9,172
6	Iran	350	610	341		1239	2,540
7	Russia	9420	1,533	47			11,000
8	Kyrgyzstan	7703	0	6			7,709
9	Ukraine	5948	44	8			6,000
10	Kazakhstan	2537	717	4			3,258
11	Philippines	12954		160			13,114
12	Singapore		2,974				2,974
13	Malaysia	193	286	1742			2,221
14	Indonesia		876	724			1,600
15	Australia	3,366	1,401	2090		143	7,000
16	USA	1,966	1539	2544	485	6,466	13,000
17	Canada	7455	248	497			8,200
18	Bangladesh	800	4215				5,015
19	Maldives		3,422	28			3,450
20	Nepal	62	2,980	185			3,227
21	Mauritius	710	465	25			1,200
22	UK	2589	1219	930			4,738
23	Italy	1116	1075	20		1,181	3,392
24	France	611	208	181			1,000
25	Spain	102	100	48			250
26	Other Countries						3,518
	Total	64,424	78671	14146	26491	9,186	1,92,968

State wise Returning Indians

S.No	State	Students	Migrants/Prof.	Tourists/Visitors	Crew	Total
1	Kerala	8282	12139	12065	580	33066
2	Tamil Nadu	5168	3442	3097	430	12137
3	Maharashtra	5134	2293	2421	2172	12020
4	Delhi (NCR)	2513	6017	3111	81	11722
5	Telangana	3284	4770	3036	750	11840
6	Andhra Pradesh	3538	4310	3025	166	11039
7	West Bengal	3088	4433	1229	166	8916
8	Punjab	3362	1081	4257	15	8715
9	Gujarat	3653	780	2351	247	7031
10	Karnataka	1660	1503	2380	557	6100
11	Uttar Pradesh	2729	2406	157	44	5336
12	Haryana	3242	280	169	2	3693
13	Rajasthan	3505	18	86	6	3615
14	Bihar	1270	1365	1117	25	3777
15	Goa	14	43	26	2976	3059
16	Madhya Pradesh	811	342	1912	1	3066
17	Odisha	204	316	1110	16	1646
18	Jharkhand	19	692	1086	6	1803
19	Jammu & Kashmir	711	83	21	1	816
20	Others + Amnesty	270	5330+28,261	7226	2484	43571
	Total					1,92,968

Measures before Arrival

- Missions to prioritize compelling cases
- Pre-arrange passengers domicile wise
- Screening/ Testing at Departure points wherever possible
- Use Non-scheduled commercial flights
- Companies to charter flights at their own expense
- State Govts. to confirm Testing at Arrival + Quarantining
- Arrangements for return of fishermen and sailors – by Ship

Best practices of Quarantine

S.No.	Countries	Screening / Testing Practices
1.	China	Thermal Screening on arrival All Passengers advised Self/Designated/Home quarantine
2.	South Korea	Mandatory home quarantine for 14 days.
	Japan	No quarantine
3.	Italy	Mandatory home quarantine for all passengers from high risk areas Even +ve cases are advised home quarantine; doctors visit them.
4.	Austria	Home quarantine for 14 days advised EU nationals are to present COVID free certificate not older than 4 days or be quarantined for 14 days
5.	Germany	Home quarantine for 2 weeks advised
6.	Malaysia	Mandatory quarantine for 14 days for all passengers.
	Singapore	Self quarantine in dedicated hotels for all passengers
7.	USA, Canada and UK	All passengers irrespective of age advised home quarantine. Only very serious cases are tested and put in hospitals

Annexure 3a: DGFT Notification on Lifting of Export Restrictions on HCQ, including for Formulations and API

(To be Published in the Gazette of India Extraordinary Part-II, Section - 3, Sub-Section (ii))

Government of India
Ministry of Commerce & Industry
Department of Commerce
Directorate General of Foreign Trade
Udyog Bhawan
New Delhi

Notification No. 13/2015-2020
New Delhi, Dated: 18th June, 2020

Subject: - Amendment in Export Policy of Hydroxychloroquine API and its Formulations.

S.O. (E) In exercise of powers conferred by Section 3 of the Foreign Trade (Development & Regulation) Act, 1992 (No. 22 of 1992), as amended, read with Para 1.02 and 2.01 of the Foreign Trade Policy, 2015-20, the Central Government hereby makes the **following amendments in the Notification No. 54 dated 25.03.2020** amending the Schedule 2 of the ITCHS Export Policy related to export of Hydroxychloroquine and its formulations, with immediate effect:

S.No	ITC HS Codes	Description	Present Policy	Revised Policy
207 E	29334900 29333990 29339900	Hydroxychloroquine	Prohibited	Free
207 F	30049059 30049099	Formulations made from Hydroxychloroquine	Prohibited	Free

2 . **Effect of this Notification:**

The Notification No. 54 dated 25.03.2020 has been amended to change the export policy of Hydroxychloroquine API and its formulations from "Prohibited" to "Free", with immediate effect.

18/06/2020
(Amit Yadav)
Director General of Foreign Trade
Ex-Officio Additional Secretary, Government of India
E-mail: dgft@nic.in

(Issued from file No. 01/91/180/21/AM20/EC/E-21154)

Annexure 3b: Words of Gratitude for Vaccine Maitri

S. No.	Country	Twitter/Phone Call/ Press Release
1	**Maldives**	"A short while ago, a flight from India with a 100,000 doses of the CoviShield vaccine arrived in the Maldives, renewing our hopes for a resolution to the Covid 19 crisis soon. Our heartfelt thanks to PM Narendra Modi, government and people of India for this most generous gift". (20 Jan 2021) *– President of Republic of Maldives Ibrahim Mohamed Solih* "Maldives is happy to receive as grant, 100,000 doses of Covishield developed by Serum Institute of India—among the first countries to receive vaccines from India. As always, India stands strong & steadfast, by our side, as 1st responder in any crisis." (20 Jan 2021) *– Abdullah Shahid, Foreign Minister of Maldives* Video Message by Abdullah Shahid, Foreign Minister of Maldives
2	**Bhutan**	"Pleased to receive additional 400,000 doses of Covishield, making possible the nationwide rollout of our vaccination program. People of Bhutan and I remain grateful @narendramodi. We pray these gestures during the pandemic turn into boundless blessings for the people of India". "Overcome with gratitude as the fog of the COVID pandemic begins to retreat in our beloved country." (22 March 2021) "As we wrap up a successful day one of the nationwide COVID-19 vaccination rollout, I would like to thank Prime Minister Shri @narendramodi and his government for the timely support and delivery of the vaccine. You played a big part in making this possible". (27 March 2021) *- Lotay Tshering, Prime Minister of Bhutan.* "Our profound gratitude to the GoI for the generous gift of 150,000 doses of Covishield vaccines that Bhutan received today. Deeply grateful to GoI for its abiding friendship and unconditional support to

		Bhutan's fight against the COVID-19 pandemic. @DrSJaishankar @RuchiraKamboj." (20 Jan 2021) "Received the precious gift of another 400,000 doses of Covidshield vaccines from our friend, India, today. Profoundly grateful to @government of India @PMOIndia @DrSJaishankar @RuchiraKamboj for the unconditional support in our fight against the pandemic." (22 March 2021) • Tandi Dorji, Foreign Minister of Bhutan
3	**Bangladesh**	A video message by Sheikh Hasina, Prime Minister of Bangladesh.
4	**Nepal**	"I thank Prime Minister Shri @narendramodi ji as well as the Governmentand people of India for the generous grant of one million doses of COVID vaccine to Nepal at this critical time when India is rolling out vaccination for it's own people." • K P Sharma Oli, Former Prime Minister of Nepal.
5	**Mauritius**	"We are deeply grateful to India for donating 100 000 doses of Covishield to Mauritius as part of its Mission" Vaccine Maitri".@PMOIndia @narendramodi @HCI_PortLouis." (22 Jan 2021) Pravind Kumar Jugnauth, Prime Minister of Mauritius • Video message by HE Eddy Boissezon, Vice President of Mauritius.
6	**Seychelles**	"My heartfelt thanks to PM @narendramodi, government and people of India for the gift of 50000 doses of Covishield Vaccine. This is a testamentto the close friendship between our two countries and comes at a critical point in our fight against the pandemic" —President Ramkalawan." (22 Jan 2021) Office of the President of The Republic of Seychelles. Video message by the President of Seychelles. "Minister Sylvestre Radegonde expressed his gratitude to the #GOI for thedonation of 50,000 doses of Covishield vaccines to Seychelles.

		He thanked his counterpart Dr. Jaishankar, for ensuring the expeditious delivery of the vaccine to Seychelles @DrSJaishankar @hci_seychelles." (22 Jan 2021) • Ministry of Foreign Affairs and Tourism- Foreign Affairs Dept the Republic of Seychelles.
7	**Sri Lanka**	"Received 500,000 #COVID-19 vaccines provided by #peopleofindia at #BIA today(28). Thank you! PM Shri @narendramodi & #peopleofindia for the generosity shown towards #PeopleofSriLanka at this time in need." (28 Jan 2021) • Gotabaya Rajapaksa, President of Sri Lanka
8	**Brazil**	"- Namaskar, Prime Minister @narendramodi Brazil is honored to have a great partner to overcome a global hurdle. Thank you for assisting us with vaccine exports from India to Brazil. – Dhanyavaad! गा5." (22 Jan 2021) – Jair Messias Bolsonaro, President of Brazil. "O @govbr receives today 2 million doses of vaccine #OxfordAstraZeneca, coming from India to fight the #COVID19. The import was made possible by coordinated actions of the #Itamaraty It's from @minsaude. Brazil thanks the Indian government for its partnership and support." (23 Jan 2021) – Ministry of Foreign Affairs of Brazil.
9	**Morocco**	"Morocco received today, January 22 2021, the first batch of the British vaccine "Astra-Zeneca" made in India, from India. The first batch of the "Sinopharm" vaccine will be delivered on Wednesday January 27, 2021 from the People's Republic of China. (Statement @Ministere_Sante)." (23 Jan 2021) - Statement by Ministry of Health of the Kingdom of Morocco
10	**Bahrain**	"HRH the CP and PM #Salman_bin_Hamad: #Bahrain thanks @narendramodi and our friends in #India for working with us to secure the delivery of the Oxford-AstraZeneca Covishield vaccine. A sign of India's global generosity and the strong partnership enjoyed between our two nations." (28 Jan 2021)

11	**Oman**	"Heartfelt thanks to our close friends in #India. We stand united against COVID-19 and this initiative is a testimony of the bonds of friendship and cooperation between our governments and peoples." (1 Feb 2021) • Sayyid Badr Albusaidi, Foreign Minister (Oman) of Oman Video message by Minister of Health, H.E. Dr Ali Bin Mohammed Bin Moosa
12	**South Africa**	"I spoke to the Prime Minister of India, His Excellency @NarendraModi this afternoon following the arrival of the first batch of #COVID19 vaccines from on Monday. I applauded the Government & people of India for its gift to the world in the form of vaccines & scientific knowledge." (4 Feb 2021) • Cyril Ramaphosa, President of South Africa
13	**Afghanistan**	"The Government of the Islamic Republic of Afghanistan is grateful for the shipment of 500,000 doses of corona vaccine to the Republic of India, which arrived at Hamid Karzai International Airport this morning. President Ghani expresses his gratitude for the timely assistance of the Government and people of India on behalf of the Government and people of Afghanistan." (7 Feb 2021) • Office of the President of Afghanistan Video message by Mohammad Ashraf Ghani Ahmadzai, Former President of The Islamic Republic of Afghanistan. My profound gratitude to my friend @DrSJaishankar, the government & people of India for assisting 500k dozes of "Made in India" vaccines to address #Covid spread in Afghanistan. A clear sign of generosity, commitment & strong partnership indeed. (7 Feb 2021) • Mohammed Haneef Atmar, Former Minister of Foreign Affairs of Afghanistan

14	**Barbados**	"India's gift of 100,000 COVID-19 vaccines arrived Barbados earlier today. This was a very special moment for all Barbadians and I want to thank Prime Minister Modi for his quick, decisive, and magnanimous action in allowing us to be the beneficiary of these vaccines." (10 Feb 2021) • Mia Mottley, Prime Minister of Barbados
15	**Commonwealth of Dominica**	"Good Morning to all Citizens and Residents, Our nation is ready to launch the largest vaccination campaign in modern history as we have received 70,000 doses of the COVID-19 vaccine from India." (10 Feb 2021) "Even though I trust every word of the bible, I must confess that I did not imagine that the prayers of my country would have been answered so swiftly. Thank You India. @narendramodi" (10 Feb 2021) • Roosevelt Skerrit, Prime Minister of the Republic of Dominica
16	**Mexico**	"We received the first shipment of vaccines against #COVID19 from India. This morning, 870 thousand doses arrived out of a total of 2 million that will arrive from the Asian country. We advance in the National Vaccination Policy." (14 Feb 2021) • Account of Presidency of the Government of Mexico. Video message by President of Mexico, Andrés Manuel López Obrador
17	**El Salvador (Stand by)**	"Tomorrow morning, a plane of @Iberia brings the first batch of vaccines against #COVID19 from @AstraZeneca, from India. The vaccination begins tomorrow with our front-line personnel. This will take a few days, vaccinating thousands of health workers daily. A special thanks to the Prime Minister of India, @narendramodi, for their indispensable support, so that vaccines could come to our country faster." (17 Feb 2021) • Nayib Bukele, President of El Salvador

18	**Argentina (Stand By)**	"Today, 580,000 doses of the Covishield vaccine, produced by the Serum Institute and developed by Oxford and AstraZeneca, arrived in the country from the Republic of India. Thanks to the chancellor @DrSJaishankar and to the entire government. Cooperation is the way to defeat this pandemic." (17 Feb 2021) • Felipe Solá, Former Foreign Affairs Minister of Argentina Video message by Ginés González García, Former Minister of Health of Argentina
19	**Dominican Republic**	"With hope and satisfaction we received the first AstraZeneca vaccines, from India. Tomorrow at 7:00 am we begin the vaccination of front-line personnel at the Ramón De Lara Hospital. In the afternoon the process continues in the other COVID hospitals in the country #VacúnateRD" (16 Feb 2021) • Luis Abinader, President of Dominican Republic Video message by Raquel Pena, Vice President of Dominican Republic.
20	**Serbia**	Today I welcomed the plane that delivered the #AstraZeneca vaccines to Serbia. Many thanks to the PM of the United Kingdom @BorisJohnson, Ambassadors @SianCMacLeod, @ukinserbia, the PM of India @narendamodi and the Minister of Foreign Affairs @DrSJaishankar. (21 Feb 2021) • Aleksandar Vučić, President of Serbia
21	**Mongolia (Stand by)**	"Excellency, the vaccines granted from India to Mongolia will tremendously help us in coping with difficulties and challenges caused by COVID-19. Sincere thanks to our Spiritual neighbor and Strategic Partner – India." (22 Feb 2021) • Battsetseg Batmunkh, Minister of Foreign Affairs of Mongolia

22	**Ukraine**	First 500K of #vaccine against #COVID19 arrived in #Ukraine. We are grateful to Indian partners for the #support. We will start vaccination ASAP. We need to fight COVID together. Oxford/AstraZeneca (#Covishield) (23 Feb 2021) • Volodymyr Zelensky, President of Ukraine Grateful to Indian friends for supplying Ukraine with COVID-19 vaccines. Let this historic step in our fight against the pandemic pave the way to new landmark achievements in our partnership #VaccineMaitri (24 Feb 2021) • Dmytro Kuleba, Minister of Foreign Affairs of Ukraine
23	**Ghana**	#Ghana makes yet another stride in its fight against the #Covid-19 pandemic as it has received 50,000 Covid-19 vaccines from the Government of #India today. (5 March 2021) • Shirley Ayorkor Botchwey, Minister for Foreign Affairs of Ghana
24	**Guatemala**	My high thanks to the Chancellor of India @DrSJaishankar for the donation of 200,000 vaccines. The people of Guatemala appreciate and value our friendship. Namaste India! (27 Feb 2021) • Pedro Brolo, Minister of Foreign Affairs of Guatemala #VacunasCovidGT we received the 200 thousand doses of the vaccine #Covishield donated by the Government of the Republic of India. Thank you for this show of appreciation and solidarity towards the Government and People of Guatemala (3 March 2021) • Ministry of Foreign Affairs of Guatemala
25	**Jamaica**	Video message by Andrew Holness, Prime Minister of Jamaica.

26	**St Lucia**	Thank you to Prime Minister @narendramodi and our friends from India for donating 25,000 doses of the AstraZeneca COVID-19 Vaccine to Saint Lucia – Allen M. Chastanet, PM of St. Lucia via Twitter on 2nd March 2021 Video Message by Allen M. Chastanet, PM of St. Lucia
27	**St. Kitts & Nevis**	Our friend #India delivers some 20,000 doses of Oxford-Astra Zeneca #Covid vaccine to save lives in #StKitts #Nevis. We say thanks to Prime Minister Modi and the government and people of India for this humanitarian gesture. A friend in need is a friend indeed! #DiplomacyMatters – Mark Brantley, Minister of Foreign Affairs and Aviation St. Kitts and Nevis and Premier of Nevis via Twitter on 1st March 2021. Video message by Timothy Harris, PM of St. Kitts & Nevis
28	**St. Vincent & Grenadines**	Video message by Ralph Gonsalves, PM of St. Vincent & Grenadines
29	**Suriname**	Video message by Chandrika Parasad Santokhi, President of Suriname.
30	**Antigua & Barbuda**	Thanking PM Modi for the 500K AstraZeneca vaccines that he generously and selflessly shared with the Caribbean to assist in the fight against COVID. – The Office of The Prime Minister Antigua and Barbuda via Twitter on 1st March, 2021 Video message by Gaston Browne, Prime Minister Antigua and Barbuda
31	**Nigeria**	Nigeria takes delivery of the first batch of Oxford-AstraZeneca #COVID19Vaccines from #COVAX. - The Federal Ministry of Information and Culture, Nigeria via Twitter on 2nd March 2021
32	**Cambodia**	Cambodia among first countries to receive #COVID19 vaccines from #COVAX Facility. A Press Release was uploaded on 3rd March 2021. – Office of Cambodian PM

33	**Kenya**	11. 100,000 doses of the Covishield (Oxford-AstraZeneca) COVID-19 vaccine donated by The Government of India has arrived in the Country Thursday evening. Health CS Mutahi Kagwe and Foreign Affairs officials were at the JKIA to receive the consignment. 12. Amb. Isiaya Kabira of Foreign Affairs speaking at the #JKIA observed that the donation by India is testament of the deep friendship and cooperation which has been the hallmark of Kenya 13. – India relations since independence. 14. Foreign Affairs further registered its deep gratitude to the High Commissioner of India and through him to the Government and people of India for the unwavering support to Kenya in the fight against the COVID-19 Pandemic, as well as in national development programs. – Ministry of Foreign Affairs—Kenya via Twitter on 11th March 2021.
34	**Rwanda**	Pleased to receive 50,000 doses of COVID-19 vaccines from India this morning. Govt of Rwanda is grateful to the Govt of India and other partner countries for their valuable contribution to the fight against #COVID19 @DrSJaishankar. Vincent Biruta, Minister of Foreign Affairs and International Cooperation, Government of Rwanda via Twitter on 5th March 2021 Minister @Vbiruta was at Kigali International Airport with Oscar Kerketta, High Commissioner of India to Rwanda to receive a donation of 50,000 doses of #COVID19Vaccine from the Government of #India #RwOT – Ministry of Foreign Affairs and International Cooperation, Government of Rwanda via Twitter on 5th March 2021

35	**Canada**	Video message by Justin Trudeau, Prime Minister Canada
36	**Mozambique**	Compilation video of receiving vaccines
37	**Guyana**	Video messages by President and PM of Guyana
38	**Belize**	Thanks @DrSJaishankar @narendramodi @ rashtrapatibhvn and the people of India for your generous contribution to the health and well-being of the people of Belize! - Johnny Briceño, Prime Minister of Belize via Twitter on 9th March 2021.
39	**Botswana**	Tsogwane said the consignment is a donation from India, and it marks the beginning of a new journey where government will be rolling out vaccination exercise. Vice President said in a weeks" time Botswana will receive another batch that has been ordered by government of Botswana. – Government of Botswana via Twitter on 9th March 2021
40	**Eswatini**	Video by Lizzie Nkosi, Health Minister of Eswatini
41	**Bahamas**	Video message by Hubert Alexander Minnis, Former Prime Minister, Bahamas
42	**Gambia**	Video by Dr Samateh, Minister of Health, Gambia
43	**Cuba**	Video Message by Ambassador of Cuba Ms Maria Estel
44	**Namibia**	Namibia extends her heartfelt gratitude to the government and people of India for the 30,000 doses Covishield vaccine donation. Your donation will make a big difference in our fight against the virus. – Ministry of International Relations and Cooperation of the Republic of Namibia via Twitter on 22nd March 2021

45	**Paraguay**	Acaban de llegar 100.000 dosis de vacunas contra el Covid-19, provenientes de la India. La prioridad es avanzar hacia la inmunisación de todo el personal de blanco y luego la población de riesgo. Gracias a la República de la India por el apoyo. Trans: 100,000 doses of Covid-19 vaccines have just arrived from India. The priority is to move towards immunisation of all target personnel and then the population at risk. Thanks to the Republic of India for the support. – Marito Abd, President of Paraguay via Twitter on 30th March 2021 Hoy arribaron al país las 100.000 dosis de las vacunas COVAXIN, donadas por #India. La República del #Paraguay agradece este gesto que fortalece aún más el relacionamiento entre ambos países que cumplirá su 60° aniversario en el presente año. Trans: Today the 100,000 doses of COVAXIN vaccines arrived in the country, donated by #India. The Republic of #Paraguay appreciates this gesture that further strengthens the relationship between the two countries that will celebrate its 60th anniversary this year. A press release link was also uploaded. – Ministry of External Relations, Paraguay via Twitter on 30th March Lazos de acero unen nuestra amistad con la República de la India. ¡Gracias querido @DrSJaishankar! Trans: Ties of steel unite our friendship with the Republic of India. Thank you dear @DrSJaishankar ! – Euclides Acevedo, Minister of External Relations, Paraguay via Twitter on 30th March 2021.

46	**Fiji**	#VaccineMaitri has arrived to Fiji with 100k doses of life-saving COVID-19 vaccines. Vinaka to my friend, @narendramodi, for helping us take this giant step towards a post-pandemic future for Fiji and for the world. – Frank Bainimarama, PM of Fiji via Tiwtter on 29th March 2021 The consignment of 100,000 doses of Made in India Covishield (AstraZeneca) vaccines was formally presented to Fiji through the Government of India. Vinaka Vakalevu India for this timely assistance. – Fiji Ministry of Foreign Affairs via Twitter on 30th March 2021 Video and Video Message by the PM and Health Minister of Fiji, respectively.
47	**UNPKF**	“India is a longstanding & steadfast supporter of @UNPeacekeeping. I want to thank the Govt and people of, who have generously donated #COVID19 vaccines to benefit our peacekeeping personnel & enable them to continue their life-saving work in a safe manner.” - Jean-Pierre Lacroix, Under-Secretary-General for Peace Operations Shared by United Nations in India via Twitter on 27th March 2021
48	**Zimbabwe**	75,000 more #COVID19 vaccines for Zimbabweans! Thank you to @IndiainZimbabwe and @NarendraModi for supplying this vital first shipment of Covaxin vaccines. – Emmerson Dambudzo Mnangagwa, President of the Republic of Zimbabwe via Twitter on 29th March 2021

Annexure 5a: East Asia Division's Inputs for Procurement Phase-I

- Department of Expenditure (DoE) vide OM No. F 6/18/2019-PPD of 27 March 2020 stated that the prevailing health emergency requires immediate procurement of certain items that may not be available in the country in sufficient quantity within the timeframe in which they are needed.
- Empowered Group (EG) for ensuring availability of essential medical equipment such as PPE, Masks, Gloves & Ventilators; Production, Procurement, Import and Distribution was constituted vide Ministry of Home Affairs (MHA) Order No. 40-3/2020-DM-I(A) dated 29 March 2020. MEA was included as part of EG for facilitation of procurement of essential medical equipment from abroad.
- EG in its first meeting on 29 March 2020 requested MEA to explore more avenues for procurement of ventilators and PPE kits. This request was reiterated in the second meeting of the EG on 30 March 2020. MEA had accordingly asked Missions abroad to send proposals for supply of ventilators, PPE kits, and masks for assessment by MoHFW/HLL. Similarly, proposals were invited for testing kits which were forwarded to ICMR/DHR for assessment.
- DoE vide OM No. F 6/18/2019-PPD dated 1 April 2020, issued further special instructions for procurement by Indian Missions. This OM noted that medical equipment and essential supplies for COVID-19 operations are currently in global short supply and are effectively in a "sellers' market". Further, in a situation of extreme urgency, it is necessary that medical equipment and essential supplies necessary to fight COVID-19 are procured and deployed quickly, and some of these medical supplies, wherever necessary, may need to be imported. The OM therefore, *inter alia,* provided that any or all of the following requirements viz. (i) consultation of Financial Advisors for full advance payment; (ii) obtaining bank guarantee from the supplier for making advance payment and (iii) performance security may be waived off by the EG on the recommendation of the Ambassador/High Commission of India in those cases where it is satisfied that it is unavoidable in the prevailingcircumstances. This was to apply only in respect of procurement of medical equipment made by Indian Missions on behalf of various Ministries/Departments under DoE OM of 27 March 2020. A specific decision was to be recorded by the EG in each case.

- The above-mentioned OM of 1 April 2020 further stipulated that the specifications, price and quantity of medical equipment and essential supplies shall be fixed in the manner prescribed in the Minutes of meeting of EG on 31 March 2020 and further modified from time to time. Paragraph 14 (i) of the said OM also noted that Department of Health & Family Welfare and Department of Health Research may authorise MEA to incur expenditure on its/their behalf through a Letter of Authorisation. The EG in its meeting of 31 March 2020 had decided that payments could be made by the Indian Missions and the concerned Ministry will transfer the funds to MEA for the same.
- In response to the request sent to all our missions, several offers were also received from Indian missions in other countries. It may be noted in this regard that due to major outbreak of COVID-19 pandemic in Europe in March-April 2020, there was shortage of medical products such as PPE, masks, testing kits & ventilators in Europe. European Union regulations had also introduced controls on their exports outside the region and therefore most of the missions in Europe had indicated that it would not be possible to source the relevant medical items from European countries. Offers that were received through some of the missions were shared with MoHFW/HLL/ICMR for evaluation. It was also found that most of these proposals were essentially from trading companies with suppliers based in China and delivery was generally from China. Most of these proposals could not be pursued further as they were not found technically suitable by MoHFW/HLL due to lack of adequate certification/clarifications; or because only limited information being available in the public domain about the companies making the offer; or since the suppliers in China were not registered with the National Medical Products Administration (NMPA) of China.[1] The proposals received for COVID-19 testing-related equipment such as testing kits, RNA extraction kits and Viral Tube Media, etc. were similarly shared with ICMR for its information/evaluation as per its requirement.
- Other facilitations by MEA: As per decisions taken by the EG, MEA requested concerned Missions to get certain medical supplies from China tested and inspected by third parties approved by technical agencies in India, as per technical parameters specified by the latter. Further, specific requests from Indian agencies and manufacturers for expediting supply

and shipment of medical products, machinery and components from abroad were pursued by MEA through our Missions, for example import of components of ventilators for BEL and AMTZ, testing inputs like RNA extraction kits, Roche Cobas testing machines, testing kits from US, Germany, China, Switzerland, Singapore for ICMR/DHR etc. In some cases of orders placed by ICMR for COVID-19 testing with Indian suppliers were facilitated by missions abroad by pursuing with their original suppliers in various countries.

NOTE

1. On 31 March 2020, Chinese Government authorities published a notice that stipulated that Chinese customs authorities would only release products for exports after checking the registration certifications for medical devices approved by the authorities of medical products. This implied that a Chinese company could only export such products if it was registered with NMPA.

Annexure 6a: LMO & ISO Containers—Arrival and Distribution

Sr. No.	Country/ Company	Destination Port	Date & Time of arrival	Remarks
33.	UAE- Arranged by DP World (private offer)	Mundra	Mid-night of 3 May 2021	34. 140 MT LMO allocated to Delhi 35. 7 ISO containers initially provided by DP World till 28 May 36. Extended retention- leased by IOCL till 30 June 2021
37.	Bahrain	Mangalore	5 May 2021; 1400 hrs	38. 40 MT LMO allocated to Karnataka 39. 2 ISO tankers for 2 months with IOCL in Karnataka
40.	UAE-Abu Dhabi National Oil Company (ADNOC)	Mundra	10-11 May 2021	41. 60 MT LMO allocated to Rajasthan. 42. 3 ISO tankers to be used by IOCL for 6 months for further refillings as per their commercial arrangements

43.	Kuwait (Total offered 2400 MT of LMO) Total offtake till date – 425 MT	Mangalore Mumbai-NhavaSheva	INS Kolkata-10 May 2021 INS Tabar & INS Kochi-12/13 May 2021 Kuwaiti commercial vessel: 14 May 2021	44. For shipment of 215 MT LMO on IN ships and Kuwaiti ship allocated to Karnataka
45.		Mangalore	INS Shardul-24/25 May 2021	46. 2 shipment 210 MT LMO -190 MT LMO allocated to Karnataka and 20 MT LMO to Kerala
47.	Kuwait		IN Ships—constraint of operations in Monsoons with loaded tanks on top decks;	3rd shipment not yet departed Reduction in demand in States. It was decided that given the low demand and ramped up production of LMO within the country, we might suspend these imports for the time being.

48.	France/Air Liquide (Filling of LMO in Qatar through Air Liquide's local partner) (Total Offered 600 MT LMO) Total offtake till date – 220 MT	Mumbai	1st IN ship-2 ISOs (40 MT) on 10/5 2nd IN ship-2 ISOs (40 MT) on 12/5 CMA-CGM Commercial ship-1 ISO (20 MT) on 21/5	49. Allocation of LMO to Maharashtra by DPIIT. Hospitals being decided by Govt. of Maharashtra 50. LMO on 10/5, the allocation is as follows: a. 20 MT to Kasturba Hospital, Mumbai b. 20 MT to Sasoon BJ Medical College, Pune
				51. LMO on 12/5, allocation: • 20 MT Jumbo Covid Hospital, COEP MaidanShivaji Nagar Pune a. 20 MT Richardson and Cruddas Mulund Jumbo Covid Centre Mumbai 52. LMO on 21/5 20 MT Sassoon General Hospital, Pune

53.	France/Air Liquide (2nd cycle of refilling) 80 MT of LMO	Mumbai	INS Trikand- 2 ISOs (40 MT) on 22/5 INS Tarkash- 2 ISOs (40 MT) on 24/5	54. Allocation of LMO to Maharashtra by DPIIT. Hospitals decided by Govt. of Maharashtra
55.	France/Air Liquide (Filling of LMO in Qatar through Air Liquide's local partner) (3 cycle of refilling)	Mumbai	The shipment did not materialise as the Navy advised not to carry the containers due to bad sea state.	56. It was decided that given the low demand and ramped up production of LMO within the country, we might suspend these imports for the time being.

Annexure 6b: Standard Operating Procedure for Handling Consignments from Abroad 27.4.21

No. 93/OSD(Covid)/MEA/2021
Government of India
Ministry of External Affairs
(Covid Cell)

27 April 2021

Subject: Standard Operating Procedure (SOP) for handling of consignment of donations/ gifts from abroad

For efficient handling offer of donations/ gifts by foreign governments, NGOs/ Associations, individuals/ companies in view of devastation caused by the second wave of Corona Virus in the country, a Standard Operating Procedure (SOP) is attached to be followed for despatch and receiving the consignments.

(Dammu Ravi)
OSD(Europe & Covid)
Tel: 49015214

To

1. All HOMs/HOP, Indian Missions abroad.
2. All Heads of Divisions, MEA
3. Secretary, Ministry of Home Affairs
4. Member Secretary, National Disaster Management
5. Secretary, Ministry of Health and Family Welfare
6. Secretary, Ministry of Civil Aviation
7. Chairman, CBEC, Ministry of Finance
8. Indian Red Cross Society, New Delhi

Annexure 6c: RT-PCR testing SoP for Crew Operating Cargo Flights arriving from Europe, MiddleEast and UK, 29.4.21

F No AV 13011/5/2020-DT
Government of India
Ministry of Civil Aviation

New Delhi, the 29th April, 2021

OFFICE MEMORANDUM

Subject RT-PCR testing for crew operating cargo flights arriving from Europe, Middle East and the United Kingdom

---

Currently, the guidelines issued by the MoHFW Dtd 17th Feb, 2021 are implemented by the stakeholders of the aviation sector for all International arrivals. According to the guidelines, crew originating/transiting from the UK, Europe, and Middle East regions have to give sample for RT-PCR testing on arrival at Indian Airports. There is no requirement of RT-PCR testing for the crew coming from any other region.

2 Meanwhile, to facilitate smooth air transportation of people and cargo, clarifications have been issued by MoCA.

i The Crew of Quick Turn Around (QTA) flights coming from Middle East, Europe and UK, who do not have a layover in the foreign stations are exempted from RT-PCR testing at Indian airport on arrival (OM dated 20th April, 2021)

ii Considering the arrival of relief flights from different countries, this Ministry has exempted the crew of international relief flights (with clearance from MEA) from RT-PCR testing at Indian airports on arrival (OM dated 27th April, 2021)

3 Considering the request of Cargo Airlines (including all type of relief flights), which are playing a significant role in transportation of medical cargo, this Ministry in consultation with Health Ministry has decided to exempt crew of international cargo flights originating/transiting from UK, Europe and Middle East (in addition to the crew of QTA flights who are already exempted) from RT-PCR testing on arrival, subject to following conditions

i Airline crew are vaccination certified

ii They plan their stay in one of the earmarked quarantine hotels near Airports

iii They will be confined to their rooms in the hotels and not interact with others, and

iv They will move from airport to hotels through earmarked cabs

(Usha Padhee) 29/4/2021
Joint Secretary
Tele 24617692

To

DG, DGCA with a request to please communicate to the cargo flights operating to India

PTO

Copy to

1 The Home Secretary, Ministry of Home Affairs

2 The Secretary, Ministry of Civil Aviation

3 Ms Arti Ahuja, Addl Secretary, Ministry of Health and Family Welfare

4 Shri Naveen Srivastav, AS, MEA

5 Shri Sanjeev Kumar Jindal, JS, MHA

6 Ms Vandana Agarwal, Sr EA, MoCA

7 Shri Lav Aggarwal, JS, Ministry of Health and Family Welfare

8 Shri Angshumali Rastogi, JS MoCA

9 Shri S K Jha, JS(Air)

10 DG, ICMR

11 Airport Operators (as per standard circulation) – to bring the contents of the OM to the notice of State Health officials deployed at airport

Annexure 6d: Standard Operating Procedure (SoP) for assisting States and UTs (4.5.2021)

Ministry of External Affairs

***

Standard Operating Procedure (SoP)
for assisting States and UTs. (4.5.2021)

The Centre has been assisting the States/ UTs with Covid relief materials coming from abroad either in the form of donations or gifts on need basis. In pursuance of Ministry of Finance Ad hoc Exemption Order No. 2/2021-Customs dated 3 May 2021, States/ UTs can procure Covid relief materials from abroad by way of purchase or donations/ gifts for free distribution. Blanket exemptions including, customs, IGST, No Object Certificates, etc. can be availed by State Government, or the entity, relief agency or statutory body, as specified in such certificate. States/ UTs shall designate a nodal officer for the purpose of coordinating such proposals.

i. On receipt of requests for procurement by States/UTs, Missions shall assist in providing appropriate information on suppliers/ vendors in foreign countries for the purpose of placing orders for procurement directly. Missions will keep MEA and MoHFW informed of such proposals.

ii. In all such proposals, consignee will be States/ UTs for the purpose of receiving customs clearance and distribution, etc. States/ UTs will designate a nodal officer for the purpose.

iii. Missions will keep informed MEA and MoHFW of any proposal of any direct purchase by States/ UTs as well as donations/ gifts to States/UTs from foreign governments, pvt individuals, Indian associations, companies and NGOs.

iv. Offers of donations/gifts by foreign governments to States/UTs should be with no pre-conditions for availing blanket exemptions. Such proposals will be cleared by GoI on a case-to-case basis.

v. For donations/gifts from private individuals, Indian associations, Companies and NGOs, Niti Aayog will be the nodal agency for handling such proposals or alternatively, States/ UTs can designate an agency for the purpose.

vi. Proposals of foreign companies that wish to donate to their employees in States/ UTs would need to seek relaxation of CSR guidelines. These proposals will be handled by NIti Aayog in consultation with Ministry of Corporate Affairs.

vii. NIti Aayog will keep MEA, MoHFW and MHA informed of all proposals received directly by it.

viii. All consignments of donations/ gifts from foreign governments or private entities seeking blanket exemptions for use by States must meet a minimum threshold as indicated.

Useful Information

Name of Organisation	Contacts	Documentation
MEA Covid Cell	Shri Jayant Khobragade Mobile: 9136550305 Ms. Vishakha Yaduvanshi Mobile: 9599638385 Tel: 011- 49016783 Email: covidcell@mea.gov.in	Link to access Indian Missions abroad: https://www.mea.gov.in/indian-missions-abroad-new.htm
Indian Red Cross Society Sansad Marg, 1, Red Cross Road, New Delhi, 110001.	Contact: Dr. Vanshree Singh Tel : +91 11 23711551 Mobile: +91 9818228394 Email: directorbloodbank@indianredcross.org	(i) Airway Bill (ii) Commercial Invoice (iii) List of items, carton-wise (iv) Donation/ Gift Certificate
HLL Lifecare Ltd.	Mr. Aroop Bose, Dy Vice President, Mobile: +91 9711996251 Mr. Sanjeev Gupta,, HCD, Mobile: 9330019140	
Niti Aayog	Shri Sudhendu J. Sinha, Advisor Mobile:8130077124 Email: sudhenduj.17@gov.in Shri Abhshek Agarwal, Sr. Specialist Mobile : 8511121023 Email: ab.agarwal@gov.in	

Threshold on priority items

Sl. No.	Item	Minimum Threshold Quantity	Minimum expected specifications
1.	Oxygen Cylinders	100	Minimum 10 ltrs
2.	Oxygen Concentrators	30	5LPM and 220 Volt
3.	Bipap/ NIV	30	N.A.
4.	PSA Oxygen Generation plants	1	At least 500 LPM capacity
5.	Ventilators	15	Should have NIV facility & inbuilt compressor
6.	Medicines: Remdesivir and Tocilizumab	N.A.	N.A.

Annexure 6e: Donations meant for the States/UTs and Organising Transportation for the Donations 12.05.21

Ministry of External Affairs

Covid Cell

12th May 2021

Sub: Letter of OSD (Covid & Europe) addressed to HOMs/HOPs on (i) procurement or donations abroad meant for the States/UTS; (ii) organizing transportation for intended donations

"With Missions' active involvement and support movement of consignments from foreign government and private entities to India are going smoothly. Based on your inputs the Inter-Ministerial Group that meets daily is able to coordinate consignments coming in from abroad. Missions may continue to to provide information on offers, including specifications and numbers etc. and also advance information on movement of flights/ships before their departure.

Since 'blanket exemptions' are also given for consignments being sent directly to **States/ UTs** either by way of procurement or donations from abroad, Missions are requested to facilitate for such offers. Joint Secretary Shri Anurag Bhushan is the nodal officer for States/UTs and information on such proposals, including from individuals, associations, NGOs may be shared with him. The simple format sent by him could be used for capturing the data which will be uploaded in the MEA Portal on a real time basis.

Several Missions have informed of the interest of local Indian associations to send Covid relief material with a request to bear **transportation** cost by the Government. As mentioned earlier, such requests should be discouraged as GoI cannot absorb transportation costs. They should be encouraged to deliver consignments CIF India. Where possible Missions could appropriately guide them to avail air cargo facility extended gratis by some airlines/agencies such as Qatar Airways, Emirates, Fedex, Maersk, etc. for delivery up to its ultimate destination".

Annexure 6f: Standard Operating Procedure for Providing Publicity on Foreign Donations/Gifts

Ministry of External Affairs

***

Standard Operating Procedure (SOP) for Providing publicity on foreign donations/ gifts

i. Missions will inform details of flights carrying foreign donations in advance to the concerned Heads of Division of MEA. HODs will liaise with Indian Red Cross Society (IRCS) and HLL Lifecare Ltd. for receiving such consignment.

ii. HODs, to extent possible, will receive the first flight on arrival carrying the donation of a country. Alternatively, HOD may depute an officer at the level of Director/Deputy Secretary for the purpose.

iii. Concerned Heads of Divisions will keep Protocol, Resident Missions and MEA Covid Cell informed of such flights.

iv. Protocol will facilitate assistance to HoDs and Resident Diplomatic Missions with airport passes and access to airport lounge. Protocol officer (s) will be deputed to assist officials and diplomats at the time of arrival of donation flights.

v. Territorial Divisions will keep External Publicity Division informed of arrival of flights, provide background information, details of consignment for tweets and photo ops.

vi. Heads of Division may share details of distribution of donations to respective Resident Missions and our HOMs abroad.

vii. Officials of Indian Red Cross Society (IRCS) and HLL Lifecare Limited (HLL) will facilitate customs clearances and take charge of the consignment.

*****

Useful information

Name of the Organization	Contacts
Indian Red Cross Society Sansad Marg, 1, Red Cross Road, New Delhi, 110001.	Contact: Dr. Vanshree Singh Tel :+91 11 23711551 Mobile: +91 9818228394 Email: directorbloodbank@indianredcross.org
HLL Lifecare Ltd. (HLL)	Mr. Aroop Bose, Dy Vice President, Mobile: +91 9711996251 Mr. Sanjeev Gupta,, HCD, Mobile: 9330019140
Protocol, MEA	Shri Sarvjeet Soodan, DCP(C) , Mobile: 9311898338 Email: dcpc2@mea.gov.in Shri Ashish, SO (protocol), Mobile: 9172572727 Email:protocol1@mea.gov.in, aptpass.protocol1@mea.gov.in
Covid Cell, MEA	Ms. Vishakha Yaduvanshi, DS, Mobile: 9599638385 Ms. Deepti Jharwal, DS, Mobile: 9821136321 Tel: 011-49016783 Email: covidcell@mea.gov.in

Annexure 6g: Standard Operating Procedure for Flight Clearances for Civilian and Military Aircraft bringing in Humanitarian Aid

Ministry of External Affairs

***

Standard Operating Procedure (SOP) for flight clearances for civilian and military aircraft bringing in humanitarian aid

For efficient handling of donations/gifts of medical assistance coming from abroad through civilian or military aircraft, MEA in consultation with MoD has proposed the following SOP for flight clearances :

(a) With regard to civilian aircraft carrying COVID-19 assistance, Indian Missions and Heads of Division concerned may advise foreign donors to submit duly filled in application form (enclosed) to DGCA. Thereafter, concerned Territorial Divisions will facilitate flight clearance.

(b) With regard to Military aircraft carrying humanitarian aid, Indian Missions and Heads of Division may advise foreign donors to submit duly filled in application form (enclosed) along with load manifest to MoD. Thereafter, concerned Territorial Divisions will facilitate flight clearance.

(c) Crew landing with medical supplies (both for civilian and military aircraft) will be given temporary landing permit and depending on the requirement of stay, visa would be facilitated on 'gratis' basis by Bureau of Immigration (BoI).

(d) In both the cases, documentation requirement such as commercial invoice, donation/gift certificate, airway bill, and list of items carton-wise is same as mentioned in the '*SOP for the handling of consignment of donations/gifts from abroad*' issued on April 27,2021.

(e) Consignee details for the assistance necessarily has to be Indian Red Cross Society (IRCS). After the arrival of the consignment, IRCS and Hindustan Latex Ltd. (HLL) would liaise with the customs for expeditious release of each consignment. MoH&FW will take possession of such consignment for further internal distribution.

(f) All International civilian airports and Air Force bases would be operating 24x7.

(g) Ministry of Civil Aviation has issued latest guidelines regarding the RT-PCR testing requirement for the crew operating international flights. Copy of the same enclosed for easy reference.

(h) Missions may note the following contact details:

Flight Clearance related queries (for civilian aircraft):

Ms. Vandana Aggarwal, Sr. Economic Advisor, MoCA,
+91-9811425500, vaggarwal@gov.in

Mr. Sunil Kumar, DDG,DGCA,
+91-9871474040, skumar.dgca@nic.in

Mr. Atul Maindola
Deputy Director, DGCA
+91-9999069074, atul.maindola@nic.in

Flight Clearance related queries (for military aircraft):

Air Vice Marshall H. Bains
+91-8130915002

Air Commodore A K Vahi
+91-9792901108

info501@nic.in

Immigration related queries :

Shri Rajeev Ranjan Verma
Commissioner (Immigration),
+91-9850255054, comm.boi-mha@nic.in

Annexure 6h: Application Form for Non-Scheduled Flight Clearances

APPLICATION FORM FOR FLIGHT CLEARANCES OF NON-SCHEDULED FLIGHTS BY FOREIGN REGISTERED AIRCRAFT

1.	**Purpose of the Flight** (VIP/Tourist/ Cargo/Ambulance/Relief/Private etc.);		
2.	Whether over-flying/technical landing or landing in India for traffic purposes;		
3.	**ATS Route(s) to be flown** (including entry and exit point in Indian air-space);		
4.	**Complete Route itinerary** of the proposed flight with dates and timings (including true origin and true destination) ;		
5.	**Arrival and departure timings** at airports in India, if any;		
6.	**Airport of last departure** before entering Indian airspace and airport of first landing after leaving Indian airspace;		
7.	**Aircraft details**		
	i)	Type	
	ii)	State of Registry/Nationality	
	iii)	Registration	
	iv)	Telephony designator (Flight Number/Call sign)	
	v)	Whether the aircraft is capable of air-dropping	Yes / No
	vi)	Whether the maximum certified passenger seating capacity of the aircraft is more than 30 seats	Yes / No
	vii)	Whether the maximum pay-load capacity of the aircraft is more than 3 tonnes	Yes / No
	viii)	Whether the aircraft is fitted with ACAS-II/TCAS-II (*NOTE: Flight clearance will not be granted to aircraft having maximum certified seating capacity of more than 30 seats or pay-load of more than 3 tonnes, unless it is fitted with ACAS-II/TCAS-II.*)	Yes / No
8.	**Pilot-in-Command**		
	i)	Name	
	ii)	Nationality	
9.	**Aircraft Operator**		
	i)	Name	
	ii)	Nationality	
	iii)	Address (with Tele/Fax Nos.)	
	iv)	Aircraft Operators Certificate/ Permit Number, if any;	

10.	**On board details**		
	i)	Number of Crew;	
	ii)	Number of passengers, if any;	
	iii)	General Description of goods carried, if any;	
	iv)	Any arms, ammunition, explosives, radio-active material, war equipment or dangerous goods? If so, attach a copy of DGCA permit.	
11.	**Any special equipment** like aerial photography, remote sensing cameras, night vision cameras on board? If so, attach a copy of DGCA permit.		
12.	**Number of passengers or tonnage of cargo** to be uplifted from and set down in India:		
13.	**Charterer**		
	i)	Name	
	ii)	Address (With Tele/Fax Nos.)	
14.	**Travel/Cargo Agent in India**		
	i)	Name	
	ii)	Address (with Tele/Fax Nos.)	

It is CERTIFIED that the information given above by the undersigned is correct.

(Signatures of CEO/ Director of Airlines/
Charter Passenger/Cargo Handling Agent)
(SEAL OF THE COMPANY)
Name and Address

Date:

Annexure 6i: PESO Notification on used/refurbished Oxygen Cylinder

तार- "विस्फोटक", नागपुर
Telegram: "EXPLOSIVES", Nagpur
Website : http://peso.gov.in
Email: explosives@explosives.gov.in
दूरभाष/ Telephone : 0712-2510248
फैक्स/ FAX : 2510577

कार्यालय उद्देश्य के सभी पत्रादि "मुख्य विस्फोटक नियंत्रक" के पदनाम से भेजे जाए उनके व्यक्तिगत नाम से नहीं.

All communications intended for this Office should be addressed to the "Chief Controller of Explosives" and NOT to him by name.

भारत सरकार
GOVERNMENT OF INDIA
पेट्रोलियम तथा विस्फोटक सुरक्षा संगठन
Petroleum and Explosives Safety Organisation
(पूर्व नाम - विस्फोटक विभाग)
(Formerly- Department of Explosives)
"ए-ब्लाक", पाँचवा तल, केन्द्रीय कार्यालय परिसर,
"A" Block, 5th Floor, CGO Complex,
सेमिनरी हिल्स, नागपुर - 440 006 (महा)
Seminary Hills, Nagpur- 440006

संख्या / No.GCR/ MISC/2021 दिनांक /Nagpur, dated 28th May., 2021

CIRCULAR

Sub: Import of used/refurbished empty gas cylinder from foreign countries for Covid management as well as trading purpose -Reg

In view of powers delegated to the Joint Chief Controller of Explosives (HOD), PESO, Nagpur by DPIIT vide order No.P-13029/6/2021 -EXPLOSIVE dated 15/05/2021 to exercise the rule 66 of Gas Cylinder Rules 2016 for Covid management, the following restriction is imposed on import of used/refurbished empty gas cylinders from foreign countries.

No person shall import any used/refurbished empty gas cylinder from foreign countries for Covid management as well as trading purpose in the interest of public safety.

However, this restriction is not applicable to the cylinders already arrived in India from foreign countries donated by missionaries/Red cross prior to 26/05/2021.

This order is valid for a period of 6 months from the date of issue of the circular.

Yours Faithfully,

(M.K. Jhala)
Jt. Chief Controller of Explosives(HOD).

Annexure 7a: Foreign Secretary's presentation at the concluding meeting of the Parliamentary Standing Committee on External Affairs (2020-21) on "COVID-19 Pandemic: Global Response, India's Contribution and Way Forward" (10 March 2021)

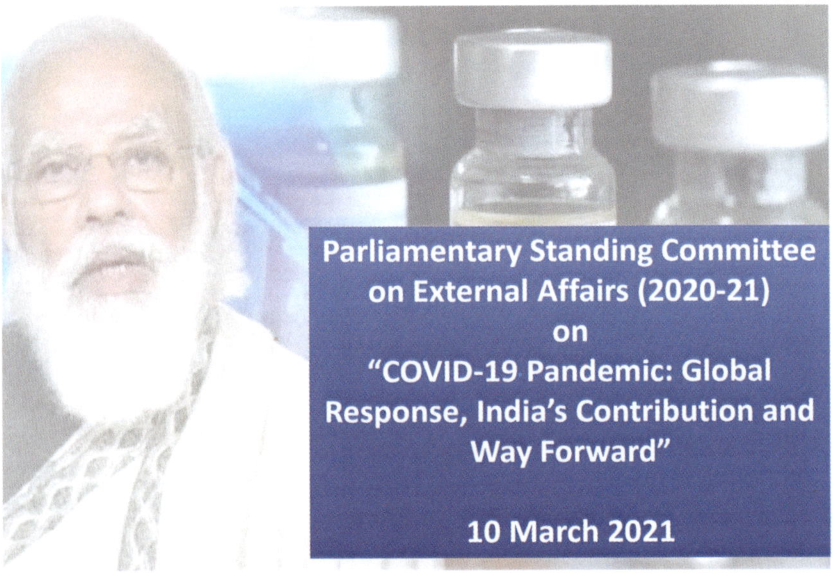

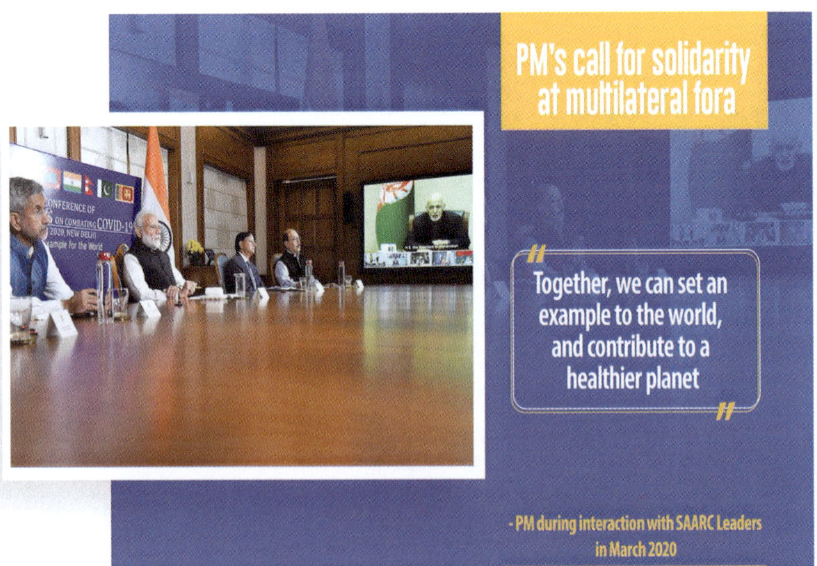

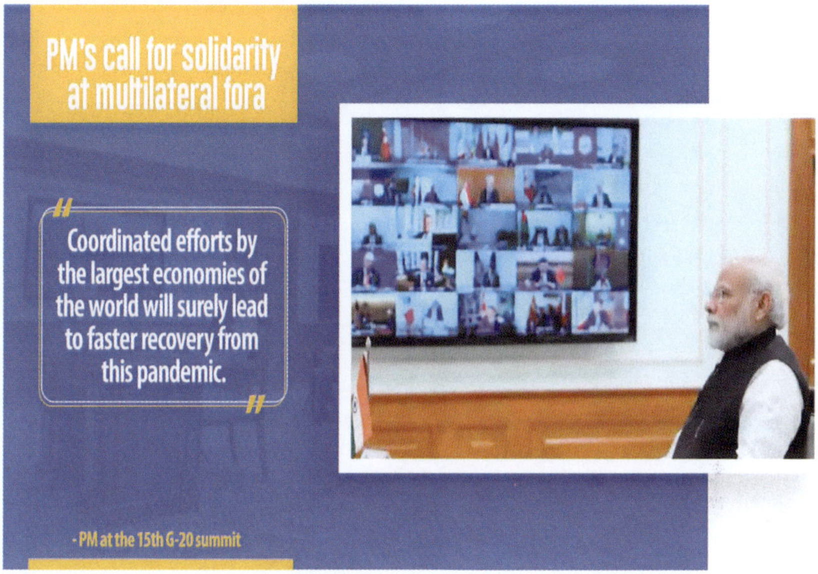
PM's call for solidarity at multilateral fora
Coordinated efforts by the largest economies of the world will surely lead to faster recovery from this pandemic.
- PM at the 15th G-20 summit

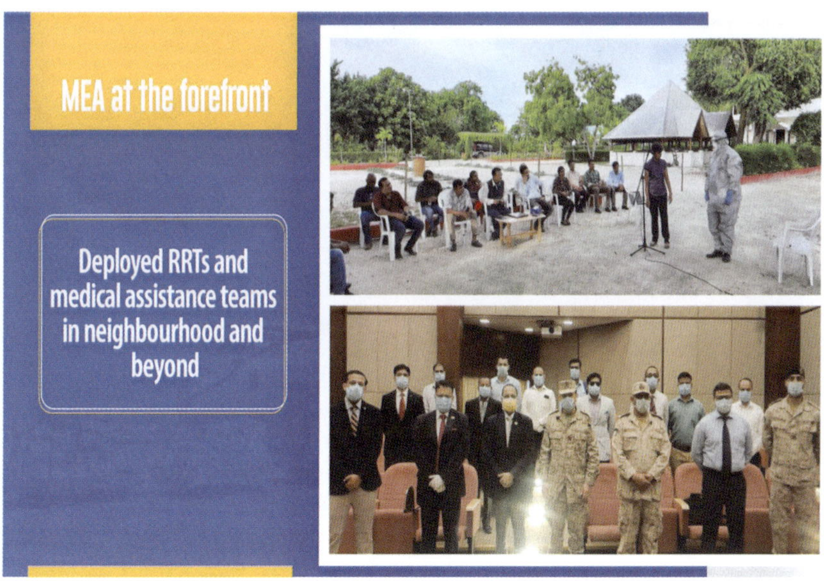
MEA at the forefront
Deployed RRTs and medical assistance teams in neighbourhood and beyond

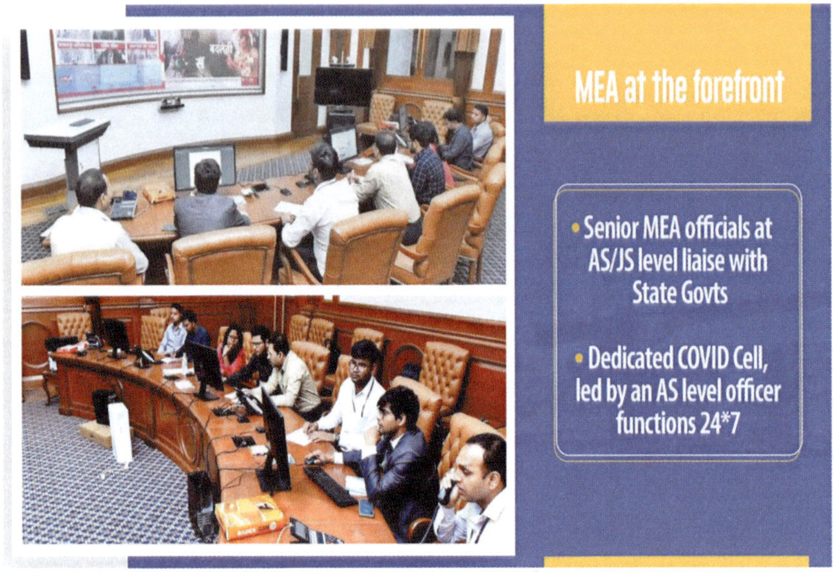
MEA at the forefront
• Senior MEA officials at AS/JS level liaise with State Govts
• Dedicated COVID Cell, led by an AS level officer functions 24*7

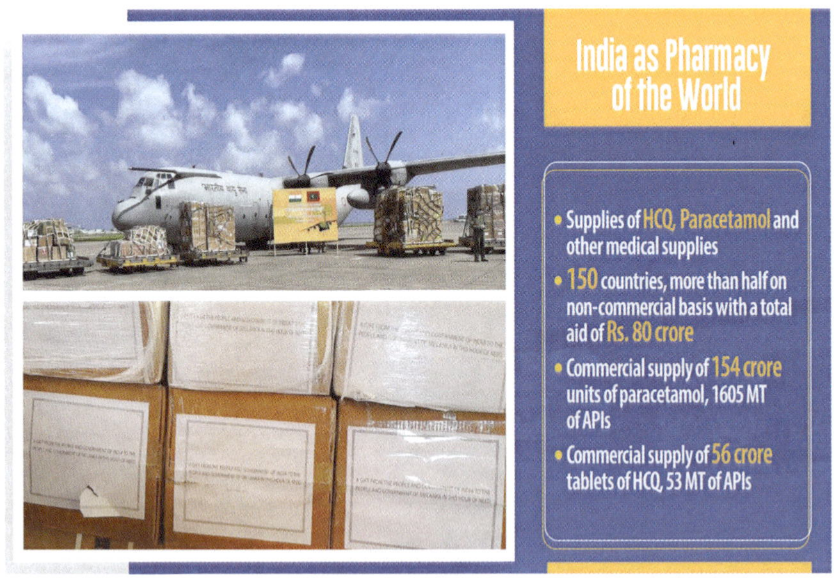
India as Pharmacy of the World
• Supplies of HCQ, Paracetamol and other medical supplies
• 150 countries, more than half on non-commercial basis with a total aid of Rs. 80 crore
• Commercial supply of 154 crore units of paracetamol, 1605 MT of APIs
• Commercial supply of 56 crore tablets of HCQ, 53 MT of APIs

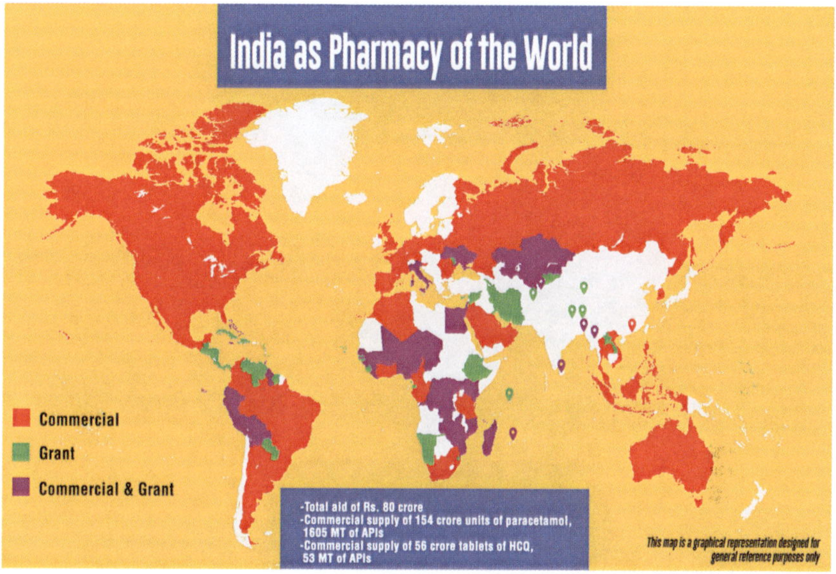
India as Pharmacy of the World
Commercial
Grant
Commercial & Grant
-Total aid of Rs. 80 crore
-Commercial supply of 154 crore units of paracetamol, 1605 MT of APIs
-Commercial supply of 56 crore tablets of HCQ, 53 MT of APIs
This map is a graphical representation designed for general reference purposes only

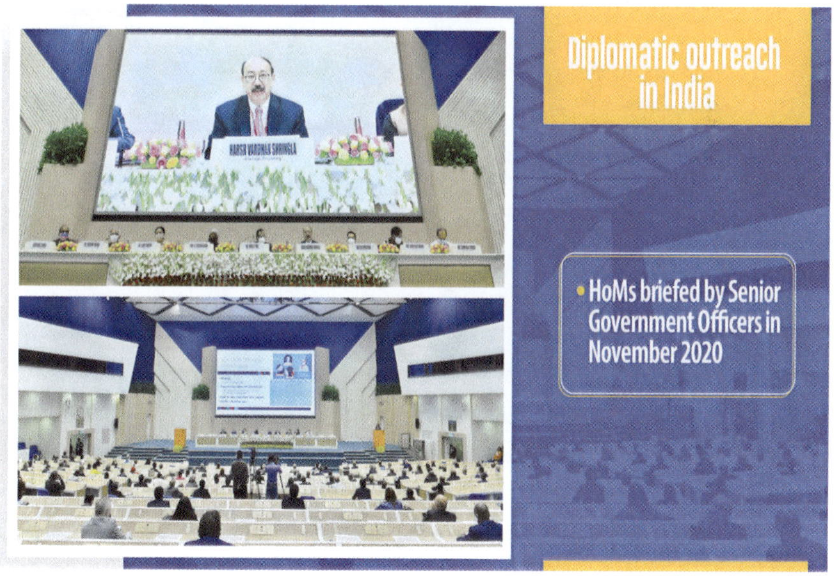
Diplomatic outreach in India
HoMs briefed by Senior Government Officers in November 2020

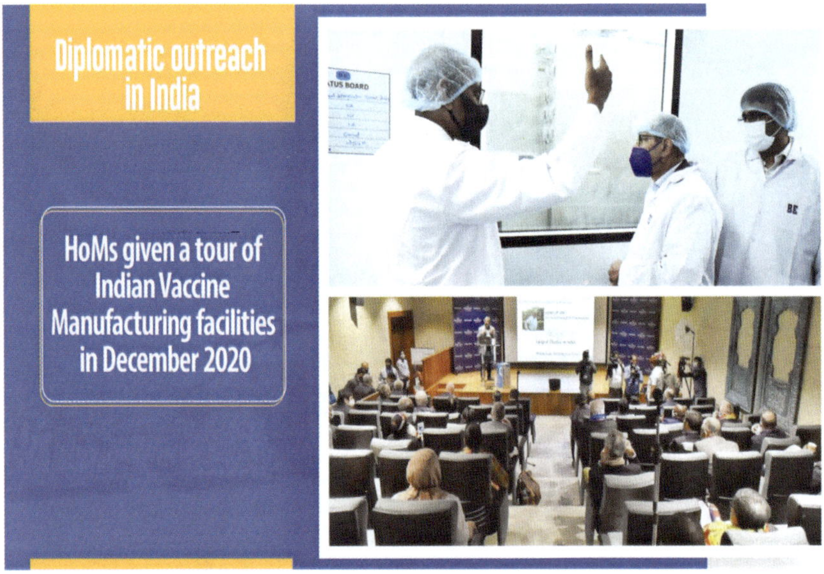
Diplomatic outreach in India
HoMs given a tour of Indian Vaccine Manufacturing facilities in December 2020

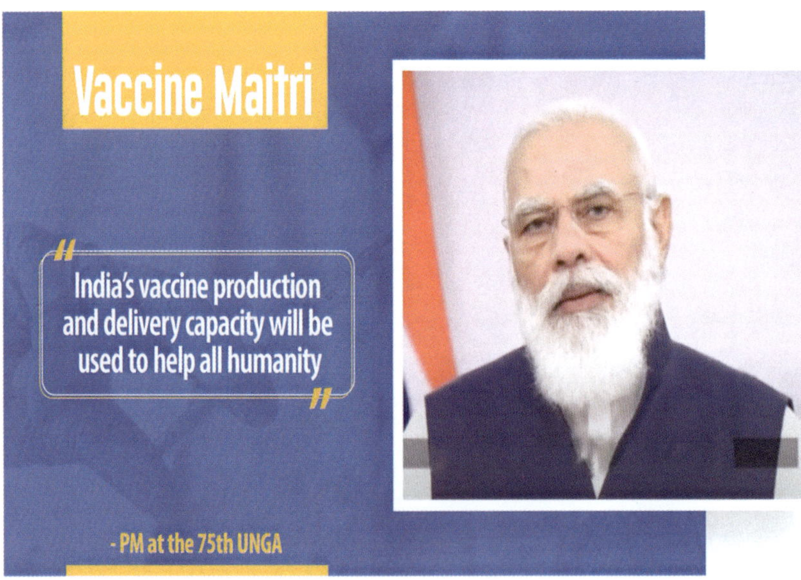
Vaccine Maitri
"India's vaccine production and delivery capacity will be used to help all humanity"
- PM at the 75th UNGA

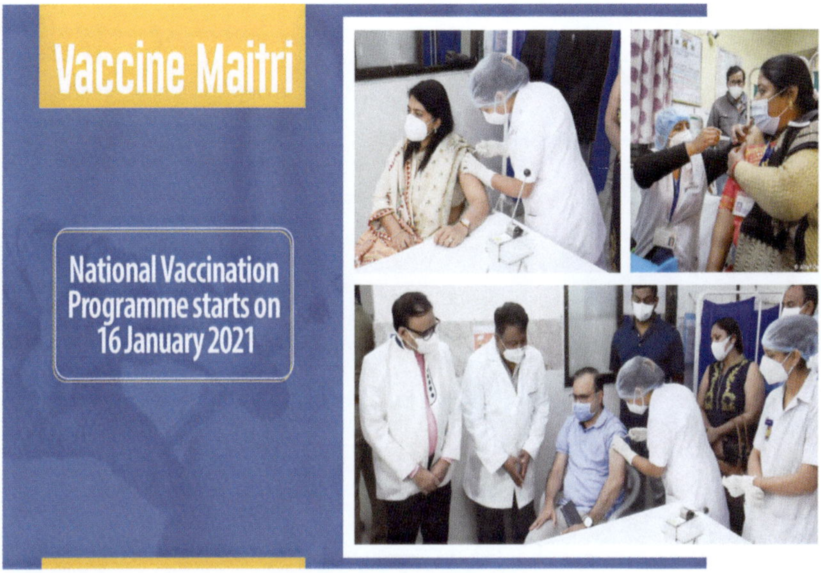
Vaccine Maitri
National Vaccination Programme starts on 16 January 2021

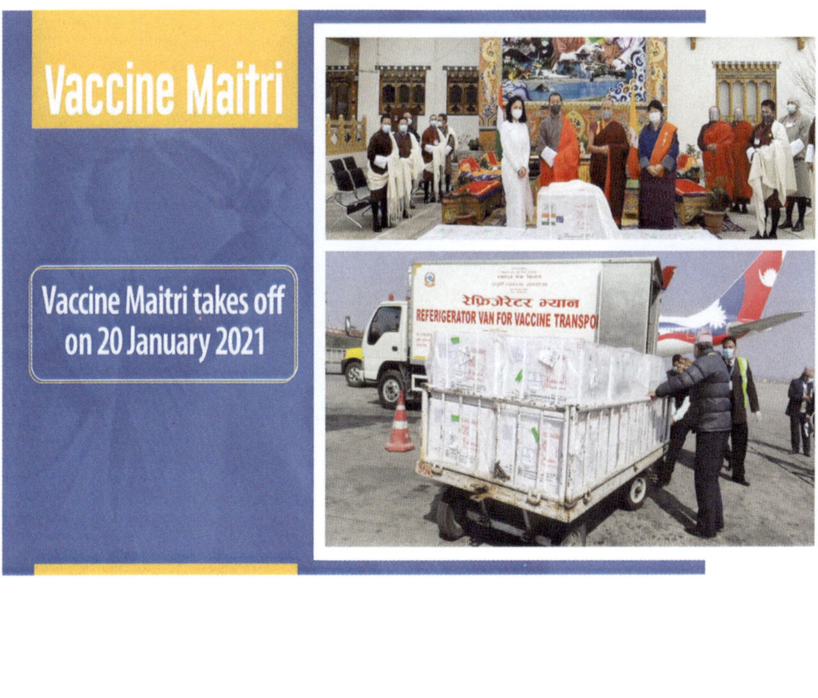
Vaccine Maitri
Vaccine Maitri takes off on 20 January 2021
रेफ्रिजेरेटर भ्यान
REFERIGERATOR VAN FOR VACCINE

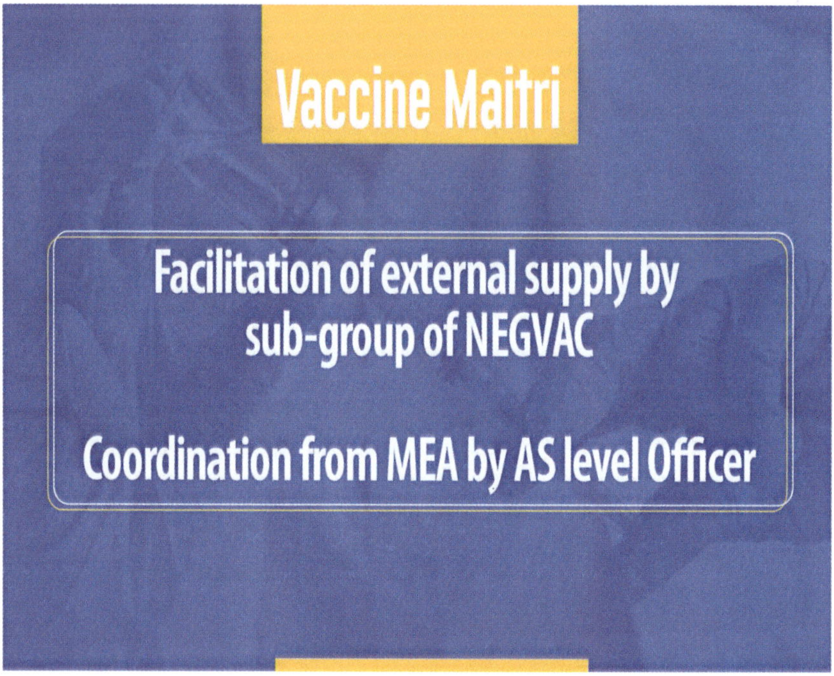
Vaccine Maitri
Facilitation of external supply by sub-group of NEGVAC
Coordination from MEA by AS level Officer

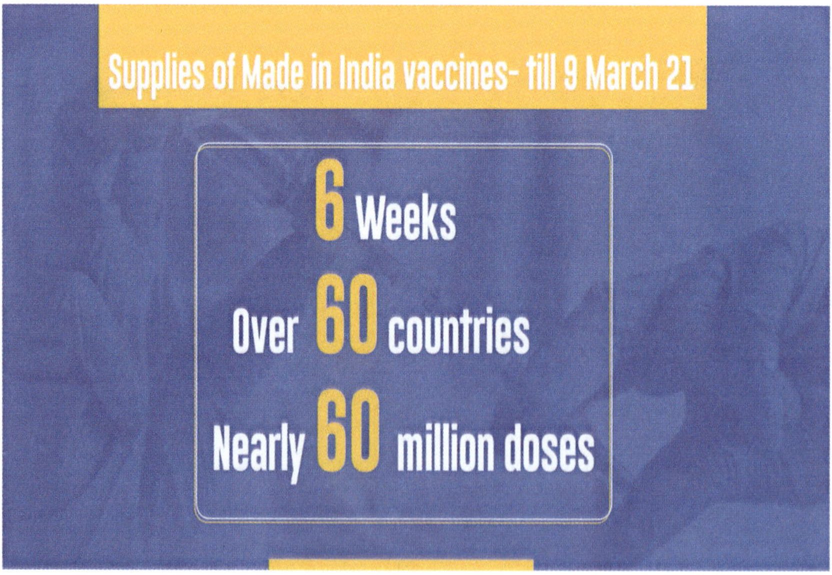
Supplies of Made in India vaccines- till 9 March 21
6 Weeks
Over 60 countries
Nearly 60 million doses

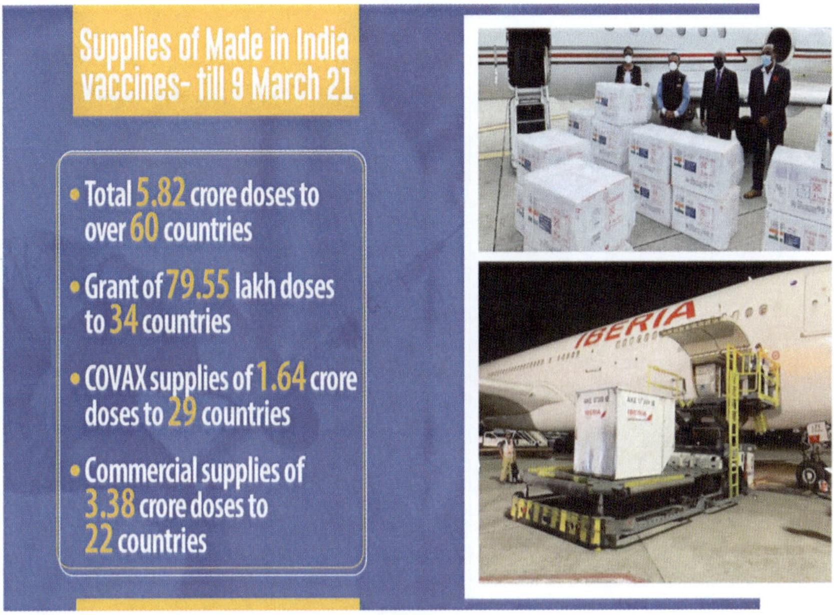
Supplies of Made in India vaccines- till 9 March 21
• Total 5.82 crore doses to over 60 countries
• Grant of 79.55 lakh doses to 34 countries
• COVAX supplies of 1.64 crore doses to 29 countries
• Commercial supplies of 3.38 crore doses to 22 countries
IBERIA

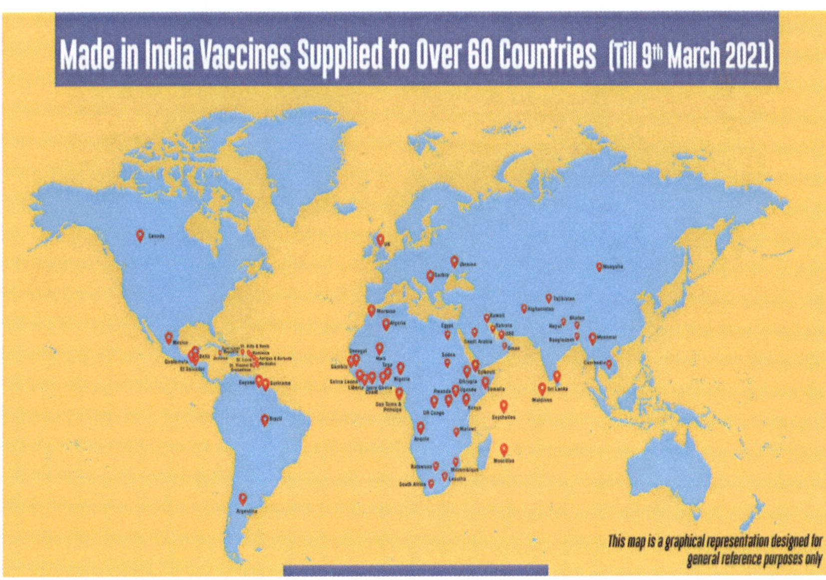
Made in India Vaccines Supplied to Over 60 Countries (Till 9th March 2021)
This map is a graphical representation designed for general reference purposes only

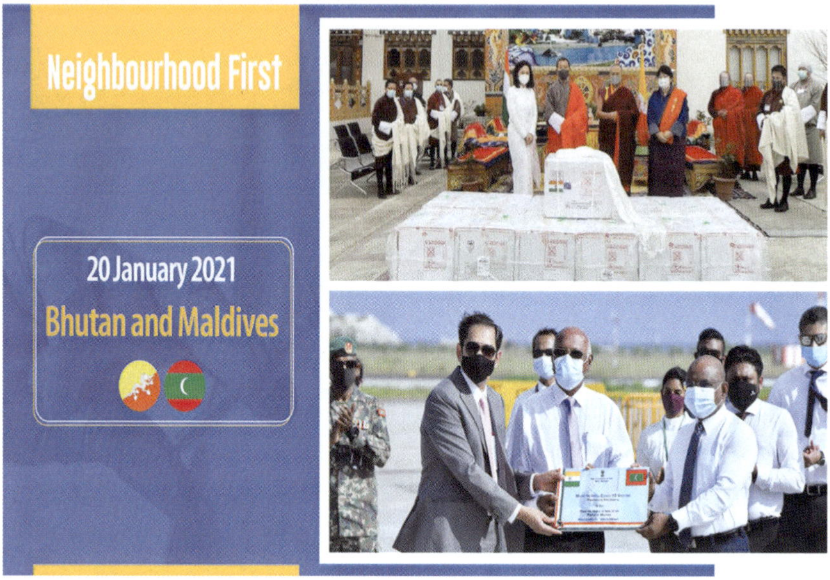
Neighbourhood First
20 January 2021
Bhutan and Maldives

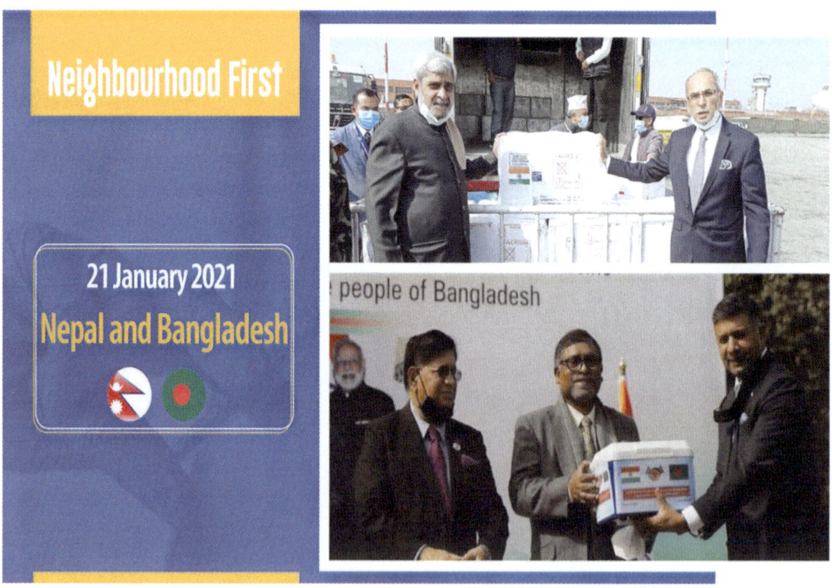
Neighbourhood First
21 January 2021
Nepal and Bangladesh
people of Bangladesh

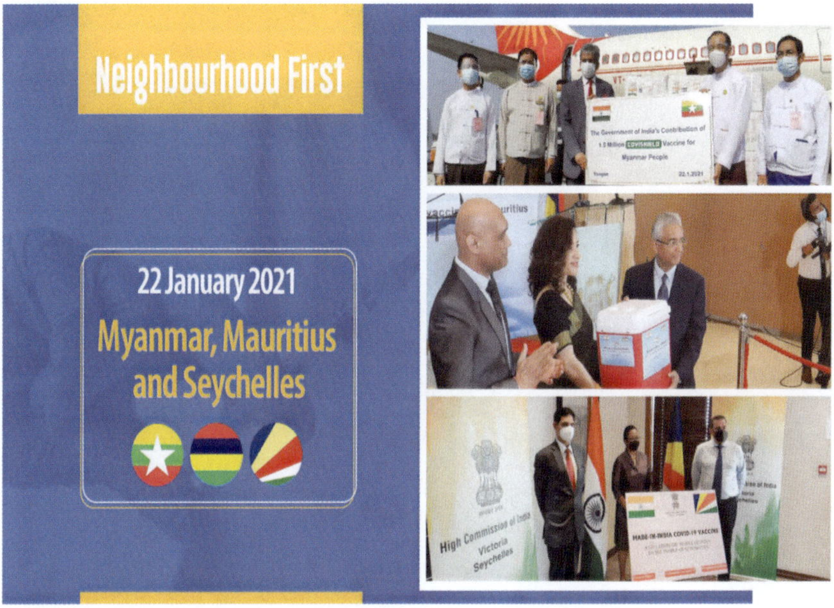
Neighbourhood First
22 January 2021
Myanmar, Mauritius and Seychelles
High Commission of India
Victoria
Seychelles

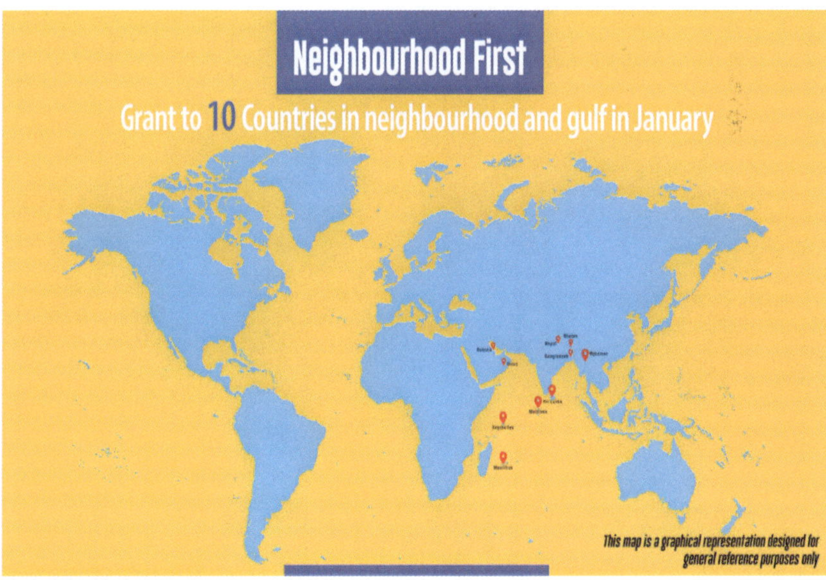
Neighbourhood First
Grant to 10 Countries in neighbourhood and gulf in January
This map is a graphical representation designed for general reference purposes only

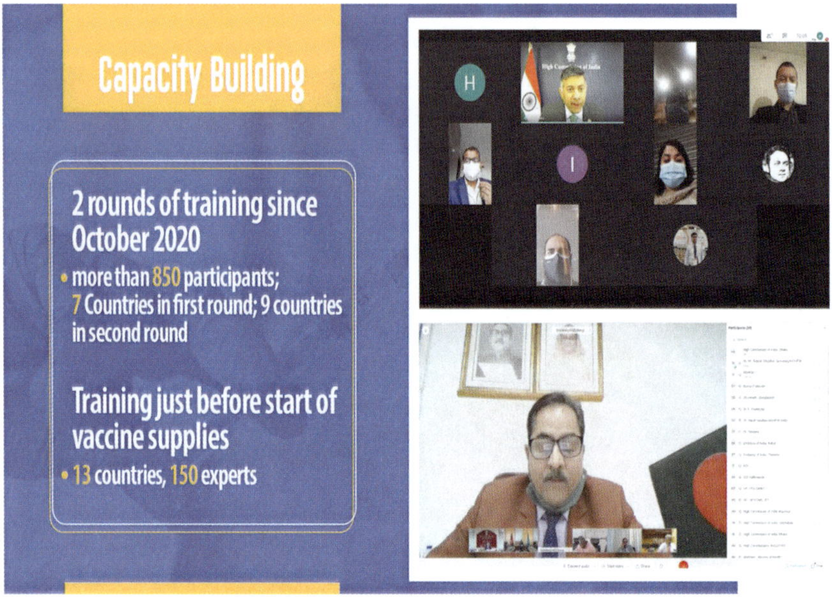
Capacity Building
2 rounds of training since October 2020
• more than 850 participants; 7 Countries in first round; 9 countries in second round
Training just before start of vaccine supplies
• 13 countries, 150 experts

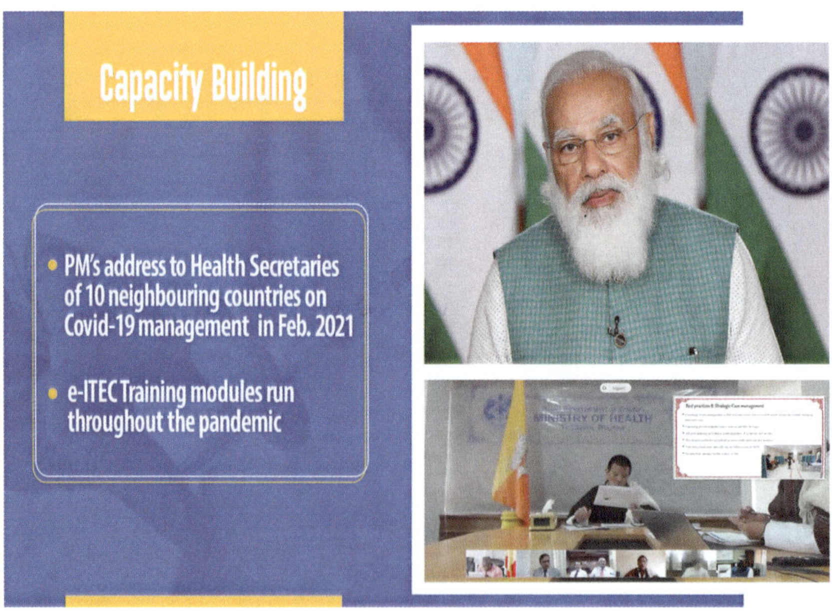
Capacity Building
• PM's address to Health Secretaries of 10 neighbouring countries on Covid-19 management in Feb. 2021
• e-ITEC Training modules run throughout the pandemic
MINISTRY OF HEALTH

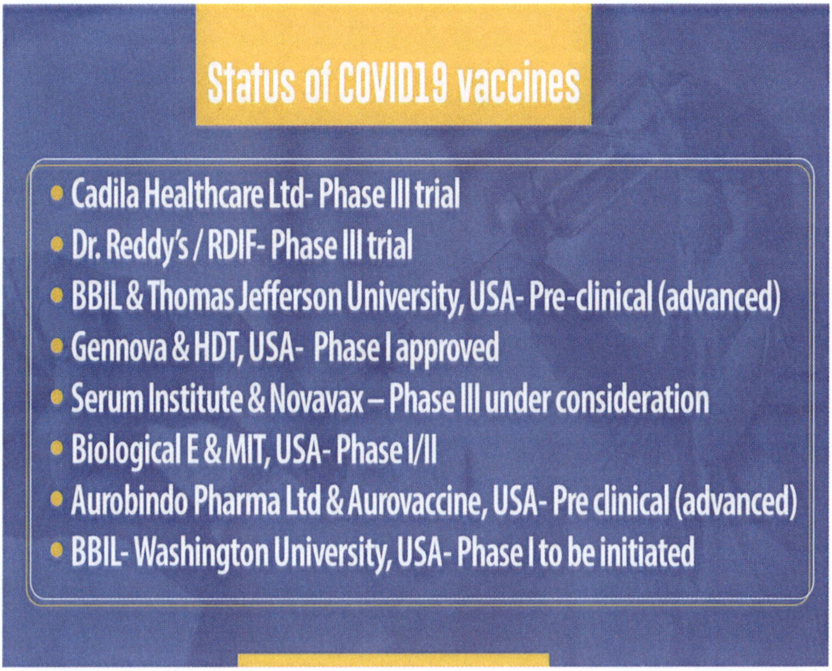
Status of COVID19 vaccines
• Cadila Healthcare Ltd- Phase III trial
• Dr. Reddy's / RDIF- Phase III trial
• BBIL & Thomas Jefferson University, USA- Pre-clinical (advanced)
• Gennova & HDT, USA- Phase I approved
• Serum Institute & Novavax – Phase III under consideration
• Biological E & MIT, USA- Phase I/II
• Aurobindo Pharma Ltd & Aurovaccine, USA- Pre clinical (advanced)
• BBIL- Washington University, USA- Phase I to be initiated

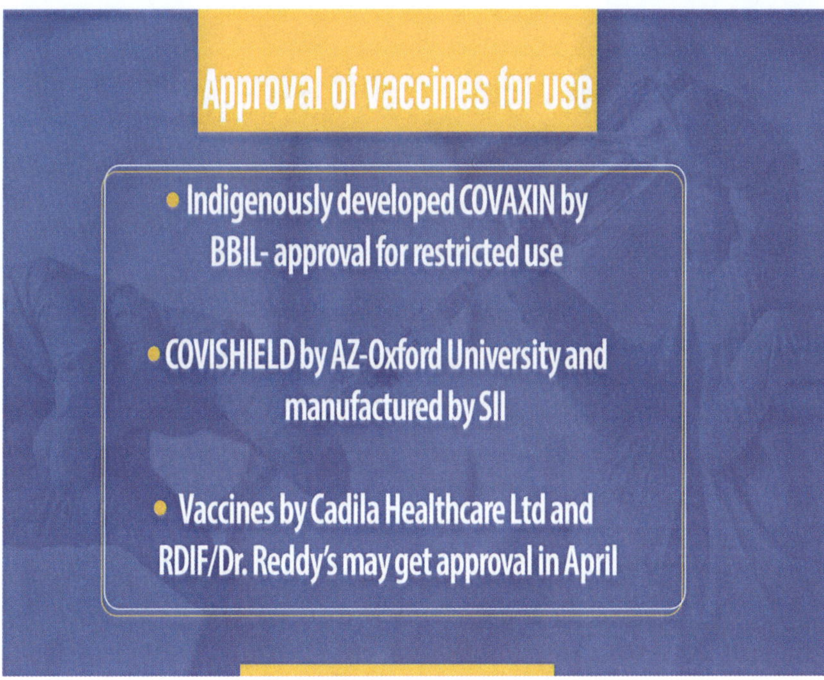
Approval of vaccines for use
• Indigenously developed COVAXIN by BBIL- approval for restricted use
• COVISHIELD by AZ-Oxford University and manufactured by SII
• Vaccines by Cadila Healthcare Ltd and RDIF/Dr. Reddy's may get approval in April

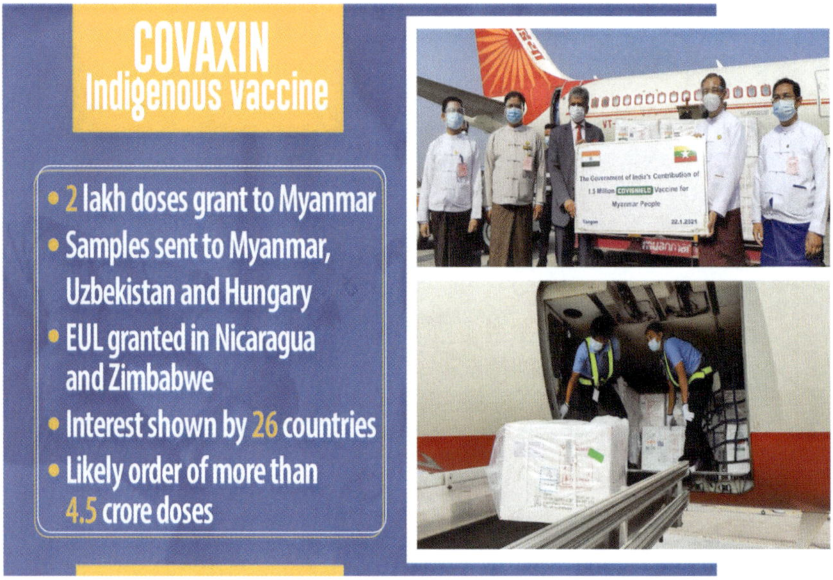
COVAXIN
Indigenous vaccine
• 2 lakh doses grant to Myanmar
• Samples sent to Myanmar, Uzbekistan and Hungary
• EUL granted in Nicaragua and Zimbabwe
• Interest shown by 26 countries
• Likely order of more than 4.5 crore doses
The Government of India's Contribution of 1.5 Million COVISHIELD Vaccine for Myanmar People
22.1.2021

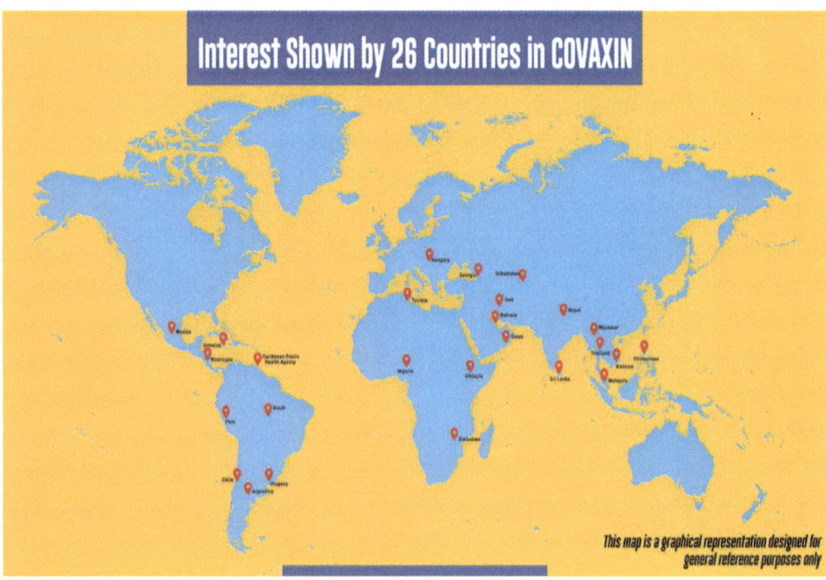
Interest Shown by 26 Countries in COVAXIN
Hungary
Georgia
Tunisia
Iran
Bahrain
Oman
Nepal
Myanmar
Thailand
Vietnam
Philippines
Malaysia
Sri Lanka
Nigeria
Ethiopia
Zimbabwe
Mexico
Nicaragua
Caribbean Public Health Agency
Peru
Brazil
Chile
Argentina
Uruguay
This map is a graphical representation designed for general reference purposes only

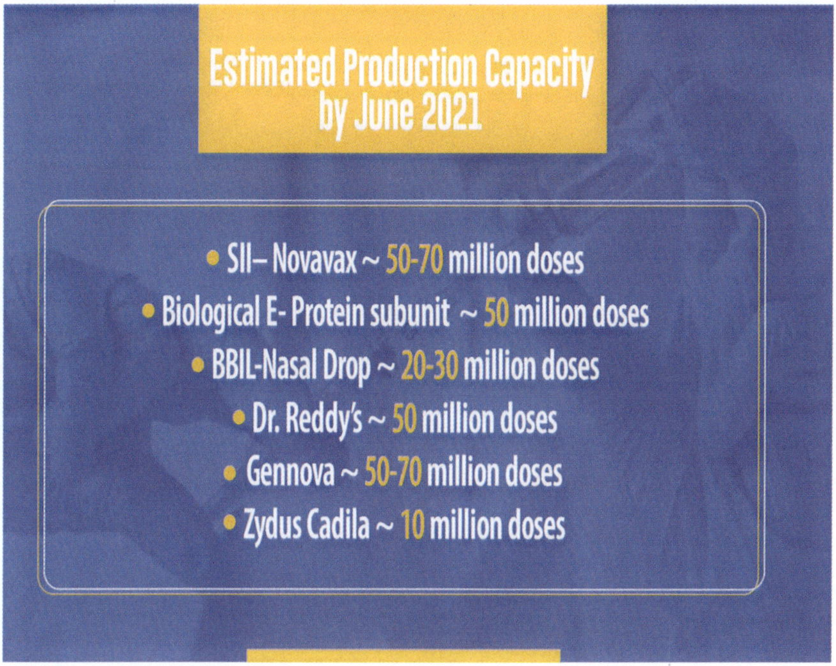
Estimated Production Capacity by June 2021
• SII– Novavax ~ 50-70 million doses
• Biological E- Protein subunit ~ 50 million doses
• BBIL-Nasal Drop ~ 20-30 million doses
• Dr. Reddy's ~ 50 million doses
• Gennova ~ 50-70 million doses
• Zydus Cadila ~ 10 million doses

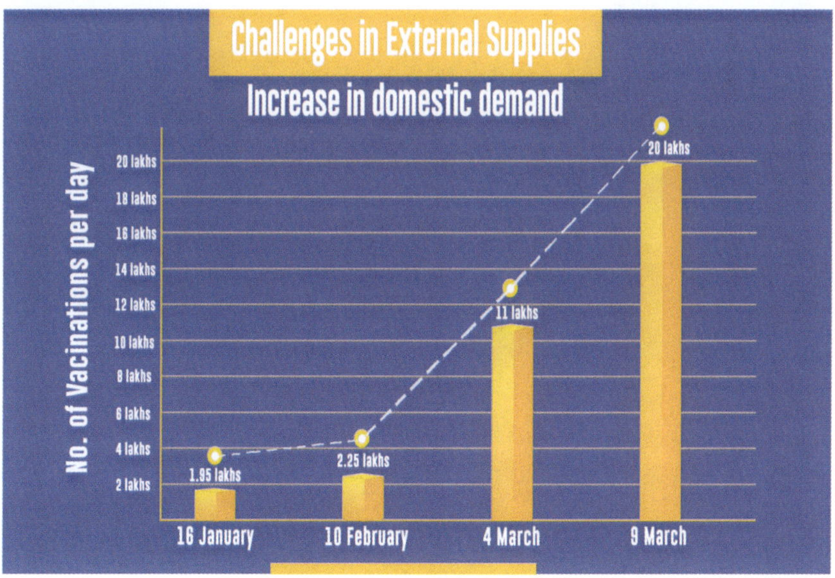
Challenges in External Supplies
Increase in domestic demand
No. of Vacinations per day
20 lakhs
18 lakhs
16 lakhs
14 lakhs
12 lakhs
10 lakhs
8 lakhs
6 lakhs
4 lakhs
2 lakhs
1.95 lakhs
2.25 lakhs
11 lakhs
20 lakhs
16 January
10 February
4 March
9 March

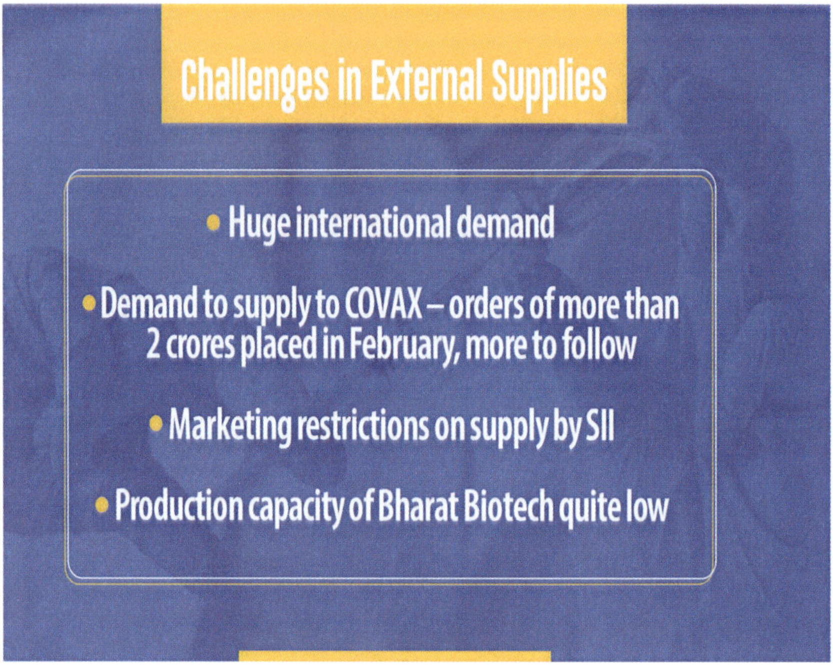
Challenges in External Supplies
• Huge international demand
• Demand to supply to COVAX – orders of more than 2 crores placed in February, more to follow
• Marketing restrictions on supply by SII
• Production capacity of Bharat Biotech quite low

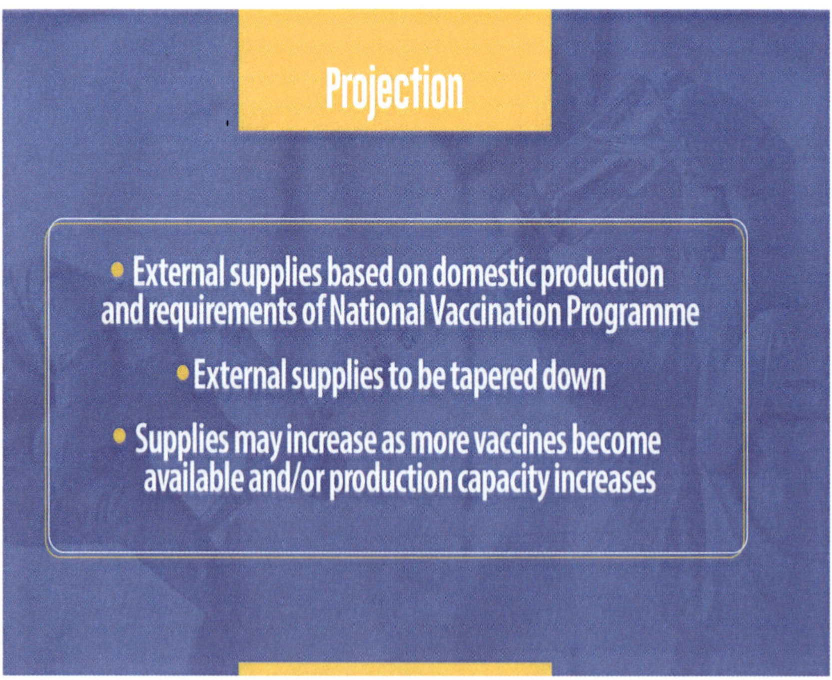
Projection
• External supplies based on domestic production and requirements of National Vaccination Programme
• External supplies to be tapered down
• Supplies may increase as more vaccines become available and/or production capacity increases

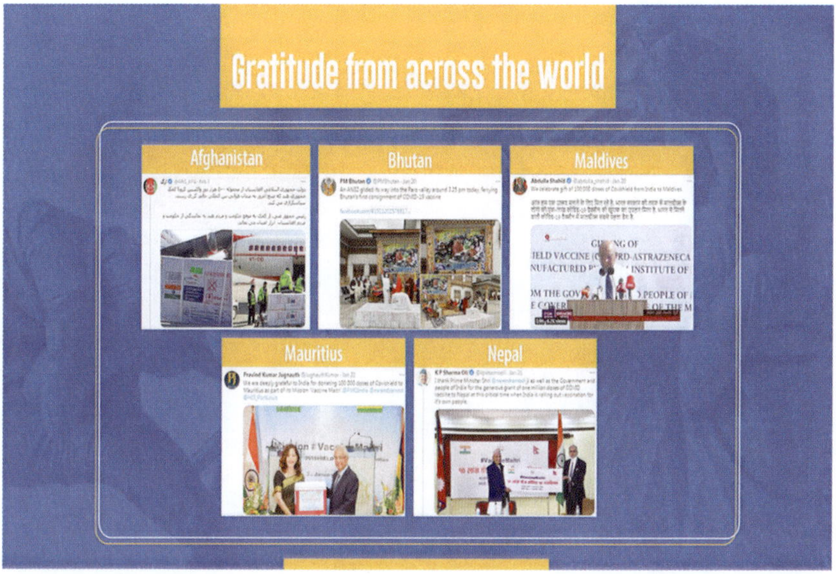
Gratitude from across the world
Afghanistan
Bhutan
Maldives
Mauritius
Nepal

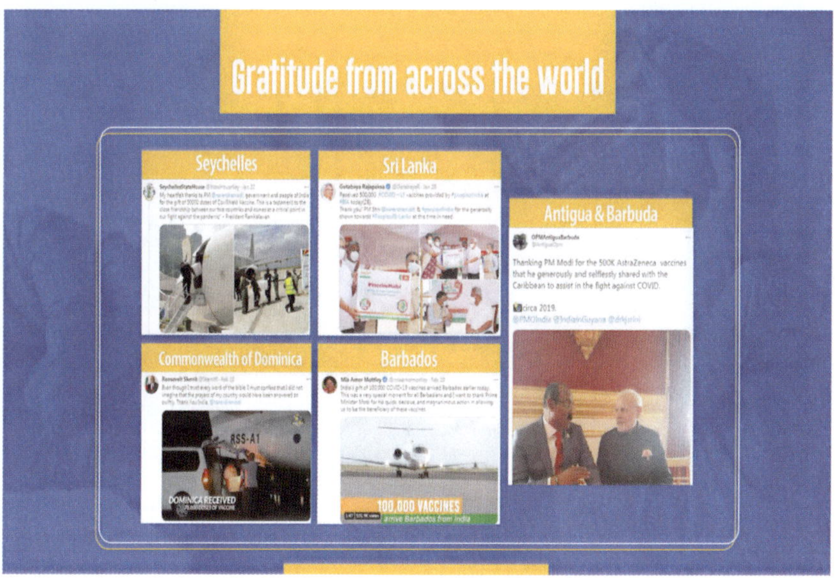
Gratitude from across the world
Seychelles
Sri Lanka
Antigua & Barbuda
Thanking PM Modi for the 500K AstraZeneca vaccines that he generously and selflessly shared with the Caribbean to assist in the fight against COVID.
Commonwealth of Dominica
Barbados
100,000 VACCINES
arrive Barbados from India

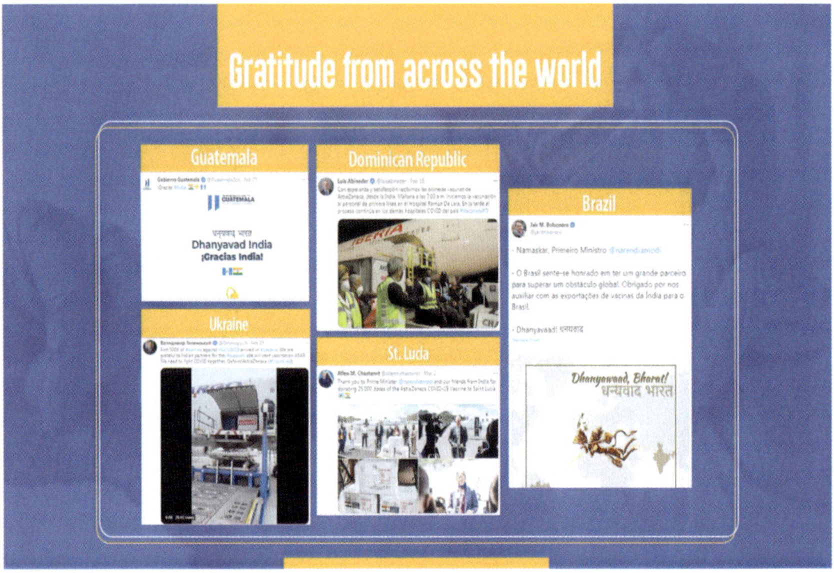
Gratitude from across the world
Guatemala
धन्यवाद भारत
Dhanyavad India
¡Gracias India!
Dominican Republic
Brazil
- Namaskar, Primeiro Ministro @narendramodi
- O Brasil sente-se honrado em ter um grande parceiro para superar um obstáculo global. Obrigado por nos auxiliar com as exportações de vacinas da Índia para o Brasil.
- Dhanyavaad! धन्यवाद
Dhanyawaad, Bharat!
धन्यवाद भारत
Ukraine
St. Lucia

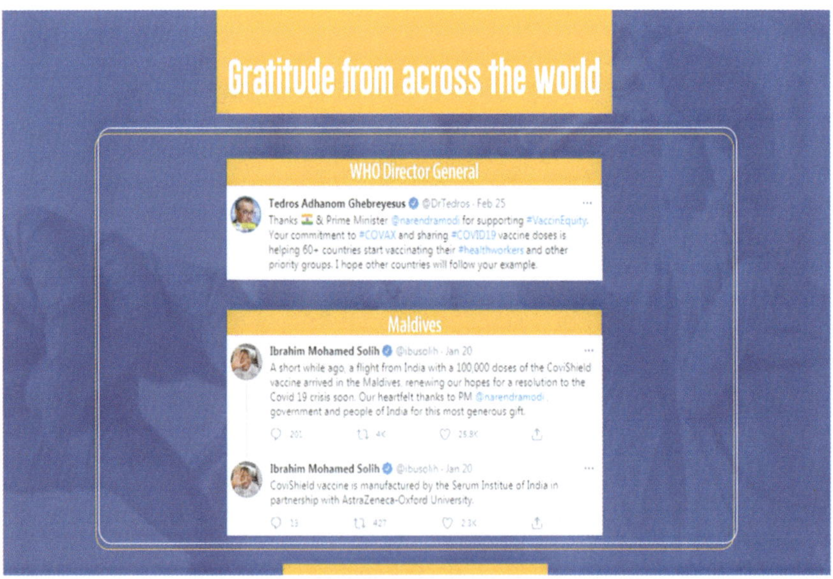
Gratitude from across the world
WHO Director General
Tedros Adhanom Ghebreyesus @DrTedros · Feb 25
Thanks & Prime Minister @narendramodi for supporting #VaccinEquity. Your commitment to #COVAX and sharing #COVID19 vaccine doses is helping 60+ countries start vaccinating their #healthworkers and other priority groups. I hope other countries will follow your example.
Maldives
Ibrahim Mohamed Solih @ibusolih · Jan 20
A short while ago, a flight from India with a 100,000 doses of the CoviShield vaccine arrived in the Maldives, renewing our hopes for a resolution to the Covid 19 crisis soon. Our heartfelt thanks to PM @narendramodi, government and people of India for this most generous gift.
Ibrahim Mohamed Solih @ibusolih · Jan 20
CoviShield vaccine is manufactured by the Serum Institue of India in partnership with AstraZeneca-Oxford University.

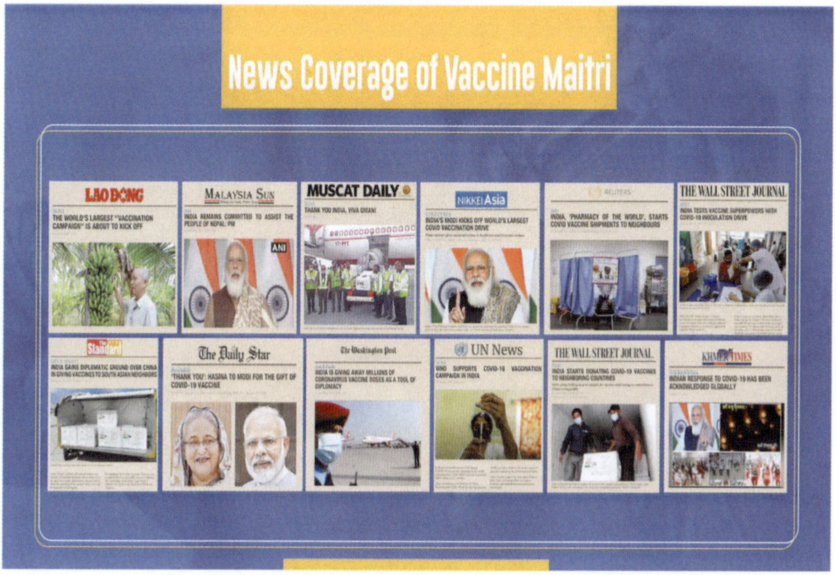
News Coverage of Vaccine Maitri
LAO ĐỘNG
THE WORLD'S LARGEST "VACCINATION CAMPAIGN" IS ABOUT TO KICK OFF
MALAYSIA SUN
INDIA REMAINS COMMITTED TO ASSIST THE PEOPLE OF NEPAL: PM
MUSCAT DAILY
THANK YOU INDIA, VIVA OMAN!
NIKKEI Asia
INDIA'S MODI KICKS OFF WORLD'S LARGEST COVID VACCINATION DRIVE
REUTERS
INDIA, 'PHARMACY OF THE WORLD', STARTS COVID VACCINE SHIPMENTS TO NEIGHBOURS
THE WALL STREET JOURNAL
INDIA TESTS VACCINE SUPERPOWERS WITH COVID-19 INOCULATION DRIVE
The Standard
INDIA GAINS DIPLOMATIC GROUND OVER CHINA IN GIVING VACCINES TO SOUTH ASIAN NEIGHBORS
The Daily Star
'THANK YOU': HASINA TO MODI FOR THE GIFT OF COVID-19 VACCINE
The Washington Post
INDIA IS GIVING AWAY MILLIONS OF CORONAVIRUS VACCINE DOSES AS A TOOL OF DIPLOMACY
UN News
WHO SUPPORTS COVID-19 VACCINATION CAMPAIGN IN INDIA
THE WALL STREET JOURNAL
INDIA STARTS DONATING COVID-19 VACCINES TO NEIGHBORING COUNTRIES
KHMER TIMES
INDIAN RESPONSE TO COVID-19 HAS BEEN ACKNOWLEDGED GLOBALLY

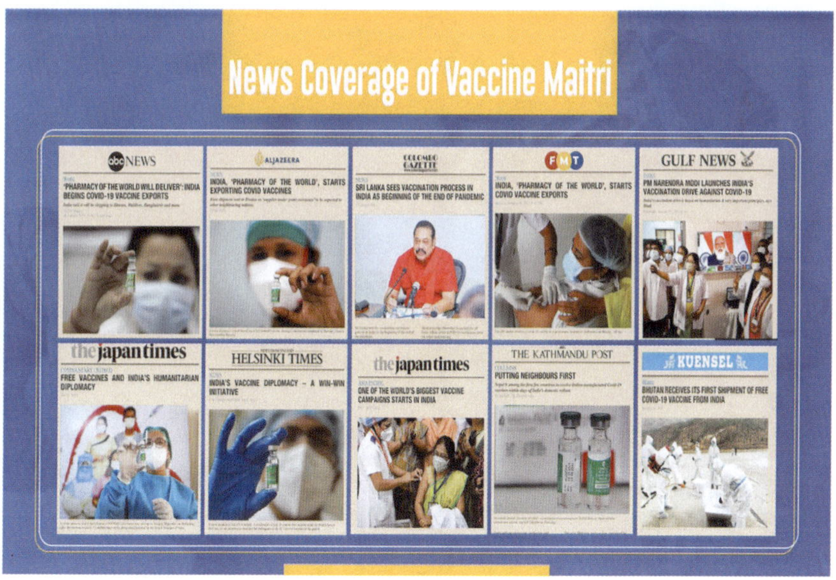
News Coverage of Vaccine Maitri
abc NEWS
'PHARMACY OF THE WORLD WILL DELIVER': INDIA BEGINS COVID-19 VACCINE EXPORTS
ALJAZEERA
INDIA, 'PHARMACY OF THE WORLD', STARTS EXPORTING COVID VACCINES
COLOMBO GAZETTE
SRI LANKA SEES VACCINATION PROCESS IN INDIA AS BEGINNING OF THE END OF PANDEMIC
FMT
INDIA, 'PHARMACY OF THE WORLD', STARTS COVID VACCINE EXPORTS
GULF NEWS
PM NARENDRA MODI LAUNCHES INDIA'S VACCINATION DRIVE AGAINST COVID-19
the japan times
FREE VACCINES AND INDIA'S HUMANITARIAN DIPLOMACY
HELSINKI TIMES
INDIA'S VACCINE DIPLOMACY – A WIN-WIN INITIATIVE
the japan times
ONE OF THE WORLD'S BIGGEST VACCINE CAMPAIGNS STARTS IN INDIA
THE KATHMANDU POST
PUTTING NEIGHBOURS FIRST
KUENSEL
BHUTAN RECEIVES ITS FIRST SHIPMENT OF FREE COVID-19 VACCINE FROM INDIA

Annexure 8a: WHO's India Situation Report

Novel Coronavirus Disease (COVID-19)
Situation Update Report – 72

World Health Organization India

June 16, 2021

HIGHLIGHTS

- 500-bed COVID hospital by DRDO operationalized in Srinagar (Link)
- CSIR and Laxai Life Sciences Pvt. Ltd. Hyderabad given regulatory approval to undertake clinical trial to assess efficacy of Colchicine in improvement of clinical outcomes during treatment of COVID-19 (Link)
- Indigenously designed and manufactured high purity oxygen concentrator being supplied to Indian hospitals (Link)
- Member, Health, NITI Aayog asserts that there is no need for immediate change in COVISHIELD dosage interval (Link)
- Press Information Bureau holds webinar to engage with public regarding post-COVID symptoms, and recovery from COVID-19 (Link)
- MoHFW emphasizes the role of Indian SARS-CoV-2 Genetics Consortium (INSACOG) in detection of Variants of Concerns (VOCs) (Link)

WHO Situation Update

India
2,95,70,881 Confirmed Cases
3,77,031 Total Deaths

South East Asia Region
33,666,359 Confirmed Cases
461,830 Total Deaths

World
175,987,176 Confirmed Cases
3,811,561 Deaths

INDIA SITUATION

- In India highest number of cases in a day were 4,14,188 reported on 7 May 2021; since then there is continuous decline in daily cases.

2,95,70,881	20,810	5,74,408	3,77,031	265	1.28
Confirmed Cases	Cases per million	Last 7 days Cases	Total Deaths	Deaths per million	CFR

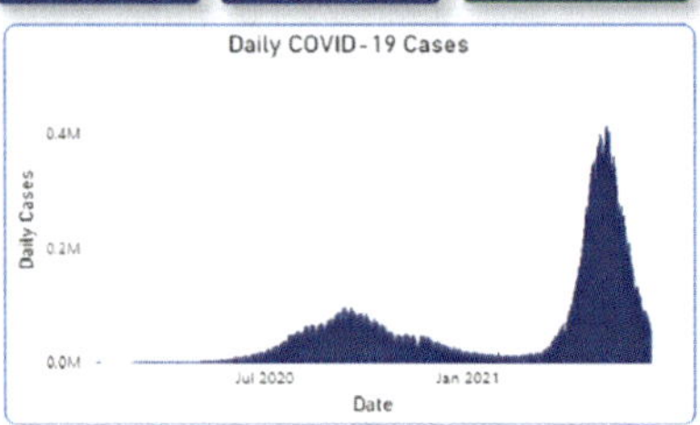

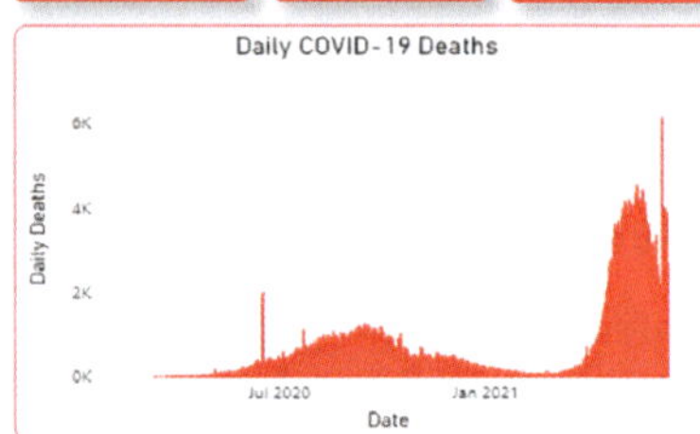

COVID-19: STATUS ACROSS STATES

- In the past week (9-15 June), as compared to previous week (2-8 June), all states/UTs have shown a decrease in cases except Andaman & Nicobar Islands and Mizoram.

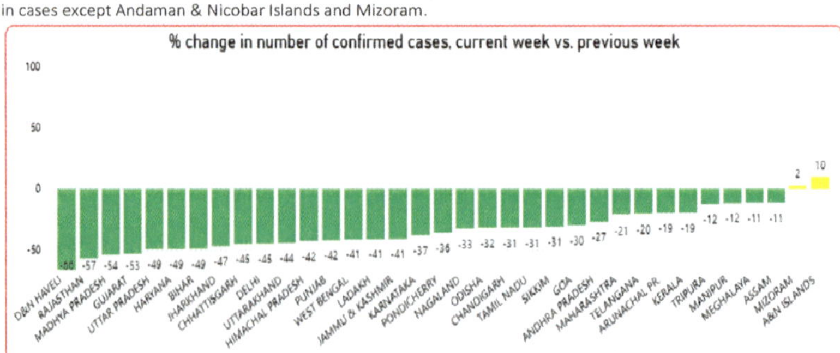

Novel Coronavirus Disease (COVID-19)
Situation Update Report – 72

World Health Organization India

June 16, 2021

- In **Kerala**, plans have been made to upgrade infrastructure of medical colleges, district hospitals, and block/ taluka hospitals to facilitate effective pediatric case management
- In **Tamil Nadu**, task force committee has been constituted for supporting surge capacity in case of a third wave
- In **Himachal Pradesh**, directives have been issued to administer second dose of Covishield between 28-84 days of first dose to facilitate smooth foreign travel for the purpose of education, employment, sports events, etc.
- In **Punjab**, the Chief Minister has asserted that a group of specialist pediatrics will develop treatment protocol for the possible third wave of COVID-19

WHO GLOBAL UPDATE

- International Coalition of Medicines Regulatory Authorities and WHO jointly issued statement for healthcare professionals regarding how COVID-19 vaccines are regulated for safety and effectiveness, details here
- Global leaders have pledged to share COVID-19 vaccine doses internationally, in support of global equitable access and to help end the acute phase of the pandemic. It will be great boost top COVAX facility, details here
- The ACT Accelerator partnership welcomes commitment of 870 million vaccine doses and calls for more investment in all tools to end the pandemic, details here
- WHO identifies young people as a priority target audience with specific concerns, experiences and behaviours regarding COVID-19, details here
- WHO issued updated recommendations for use of Pfizer–BioNTech, Moderna and Janssen vaccines against COVID-19, details here

WHO COUNTRY UPDATE

Coordination

- WCO continues to provide technical support to MoHFW, NCDC, ICMR and NDMA at the national level and through task force/control rooms at the state and district level in **Andhra Pradesh, Karnataka, Kerala, Tamil Nadu, Telangana, and Puducherry**
- WHO field staff participated in meetings on response, preparation for addressing any future surge, vaccination; chaired by Chief Ministers, Health Ministers, Chief and/or Health Secretaries, MDs – NHM, etc in **Karnataka, Kerala, Lakshadweep, Puducherry, Tamil Nadu, Uttarakhand, and UP**
- **Odisha** has set up Auxiliary Health Facility with WHO provided tents in Balasore district. The facility is functional and is helping in reducing pressure on district hospital.

COVID-19 vaccination

- High level oversight during vaccination is provided by WHO teams at district and state levels
- WCO is supporting monitoring of vaccination sessions across the country and continues to provide surge support for training, microplanning and monitoring

Contact Tracing, Containment and Surveillance

- WHO Country office and field offices are providing supportive supervision to monitor contact tracing; identify containment zones and sharing regular feedback with government health officials on regular basis

Information and Planning

- Supporting facilitation of sensitization meetings of doctors and local practitioners of North East district in **Delhi** regarding COVID response
- Supporting **Kerala** with development of guidelines for vaccinating bed-ridden and palliative patients at their place of stay
- Facilitating lab strengthening activities in **Andhra Pradesh** to initiate DPT surveillance
- Supporting implementation of serosurvey in **Maharashtra**
- Supporting **Rajasthan** with death audit and analysis

Novel Coronavirus Disease (COVID-19)
Situation Update Report – 72

World Health Organization India

June 16, 2021

IPC

- Supporting training of health workers in public and private hospitals in **Delhi** on IPC protocol
- Supporting capacity building of Medical officers and ANMs on IPC in **Andhra Pradesh, Delhi, Haryana, Himachal Pradesh, Jammu and Kashmir, Ladakh, Punjab, and Rajasthan**

Essential Services

- Efforts to strengthen VPD surveillance and immunization are underway in **Andhra Pradesh, Karnataka, Kerala, Lakshadweep, Puducherry, Tamil Nadu and Telangana**
- Supporting **Chhattisgarh and Puducherry** with sensitization efforts for surveillance of AFP/ MR/ DPT
- Supporting **Gujarat, Haryana, Himachal Pradesh, Jammu and Kashmir, Maharashtra, and Punjab** with fever and rash surveillance

As of 15 June 2021, India has tested more than 373 million samples. Tests include both, RTPCR and Rapid Antigen. India's current test positivity rate (7DMA) is 4.38%.

Testing - National Level

37,37,28,224 *
Cumulative Tests

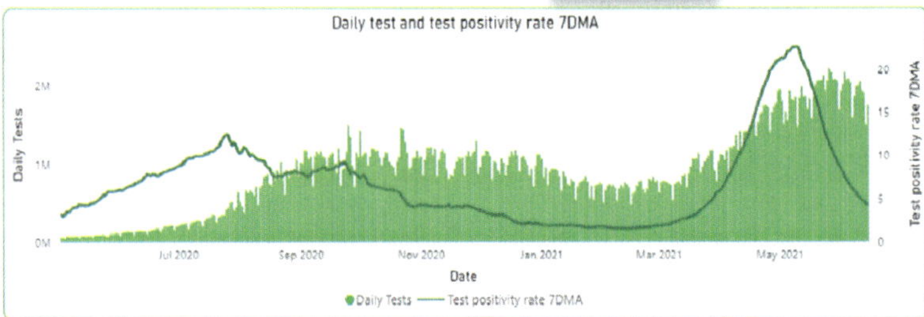

India continued to drive Covid-19 vaccinations among various age group with preconditions, details here.

Cumulative Coverage Report of Covid-19 vaccination (as on 16 June 2021, 07:00 AM)

	Beneficiaries vaccinated		
	1st Dose	2nd Dose	Total Doses
India	21,26,81,921	4,92,90,093	26,19,72,014
	24,02,842 in last 24 Hours	3,97,616 in last 24 hours	28,00,458 in last 24 Hours

IMPORTANT GUIDELINES/TECHNICAL PUBLICATIONS THIS WEEK

- Young people and COVID-19: Behavioural considerations for promoting safe behaviours [LINK]
- COVID-19 Vaccine Introduction and deployment Costing tool (CVIC tool)- Version 2.2 [LINK]
- Technical specifications for selection of essential in vitro diagnostics for SARS-CoV-2 [LINK]
- Considerations for implementing and adjusting public health & social measures for COVID-19 [LINK]
- Guidelines on Operationalization of COVID Care Services for Children & Adolescents [LINK]

FOR MORE INFORMATION CONTACT

In case of any queries on COVID-19, call +91-11-23978046 or 1075 (Toll-free). State Helpline here.
WHO Country Office for India I Telephone number: +91-11- 66564800 I Email: wrindia@who.int

Annexure 9a: List of COVID related Supplies from Canada to India

- Federal government donated C$ 10 million to Canadian Red Cross to assist IRCS.
- Federal government supplied 350 Oxygen concentrators to IRCS.
- Federal government supplied 25,000 doses of Remdesivir to IRCS.
- Federal government supplied 16 Oxygen generating plants through Canadian Red Cross.
- Ontario government donated 5000 ventilators, 500 oxygen concentrators, 80 cylinders and 7 mini oxygen generators to IRCS.
- Saskatchewan government donated 100 ventilators to IRCS.
- British Columbia government promised C$ 500,000 to Canadian Red Cross.
- Yukon territory donated C$ 25,000 to Canadian Red Cross.
- Canada India Foundation has offered three Oxygen Generation plants
- M/s. InkSmith offered to donate 500,000 face shields to IRCS.
- M/s. David McAntony Gibson Foundation – Global Medic offered 42,000 face shields.
- Two private individuals (Nitin Thakur and Anil Sedha) sent oxygen concentrators to IRCS.
- Vraj Community Services (Indian community members in Toronto) offered to supply 1000 oxygen concentrators from China.
- M/s. Tech Resources Ltd., Vancouver donated C$50,000 through UNICEF Canada.
- Mr. GodupTsering, North America Representative of His Holiness & Central Tibetan Administration conveyed that Tibetan people in Canada have sent a donation of CAD 90543.25 to PM CARES through Central Tibetan Administration, Dharamsala.
- Mr. Norton Kothari from Trillium Health Partners Foundation agreed to match all community gifts up to C$250,000, to raise $500,000/- to help India.
- A.K. Taploo Foundation, Ontario sent 30 Oxygen concentrators to IRCS.
- IndiaO2.org donated 200 oxygen concentrators to IRCS.
- Steve Gupta Foundation donated 300 oxygen concentrators.
- Trillium Health Partners raised an amount of C$ 597,000 from community members with contribution of C$250,000 from Kothari Group.
- Government of Quebec donated C$ 250,000 to Oxfam in India.
- M/s. Fairfax Holdings announced a donation of C$ 5 million for relief in India.
- M/s. McCain Foods Ltd. donated C$ 250,000 to Canadian Red Cross.

Annexure 9b: US Government COVID Assistance received in India

The seven emergency airlifts to India deployed, starting 30 April 2021, delivered:

- 20,000 courses of Remdesivir (125,000 vials)
- Nearly 1,500 oxygen cylinders
- Nearly 550 mobile oxygen concentrators (Arrived but later recalled)
- One million rapid diagnostic tests
- Nearly 2.5 million N95 masks
- One Deployable Oxygen Concentration System
- 210 pulse oximeters

The Global Task Force on Pandemic Response assistance received in India

By 17 June 2021, the following items were received from Global Task Force via USIBC and USISPF (P2G):

- 1,000 ventilators.
- 8160 Oxygen Concentraters received. *They are aiming at supplying 100,000 concentrators in aggregate.*
- One million Rapid Test Kits
- 4.6 million RT-PCR kits
- 10 million swabs
- Airlifting 4 large Oxygen trucks from Germany

Annexure 11a: Statements on COVID-19 Second Wave by the Leadership

Prime Minister participates in the first Outreach Session of G7 Summit

(12 June 2021)

Prime Minister Shri Narendra Modi participated in the first Outreach Session of the G7 Summit today.

The session, titled "Building Back Stronger—Health", focused on global recovery from the coronavirus pandemic and on strengthening resilience against future pandemics.

During the session, Prime Minister expressed appreciation for the support extended by the G7 and other guest countries during the recent wave of COVID infections in India.

He highlighted India's "whole of society" approach to fight the pandemic, synergising the efforts of all levels of the government, industry and civil society.

He also explained India's successful use of open source digital tools for contact tracing and vaccine management, and conveyed India's willingness to share its experience and expertise with other developing countries.

Prime Minister committed India's support for collective endeavours to improve global health governance. He sought the G7's support for the proposal moved at the WTO by India and South Africa, for a TRIPS waiver on COVID related technologies.

Prime Minister Modi said that today's meeting should send out a message of "One Earth One Health" for the whole world. Calling for global unity, leadership, and solidarity to prevent future pandemics, Prime Minister emphasised the special responsibility of democratic and transparent societies in this regard.

Prime Minister's Keynote address at the 5th edition of VivaTech

(16 June 2021)

Friends, I believe where convention fails, innovation can help. This has been seen during the COVID-19 global pandemic, which is the biggest disruption of our age; all nations have suffered loss and felt anxiety about the future.

COVID-19 put many of our conventional methods to tests. However, it was innovation that came to the rescue. By innovation, I refer to innovation before the pandemic, innovation during the pandemic. When I speak about innovation before the pandemic, I refer to the pre-existing advances which helped us during the pandemic. Digital technology helped us cope, connect, comfort, console. Through digital media we could work, talk with our loved ones and help others. India's universal and unique biometric digital identity restream, Aadhaar, helped us to provide timely financial support to the poor. We could supply free food to 800 million people and deliver cooking fuel subsidies to many households. We in India were able to operationalise two public digital educational programmes, SWAYAM and DIKSHA, in quick time to help students.

The second part innovation for the pandemic refers to how humanity rose to the occasion and made the fight against it more effective. In this, the role of our start-up sector has been paramount. Let me give you India's example. When the pandemic hit our shores, we had inadequate testing capacities and shortage of masks, PPE, ventilators and other such equipment. Our private sector played a key role in addressing this shortage. Our doctors adapted telemedicine in a big way so that some COVID and other non COVID issues could be addressed virtually. Two vaccines are being made in India and more are in the development or trial stage.

On the government side, our indigenous IT platform, Aarogya Setu, enabled effective contact tracing. Our Co-WIN digital platform has already helped ensure vaccines to millions. Had we not been innovating, then our fight against COVID-19 would have been much weaker. We must not abandon this innovative zeal so that we are even better prepared when the next challenge strikes.

Transcript of Interview of External Affairs Minister with ANI during his visit to the United Kingdom

(5 May 2021)

As Foreign minister, I'm very involved in harnessing the enormous good will that we have in the world and UK has been really a very solid friend. We are getting oxygen plants, concentrators, cylinders to address the oxygen challenge, cryogenic tanks and you of course know the vaccine collaboration we have, covishield is the outcome of that which is the main vaccine that is made in India. Our scientists are working together on sequencing as well. So it's an important day today for the relationship, but it is also a day today when I feel sitting in UK the enormous support and feeling which people in UK, Indian community here has for the covid situation and how much would they like to contribute to our efforts to deal with.

Journalist: Jaishankar Ji, Now you will be moving to G7 meetings after this. And as you mentioned in your answer that this is very serious Covid situation so what will be your agenda in G7 vis-à-vis covid situation? Will you be raising this issue with them? Will you be seeking help from them? Can you give us a brief outline?

External Affairs Minister, Dr S Jaishankar: G 7 had its own agenda. It's G7 and there are four of us who are guests, ourselves, Australia, South Korea and South Africa. The agenda already had covid very much in it, because it is today the biggest challenge which not just India but the entire world faces. Now when it comes to G 7 Foreign Ministers, bear in mind I am pretty much in touch with all of them. They actually have been through it, many of them. The US has been through it, UK has been through it, Germany, France Italy and not just been through it, they have been through very severe form of it last year and the beginning of this year. In fact if you look at it proportionally in many cases their intensity is as much as we are going through it in India. Some ways it is even more than what we are going through and a lot of our situation and our stresses today, you know the hospitals situation, oxygen situation, New York has seen it, France has seen it, Italy has seen it. I was in fact, though he is not here, just while coming in was talking to my counterpart in Portugal, he was telling me, he said just a few months ago we went through it, we had the highest per capita cases and fatalities but we have come through it. So my message going to G 7 is this is a global challenge and everybody knows that all of you have been through it, we are going through it right now, there are various factors and reasons why it is serious and severe as it is and global pandemic requires global effort and in the past we have contributed to that global effort, being part of other people solution and I am sure beginning with the meeting that I already had with Secretary Blinken yesterday, I think rest of the G7 feels the same.

Journalist: Sir will you be talking about the aid? The material aid which these countries are giving and Sir, is it a shift in our policy because I think we are asking for aid after some decades and aid is coming in from foreign countries. Can you just touch on this topic?

External Affairs Minister, Dr S Jaishankar: I think quite honestly to my mind this is not the accurate way of projecting the situation, as I said covid is a shared problem for the whole world. Now just look at last year or even this year, when it came to medicines we gave hydroxychloroquine, paracetamol, we gave to US, we gave to Singapore, we gave to European countries, we sent medical team to Kuwait, we gave vaccines to some countries in the Gulf. Now what you describe as aid we describe as friendship and as support. I think we have to understand the uniqueness of the problem we are facing today, so when you say it is not like what it was before, look there was no covid before, we never really had it. In my lifetime, I'm older than you, I have never seen a global crisis of this proportion. A global crisis require people to come together so I think this kind of aid and this kind of argument, this is sort of point scoring. I think people are not connecting conceptually to the problem; they are not connecting emotionally with the suffering and the danger happening in India. The kind of situation which I am seeing and you are seeing in Delhi, I will do everything in my power to get help to our people. So I will leverage all my relationships, I will call in every I owe you I have and I have many because I have done my shift in the past and people know that. I had foreign minister saying this I would like to do this. There are people who say at least I am morally with you, I feel I like to do something, I have limitations. You must understand to say this is aid, this is different, have you gone down in life because we are getting support from outside, I don't think so. For me, I have one objective; my people are going through a very difficult phase of covid in the second wave. As Foreign Minister, as someone heading a Ministry which has relationships around the world, I will do everything which I have accumulated in many years to help my people, its natural.

Journalist: Sir, there is also a political angle. A lot of foreign media coverage covering this pandemic in India in a different manner. You are representing the entire country here in abroad so how do you defend this? There is some sort of politics around this covid situation in India, How do you look at it?

External Affairs Minister, Dr S Jaishankar: Sadly you are right, I wish it wasn't so but what I can say is when it happened in other countries including UK, when Pandemic hits our society very hard, there are questions, there are arguments, there is a lot of second guessing, you should have seen it coming, we could have told you so etc and it is not unique to India, it happens in other societies as well. In our case, yes I'm very conscious of our own debate that's something I hear and involved in everyday. People have spoken about elections, now, obviously we are a democratic country you don't stop elections in a place like India, the only time I remember we stopped elections is a era some decades ago when I was pretty much younger, where none of us really want to be associated with that kind of memory. Now, we are a democracy, we are very argumentative society, there will be this kind of point scoring. Somebody will say this crowd contributed to it, somebody else will say well that crowd contributed to it, somebody will say that some individual or leader A somebody will say leader B didn't wear a mask there. So I would say when I go out, in my sense and my view, I think we need to put a pause to it. We have a serious national crisis. The fact is that societies are defined by their ability to come together when you deal with the crisis of this magnitude, it's like a war, what happens when there is a war, people come together as a society. So I would hope very much that we should do. I realise when it comes to the press, our press, foreign press, people will focus on us, it's natural. People in governance would understand the problem, because everybody has been through it or say well that could be me tomorrow. I think people of Indian community will get it because they are worried about their relatives and friends but when it comes to the media, there would be media where editorial lines are very strong. When I see comments, very frankly, I see a lot of analysis by people who write fiction, by people who are political commentators. I am not saying they shouldn't have a view, everybody has a right to view this country. But I would rather take very seriously public health people who would sit very objectively and diagnose and analyse why we are facing this problem we are and the fact is that we are facing this problem due to two variants 117 and 1,617, they have really hit us very very hard and they are far more virulent than the virus strain we saw last year. Just look at our numbers, I remind you where we were in February. At the end of February we were less than 10,000 cases a day, today we have 350k cases a day. Today you can say well you should have seen it coming but let us face it you and I live in the same society; we saw societal fatigue with a lockdown. Today people are urging lockdowns, who are opposing lockdowns earlier. So I would say at the end of the day when I go abroad, I would try to make people understand that these are my challenges, this is where international partnerships come into being and yesterday most of my meeting with Tony Blinken was actually devoted to what would be the solutions, the solutions in India and solutions abroad and the heart of the matter will be vaccines and how will we get that kind of vaccination scales which means vaccination production and we can't do it right now by ourselves. We are part of global pharmaceutical chain so we all need to sit and work this. So when I go outside, I'm not impervious to the debate at home, that's part of vey effervescent society like India would be. I go out, look at what will be our national requirements today, but also make the case to people that I am part of global solution, today I'm going through this crisis, tomorrow someone else will be going through crisis and just as I get support from world today, I will be offering support to the world tomorrow as I did yesterday when my situation was better.

Journalist: After the second wave has struck, this is your first visit abroad. What is the kind of message you want to convey to our missions all over the world because there is a lot to be done and a lot is done by these missions abroad, so what are you telling them ?

External Affairs Minister, Dr S Jaishankar: To some extent it would depend on the mission. But I would say as a general message, there will be people who will be naturally be worried about what's happening in India and understandably so. Some of it would be to explain to them what is happening but the key message would be, look, there will be debates in India, filter the noise, do what you have to do as a mission, do your job and what's your job right now? Your job is to ensure that the key requirements, today oxygen is the major requirement, pharmaceuticals, remdesivir, other medicines are a requirement, vaccine supply chain is a requirement, so logistics for all of this is a requirement. I have embassies who are working with shipping lines, with airlines, different countries creating hubs, you know how big the oxygen challenge is, so we are getting liquid medical oxygen, we are getting cryogenic tankers, we are getting oxygen tanks, oxygen cylinders, you have to locate them, organise them, send them and you have seen now that support is flying in from different countries, all of that requires coordination. Now my message to Embassies is keep your eye on that and don't get distracted by the rest of debate, that's not relevant to what your focus should. Your focus should be right now a very serious situation back home, just like government is focused in addressing the pandemic at home single mindedly, you also please do that, we will deal with argument down the road, at the moment keep your eyes and energy focused on this.

Keynote Address by External Affairs Minister at Policy Ex-change, London on "India & U.K. in the post-Covid World"

(6 May 2021)

The Covid era has accelerated many of the changes in the making. Indeed, whether it is our scientists working together, our pharma business producing in collaboration or the generosity of the support the

U.K. has currently extended to India in an hour of need, there are larger lessons from each experience. Covid has also brought to the forefront globally issues of trust and transparency, in fact, I would say of reliability and resilience as well. The pandemic has highlighted the risks of globalisation, even though it has driven new opportunities for cooperation. It has helped make a more compelling case for working together, obviously in public health and R&D, but equally so, for secure supply chains and in global governance. Our partnership was even otherwise getting ready for an upgrade; the new context has given it a greater urgency.

Speech by External Affairs Minister at the "Future of Asia" Conference organised by Nikkei

(20 May 2021)

Thank you.

Mr. Naotoshi Okada, Nikkei Chairman & Group CEO,

Mr. Tsuyoshi Hasebe, Nikkei President & CEO Distinguished Guests, Ladies and gentlemen,

1. I have great pleasure in addressing the 26th "Future of Asia" Conference organised by Nikkei on shaping the post-Covid era with a specific relevance to Asia's role.
2. A year and a half ago, as the enormity of the Covid-19 pandemic dawned on the world, we were truly confronted by a black swan event. Since then, even though we may have addressed some facets of a very complex challenge, it continues its devastating course across geographies. We, in India, are going through a particularly difficult situation right now. Understandably, the world's attention is focused primarily on the public health response. The economic consequences of the pandemic were of course immediately felt, though its social ones are now also starting to be realised. What perhaps is yet to be fully comprehended is its long-term impact on the global order, including on the future of Asia.

3. How is the Covid-19 reshaping the world? Amongst others, by changing the perceptions and calculations of nations about each other and the world. Specifically, by:
   (i) Bringing out the value of trust and transparency and the importance of reliable supply chains,
   (ii) Heightening risk aversion in a world now clearly more insecure and encouraging strategic autonomy to address over-dependence,
   (iii) Focusing on the need to create greater global capacities so that pandemic-scale challenges are more effectively met, and
   (iv) By doing so promoting decentralised globalisation and establishing resilient supply chains to de- risk the world economy.
4. This pandemic may be the most serious in living memory; but it should be seen as a recurring challenge and not as a one-off. It demands international cooperation on a scale that could not have even be conceived of earlier. No national capacity, however large, can be adequate. And just overflows from such capacities are clearly not enough to address global needs. Even a collective response, by itself, could fall short if it is just an aggregate of the present capacities. What we will now have to conceptualise is re-engineering the way the world works to prepare for and mitigate such cataclysmic events. Covid-19 has certainly triggered debates on issues like supply chains, global governance, social responsibility and even ethics. But for many of us gathered here today, it equally encourages an objective assessment of the contemporary world so that we are better prepared for tomorrow.
5. As nations contemplate the world, there is no question that Covid-19 has moved the needle in the direction of risks as opposed to opportunity. This is reflected in national security acquiring a more expansive definition. In the past, defence, politics and intelligence drove calculations, with some extrapolation into domains like resources, energy or technology. With some notable exceptions, its demands were balanced out by the requirements of global exchanges, economic efficiency and perhaps by social habits. These trends, in fact, became stronger as the globalisation mantra took deeper root. The pandemic, however, saw capabilities leveraged, commitments dishonoured, supply chains blocked, logistics disrupted, and shortages created, with all the accompanying anxieties. When this applied to PPEs, medicines or ventilators, we all woke up to health security. Those who

saw their essential supplies under threat now realised the value of food security. When economies slowed down due to material disruptions, we now understood the need for manufacturing security. Call it buying nationally, middle-class concerns, dual circulation or self-reliance, there is no question that many polities are seeking to hedge against excessive exposure internationally.

6. In parts of the world previously more sanguine about their own globalisation, the concept of strategic autonomy has started to gain more traction. The efficiency of others may have strengthened bottom-lines in good times; they are now seen as too vulnerable in difficult ones. Disruptions also raised natural concerns about long-term reliability and resilience. In many areas, it became apparent that the global economy was dangerously dependent on specific production centres. Even the world of services is understanding the consequences of over-reliance on limited sources. Whether it is tourism or travel, mobility or off-shoring, the value of multiplicity and redundancy is realised more than ever before.
7. The nature of the Covid experience has also brought to fore concerns of trust and transparency. Opacity can no longer be overlooked; it has real implications for the rest of the world. It was bad enough to be confronted with shortages and disruptions; worse that they could become pressure points. There are also worries that the financial distress caused by the pandemic could lead to new vulnerabilities. Consequently, strategic autonomy is now being debated as greater self-sufficiency, stronger partnerships and multiplicity of options—all of which are perceived as integral to risk mitigation. These of course could have geo-economic implications in the days ahead.
8. Behavioural aspects have also played their part. Stresses induced narrower definitions of self-interest and departures from collective endeavours. Few practised what they preached; some even stopped preaching altogether. Inadvertently, insights emerged on the interplay of culture, interests and values. Pluralistic societies remained more engaged with the world and international solidarity was stronger in the South. Those who saw the world also as a work-place rather than just a market-place had a deeper interest obviously in remaining connected.
9. Given that interests are the primary driving-force, global outlook of nations reflects their exposure to global supply chains. This holds true as much for

priorities like vaccine production as for the larger economic routine. But somewhere, there are factors beyond comfort and gains at play. An outlook that envisages the world as a family—where exceptionalism is not the main prism—will encourage a shared approach. And that is important because the pandemic is a global challenge that requires nothing less than global solutions. If its overall result is to compel us to approach the big issues of our time with greater unity and cohesion, it may well have done us more than a small favour.

10. Changes within societies are also important to recognise. Many societies—and I can certainly speak for India in this regard—have discovered the real potential of the digital in this process. Whether it was in terms of government or business or indeed education and health, the digital medium helped provide better and more effective solutions. Few believe that they will come through the Covid experience unaffected in their decision-making or indeed in their debates.
11. But traumatic as it has been, the essential realities of our times cannot be denied. Our globalisation is deep and pervasive and will continue to shape activities and strategies. What the Covid has brought out are some of the particular risks of its current incarnation. The task before us is therefore to de-risk that, even while pursuing other objectives, including rapid economic recovery. In doing that, we should take into account that this is both a more multipolar world and a more rebalanced one. In plain words, that means more players and greater capabilities whose full potential needs to be aggressively explored. It is only then that we can strengthen global resilience and confidence. Clearly, that means de-centralised globalisation, with multiple supply chains and more engines of growth. It is only with such redundancy that the world can face the next pandemic better than we are doing the current one.
12. Making that happen requires decisions, initiatives and consultations at many levels. India, on its part, can help strengthen and de-risk the global economy through more effective partnerships. With Japan and Australia today, we are working on a Supply Chain Resilience Initiative. Where the Quad arrangement that also involves the United States is concerned, its agenda today covers vaccine collaboration, critical and emerging technologies, semi-conductors, supply chains, critical materials and of course connectivity, amongst others. Recent Indian summits with the European Union and the

United Kingdom, that saw advancement on FTAs, are also noteworthy in that regard.

13. Meeting the health and medical requirements of the world effectively requires a mature recognition of the global nature of the underlying supply chains. Barring a select few, it cannot be addressed purely nationally and in fact needs a collaboration of a very different order. The answer to the pandemic challenge is to expand and smoothen global flows, while creating confidence that its outcomes are for the benefit of the entire world.

14. Better international cooperation can also be facilitated by improved national capacities. So, if India is to make a real contribution to Asian and global economic recovery, it can start by helping itself. Even while the Covid-19 was ongoing last year, bold reforms were undertaken in industry, agriculture, labour and education. Perhaps most relevant to this audience are the Production-Linked Incentive (PLI) schemes to attract and encourage manufacturing in 13 sectors which include mobiles and electronic components, KSM and APIs for pharmaceuticals, medical devices, electronic and technology products, drugs, telecom and networking products, food products, white goods, high efficiency solar PV models, auto and auto components, ACC battery, textile products and speciality steel. We aim to make manufacturing in India globally competitive by removing sectoral disabilities, creating economies of scale and ensuring efficiencies. By creating a level-playing field and encouraging a component eco-system, it will integrate India deeper into the global supply chain. Already, the global response to the PLI initiative has been strong. Coupled with an improvement in India's position in the World Bank's Ease of Doing Business rankings—last year we were 63, we used to be 142 in 2014—this would enhance our economic relevance.

15. But, beyond this, the world also has a natural interest in the direction, pace and quality of India's development. Much of what India is to build still lies ahead of us. We thus have a unique opportunity to embrace a greener and more technology-driven future. But this needs the requisite global partnerships and resources. Let us appreciate the implications of 140 million households moving into the middle class, even as another 20 million reach the high-income bracket. The winds of change have been blowing harder in India, especially in the last seven years. They can make

universal access to power, piped water and affordable housing realisable goals within a generation. As India urbanises like the rest of the world, a Smart Cities Mission covering a hundred locations is addressing challenges holistically through retro-fitting, re-development, green field and pan-city development.

16. And as I have stressed, even as India builds more, it builds greener. A renewable target of 450 GW by 2030 seeks to transform its energy profile. As one of the few G20 economies adhering to its Paris commitments, its 15 per cent energy efficiency savings, its shift to LED lighting with more than 367 million bulbs, moving 80 million households from bio-mass to LPG cooking and being among the top three nations to expand forest cover in the last decade are examples of its seriousness.
17. The changes in the environment are paralleled by progress in human resources. National campaigns of financial inclusion, educating daughters, Digital India, Clean India, Skill India, Water Mission, etc. enable us today to directly fund 400 million vulnerable citizens and provide food support to 800 million during the Covid challenge. I would urge you to look at these trends not just as a national accomplishment in the making but as improving global human resources.
18. In ensuring economic recovery, Indo-Japan relations have a notable role, in fact one I would argue even beyond Asia. Our partnership is seen today as among the most natural in the region. Japan is a valuable partner in these national campaigns that I have spoken about. And consistently supportive of our infrastructure development, including through ODA loans. In fact, Japanese-supported projects are among the most successful infrastructure examples, most recently the Delhi-Mumbai Industrial Corridor and the Dedicated Western Freight Corridor. Its long-standing FDI footprint in India is steadily expanding, covering 1455 companies as of 2021, and more than half of them are in manufacturing. New industrial collaborations are in the making even as we speak. And Japan's contribution in skills enhancements is visible in 16 Japan-India Institutes for Manufacturing and 5 Japan Endowed Courses.
19. Japan is of course closely associated with the growth of our auto sector and in fact also with the introduction of Metros in India. The bullet train

initiative is the current flagship project. Our cooperation reflects the needs of the time, whether it is through a fund to support start-ups or an agreement to receive skilled workers from India. Our strong strategic convergence is evident in our Annual Summit, 2+2 meetings, defence and military activities as well as cooperation at regional and multilateral forums.

20. Distinguished guests, the Covid challenge has certainly created a stronger case for greater international cooperation, be it in vaccine production or to facilitate economic recovery. Those with shared interests and common values will find it easier to forge stronger partnerships. To make a real difference, the global order must address the concerns and issues that the pandemic has thrown up. I thank this conference for the opportunity to share my thoughts in that regard and I am confident that its deliberations will help us find pathways to better solutions.

Opening keynote interview by External Affairs Minister at the FT-Indian Express Webinar

(20 May 2021)

It is also not today, an issue of nationalism and internationalism. I think, a lot of things have become so much clearer in the last year in terms of the behaviour of states. And I would also caution against, analysing the world, in western and non-western terms. I think the West isn't cohesive, and the non- west is so differentiated, that there is no such concept, really. So what is it? I would say it's a paradox. It's a paradox of sharpening geopolitics, as Raj you mentioned, where values, systems, beliefs, freedoms, have kind of come back into the debate. But that is set off against a very deep interdependence, which has been fostered by 40 years of developing globalisation. And, in fact, there's nothing really like the COVID challenge to remind us of actually how interconnected and interdependent the world has become, but it's not just COVID, I would argue climate change is another example. So, you have a situation where at one level national divisions could be sharper, but at another level global compulsion is greater. So even with COVID, for example, the issues of trust and transparency that they have raised, they reflect both because there is today, an urge to secure yourself, but also an understanding that you have to work with others to make supply chains more resilient and reliable.

External Affairs Minister in conversation with General HR McMaster in Battlegrounds session on 'India: Opportunities and Challenges for a Strategic Partnership' (26 May 2021)

(27 May 2021)

I don't want to make this about country A or country B, however big the country maybe. I mean, to my mind, this is the big issue. The world's not going to be the same after the COVID whenever that after is. It's not going to be the same because we are, as I said, all of us, in different ways, are going to worry about our international exposure. Historically, you know, when times are good, you tend to see international relations as endless opportunities, sort of waiting to be exploited. When times are tough, you realise that those opportunities come mixed with a lot of risks, which take place and we are going through one of them which is the pandemic. So, as I said, what's the big takeaway, the big takeaway is we need a better world, the safer world, the less risky world, something which by the way, works for everybody. Because that too, is an issue, if we construct a world order, in the name of globalisation, but it works for some countries at the expense of others, it works for some people in some countries at the expense of others, we're going to have a frankly, dysfunctional international relations and dysfunctional societies. We've seen that in the last decade. So I would argue that in many ways international equity and fairness are not just noble principles, they are a practical common sense. It's like creating a broader stakeholder ship in the world, so that the totality of the world is better balanced. And then you apply that in different ways. I mean, we are going through a pandemic, today. Okay, the key question, the number one question on everybody's mind today is COVID. And the worry which people had, and I have heard this expressed by many countries, do we have accessible, affordable vaccines? Now, we can't have a world which is part vaccinated and part neglected, because that was not going to be safe. So how do we get through the global challenges in a global way? I think that's the big question and here the importance of countries willing to harmonise their national interest with global good. If countries, especially large countries, pursue their national interest, disregarding everything else, I think the world is going to have some big problems.

Virtual Address by External Affairs Minister to the Indian Community in Kuwait (11 June 2021)

(12 June 2021)

...But my visit, and my talks with Foreign Minister Ahmed were actually focused on how do we find new areas of cooperation, as keeping in mind both the immediate impact of the COVID, because I think all of us have learnt many things from the COVID experience, as well as the longer term changes which are happening, the growth in India's capacities, its influence, what you might call the rebalancing, in a way of the global order. And what does that really mean in practical terms for India and Kuwait? I think some of it we are seeing, even as we speak, I would say today, in an environment which is very dominated by COVID concerns, health issues have become very important for every society. In fact, we look at health very much today as part of our national security. And we discussed really, how we could work more closely. I think, last year, many of you would remember that we had sent out military medical team to be with the Kuwait health authorities as they coped with the COVID. We also supplied some Made in India vaccines earlier this year. So it's very clear with the kind of impact that this pandemic has made, with the expectation, that this is not a one of affair, but going to be something recurring, something we need to factor in. Clearly health is a big issue. Food Security is also another issue.

Again, I think COVID has heightened concerns, there were anxieties expressed in Kuwait and in other Gulf countries, because many of them source their essential supplies, especially food from India. And I think you would know that we made exceptional efforts to ensure that the supply chain, the food supply especially was kept open, kept undisrupted through last year.

We also discussed education because I think people do see India today as not just a source of skills and talents but as a country, which is being very creative about growing its educational capacities. And again, during the COVID period, we've had a lot of exposure to distance education. But most of all, I think we focused heavily on the digital aspect, because the COVID has accelerated the digitisation of our daily existence. We all do more online shopping. But I think there was a lot of interest in Kuwait to understand how, for example, our contact tracing was done through an app, how our vaccine registration is done through a portal, how, in fact, whether it is payment of money into the accounts of vulnerable sections of society, or providing rations for people, again during the time of COVID, how all of this was done using digital mediums and in a very seamless manner without any leakages. So the overall sense really was that, even as we deal with COVID, as we battle challenges to our health and to our social fabric, the experience has actually brought to forefront a new agenda in a way.

... Since I was speaking about the COVID, and I mentioned to you that we had sent the medical team and also ensured the food provision. I think it would be right for me also to bring out the importance of the effort that Kuwait has made, in fact, is still making as we speak, in terms of providing medical oxygen to India. You all know that we had a very severe second wave, nationally, of COVID. The variants in question were exceptionally virulent. So even though people had debated and modeled what could be a second wave, I think the reality was far bigger. It was more than four times what the first wave of the COVID was. And one of the immediate implications of that was really a large number of people who were in hospital with respiratory issues, who required oxygen, and in fact, the demand for medical oxygen went up from more than 1,000 metric tonnes which is what it was last year, to 8,000, almost 9,000 metric tonnes. And we of course, expanded our own capacities nationally. But it was very helpful for us to get oxygen supplies from abroad. And among the countries which actually took the lead, I would particularly single out Kuwait in this regard, they provided us more than 500 metric tonnes, and they're very prompt and very efficient in that regard. So, to me, it is actually a proof that international partnerships and cooperation, these are not just phrases, they actually make a difference when countries face challenges and what we have done for each other during the COVID period, to my mind is a very good example of the trust and confidence but also the new vistas of cooperation that today we need to address.

... And to do all that, of course, we need to have flights coming in from India. These as in many cases have been temporarily suspended because of COVID. So as the numbers go down, I obviously would like very much to see a resumption of flights. And definitely, I think this situation has also opened up opportunities for our businesses, for more exports to this region, and for a role for the Indian community, in enhancing the economic contacts between us.

... I think it's clear by now that the second wave of the COVID has started to definitely deceit, the numbers, the daily numbers, you can see of people who are newly infected is now one quarter, 25 per cent maybe even less than what it was in the peak in early May, the positivity rate has also come down very dramatically in most population centres. And a large part of that has been made possible by a very, very vigorous government response to the second wave. I can tell you that as someone who's been in government for many decades now, the kind of effort and energy that I saw, the long hours that people put in, people really moved mountains to respond to what was an unprecedented situation. We were talking about oxygen, we ran really hundreds of oxygen trains to ferry oxygen from the production centres to the major cities, all our planes were mobilised including the Air Force planes for the oxygen cylinder tanks to be moved, both within the country and from abroad to India. We procured medicines which were essential for COVID treatment, many of them from abroad. We also ensured that the domestic production of medicines was enhanced. And, of course, where the vulnerable sections were concerned, many of you would know that we've actually ensured that as many as 800 million people get rations from the government and 400 million people have actually got funds put into their account in terms of support. Vaccination is of course, a big issue. Again, it has picked up, we are currently vaccinating more than 3 million a day. Our expectation is that this will go up as the vaccine production increases. We have cumulatively vaccinated about 245-246 million so far. And the confidence is there, that as more vaccine comes into production, as the production of even the existing vaccine scales up, that as the year progresses, we will actually be able to vaccinate all our people. Along with the health situation of course, there is a natural worry, what is the state of the economy and there I want to share with you that the picture has been quite confident in some ways, we saw a strong recovery in the early months before the second wave. But during the second wave actually, the lockdowns have been local, interstate traffic, interstate movement has not been disrupted at all, I think a lot of the logistics has kept going. So, there is a sense that the economic impact of the second wave would be far less than what happened last year. So, the belief we have that India will pick up, that India will recover rapidly, that what we have seen in the last few years as the steady rise of India and its economy and its influence in the world, that would continue.

... So as I conclude, I want to come back to all of you because while I have appreciated what the Government of Kuwait did, I particularly want to emphasise that we very much recognise what the Indian community in Kuwait did. I know that many of you have helped to acquire oxygen cylinders; it is both the practical relevance of what you did as well as the feeling for your motherland, which this expresses, that is deeply appreciated by us. So, I thank you here.

External Affairs Minister's virtual interaction with the Indian Diaspora in Kenya (13 June 2021)

(15 June 2021)

So, let me share with you also what is happening in India, because I think that is something which is of natural concern for all of you. You all know, we went through a very severe second wave of the COVID. In fact, we're still going through it but from the peak of where it was which was about a month ago, today if you take the number of new cases as a index, we are down to about 20 per cent of what the peak was. I think the general sense, looking at the positivity rates coming down, the pressures on the hospital, I mean it is clearly now very much on the decline. There was no question that this was a very, very severe public health challenge to us.

Regarding what was sent from Kenya during the second wave of the COVID. Look let me say this, the entire international community across the world responded to what happened in India, they did so, because, on the one hand, people recognise this was something very intense, very serious. On the other hand, there's a very good feeling for India, there's a lot of affection for India, for its people. People saw India had also done things for the world. So, to me, when someone feels for you, everybody expresses it in their own way. I take the feeling. For me, it was an expression of affection or of sentiment I value it. I can tell you, I value it. I know my government values it and I'm very confident my people value it. I have had occasions where actually, Foreign Ministers have called me up and said, look, we don't have anything practical to do we just want to call you up and tell you we feel free for you. I value that also. So please be assured that whatever concern there was in Kenya, whatever manner Kenya wanted to express its friendship and his affection for India, the people in India fully understand that. So take that from me.

Statement by Shri V. Muraleedharan, Minister of State for External Affairs at 20th Session of High-level Committee on South-South Cooperation (1 June 2021)

1. The COVID-19 pandemic is threatening to setback decades of progress made by developing countries and push millions back into poverty. We need

to raise our collective voice for recovery, resilience and reform to ensure that we go back to the path of development and to the path of achieving the SDGs. The outcomes of the BAPA+40 should lay the foundations for our efforts.

Mr. President,

2. COVID-19 pandemic has laid bare the shortcomings of multilateral institutions. It has taken time for multilateral institutions to react to the pandemic and cater effectively to the Global South. We have realised that during the pandemic, even the traditional North-South paradigm has not worked well and the Global South have been left largely to fend for themselves. It is here that South-South Cooperation becomes necessary, even crucial.
3. India reached out to 150 countries in a spirit of solidarity to supply medicines, medical equipment and other urgent requirements when the pandemic began. When we produced COVID-19 vaccines, we reached out to some of the most vulnerable countries first to provide these vaccines. We have done this in a spirit of South-South Cooperation and in the recognition that "no one is safe till everyone is safe".

Remarks by Minister of State for External Affairs at the Inaugural Ministerial Session of India-New Zealand Business Summit

(23 June 2021)

1. COVID-19 pandemic calls for global action. This has been articulated by Prime Minister Shri Narendra Modi most recently in his address to the G-7 leaders. He called for a "One Earth One Health" approach for global recovery, while synergising the efforts at all levels of the government, industry and civil society to "Build Back Stronger". I commend the organisers of this event for their efforts in bringing together the key stakeholders from the spheres of politics, business and academia for this deliberation. I am happy to note that both FICCI and CII are strategic partners for this event.
2. I thank the Government & the people of New Zealand and the Indian Diaspora for their support and solidarity during the second wave of COVID-19 pandemic in India.

Foreign Secretary's Remarks on "India's Foreign Policy in the Post-Covid World: New Vulnerabilities, New Opportunities", Public Affairs Forum of India (18 June 2021)

1. The Ministry of External Affairs, like the entire Government of India, adapted to respond to the new realities of the pandemic. Our Ministry created a de novo vertical, the COVID Cell that worked 24×7 to coordinate our COVID related operations. This was resourced appropriately with some of our best officers and was able to scale up rapidly on demand.
2. Our network of diplomatic Missions played a key role in organizing the Vande Bharat Mission, the largest logistical mission of its type ever undertaken. This has facilitated the movement of more than 7 million people through lockdown and post-lockdown periods.
3. Indian HADR operations, which are complex inter-agency operations requiring detailed planning and efficient execution, acquired global dimensions with the deployment Rapid Response Teams to Maldives, Kuwait, Mauritius and Comoros and with Mission SAGAR to Maldives, Mauritius, Madagascar, Comoros and Seychelles. India also supplied healthcare products to over 150 countries in the face of daunting logistical challenges.
4. MEA has acted as the global arm of the Government of India's Empowered Group system to procure essential medical supplies for COVID-19. We have, throughout the pandemic, identified and connected with potential suppliers of essential medical equipment across the world. During the first COVID wave last year, a global sourcing operation was launched to procure ventilators, PPE kits, N95 masks, 3-ply surgical masks and testing kits. These helped us to tide over the situation till domestic manufacturing scaled up to meet demand.
5. We also intervened to source medical products, machinery, and components that were vital for enhancing our domestic manufacturing capabilities. MEA facilitated the import of components for ventilators, testing inputs such as RNA Extraction Kits, Roche Cobas testing machines and testing kits from the US, Germany, China, Switzerland and Singapore.
6. Our Missions abroad, where required, also reached out to original suppliers in various countries to expedite shipments of critical items.
7. This effort to procure essential medical supplies intensified during the second wave. We worked closely with other Ministries and agencies, our Armed Forces and State governments, during the massive procurement and logistical operation to secure supplies of critical items.

8. The immediate need during the second wave was to ramp up oxygen supply in thousands of hospitals spread across India. One of the challenges was to transport medical oxygen to the places of need from distant places of production within India. MEA and our diplomatic Missions reached out to suppliers and Governments and arranged cryogenic tankers, which helped with quick transportation of medical oxygen in the country. Our Missions in the Gulf countries worked with the Indian Navy for the supply of medical oxygen from those countries. Our Missions worked with the Indian Air Force in arranging the airlift of cryogenic tankers from Singapore, Thailand and other South East Asian countries. We also facilitated the supply of oxygen plants, large number of oxygen cylinders and concentrators from Governments and private organisations.
9. We facilitated procurement of critical drugs such as Remdesivir, Tocilizumab, Favipiravir and Liposomal Amphotericin-B. When demand for Remdesivir shot up in the country, we had to ensure that our domestic manufacturing capacity for this vital drug was significantly augmented. This required enhanced supplies of raw materials which were facilitated by our Missions from diverse locations such as the US, Europe and China. Another example is the case of Tocilizumab which is not currently manufactured in India. Roche Pharma, Switzerland is the sole supplier of the drug. We reached out to the leadership of the company and, through consistent efforts, supply to India increased significantly over the last year. We also scouted for alternate sources and were able to get supplies through foreign assistance. We were also able to secure supplies of antibody cocktails from Roche.
10. Another important aspect of our efforts was to facilitate supplies of essential raw material and components. For instance, CSIR, DRDO and several of their industry partners were provided assistance in procuring zeolite molecular sieves, which is a critical component of oxygen generators and plants.
11. India received extensive support and assistance from its partner countries around the world during the second wave. This reflected the goodwill earned by India for the assistance extended by it to other countries when they needed it. The COVID cell within MEA handled the complexities associated with the delivery of foreign support. In close collaboration with other stakeholders in the Government of India and State Governments, the cell facilitated the arrival and distribution of critical items such as medical

oxygen, oxygen cylinders and concentrators, oxygen plants, medicines and other equipment received from our partner countries.

12. Our Embassies in Russia and USA facilitated discussions with major vaccine manufacturers about procurement and possible local manufacturing of their vaccines. For example, we have been involved in the introduction of Sputnik-V into India.
13. Vaccines have complex supply chains. We have worked to ease regulatory disruptions to these supply chains by diplomatic interventions with some of our key partners.
14. We have adapted rapidly to virtual diplomacy. Our high level engagements at the bilateral, plurilateral and multilateral levels have continued in the virtual mode. In recent months, the Prime Minister has participated in the G7 Summit; India-EU Leaders' meeting; first Quad Summit; and Leaders' Summit on Climate. These engagements have been accompanied by regular virtual and telephonic conversations with leaders of partner countries, including the US, Russia, UK and Japan.
15. Indian diplomacy as you can see is adjusting to this complex and uncertain environment. It is doing so with agility and flexibility. We have to think and act innovatively and to adapt at the conceptual and operational levels.
16. The challenge before us is to create capacities to deal with unexpected and catastrophic events. We have to be able to repurpose organisations at very short notice to deal with unexpected challenges. Existing hierarchies and structures are often unable to cope with such challenges and may require re-engineering.

Foreign Secretary's Remarks at the Thematic Discussion on "Growing Role of Asia in International Affairs and Related Adaptation of Conference on Interaction and Confidence-Building Measures in Asia (CICA)"

(23 June 2021)

The COVID-19 pandemic has brought about unprecedented global challenges, exposing vulnerabilities and underscoring our interdependence in Asia and across the world. This interdependence has also been our greatest strength as we collectively battle this crisis. Over the past year, India has provided COVID-19 related pharmaceuticals, vaccines and medical equipment to more than 150 countries, including to CICA member states. In that same spirit of friendship and solidarity, we extend deep appreciation to those that have provided us with some priority requirements to battle the second wave of the pandemic in India in the preceding months.

Annexure 13a: Handling of Cargo, Customs and Clearance-Major Donation Items Received—HLL

The Major Donation items received through 402 shipments as on date are:

1. **Equipment**
    - Ventilators
    - Oxygen Concentrators
    - Oxygen Generation Plants
    - Oxygen cylinders
    - C Pap Equipments
    - Bi Pap Equipment
    - ECG Machines
    - Cots
    - Bedside Monitor etc.
2. **Medicines**
    - Remdesivir
    - Tocilizumab
    - Fabipiravir
    - Fragmin
    - Casivirimibab
    - Other—Azythromycin, Paracetamol, etc.
3. **Consumables**
    - PPE Kits
    - Gowns
    - N 95 masks
    - 3 ply masks
    - Face masks
    - Face Shields
    - Goggles
    - IR Thermometer
    - Hand Sanitizer
    - Blanket
    - Mattresses
    - Oxygen masks
    - Body bags

Annexure 13b: Handling of Cargo, Customs and Clearance-Warehousing—HLL

- HLL operated 7 non-cold chain warehouses at different locations in India of which the main warehouses rented for the longest period of time were:
  - a. Gurgaon - 1 No
  - b. Kolkata – 1 No
  - c. Mumbai – 1 No
  - d. Visakhapatnam – 1 No
- Other locations where HLL has rented for smaller durations are:
  - e. Mangalore – 1 No
  - f. Chennai – 1 No
  - g. Bangalore
- HLL also operated 4 cold chain warehouses at the following locations for the storage of medicines at 2-8 deg Celsius or at 15-25 deg Celsius as per the requirement:
  - a. Kolkata – 1
  - b. Mumbai – 2
  - c. Delhi – 1

INDEX